T0132974

Making and Unmaking Public Health in Africa

CAMBRIDGE CENTRE OF AFRICAN STUDIES SERIES

Series editors: Derek R. Peterson, Harri Englund, and Christopher Warnes

The University of Cambridge is home to one of the world's leading centers of African studies. It organizes conferences, runs a weekly seminar series, hosts a specialist library, coordinates advanced graduate studies, and facilitates research by Cambridge- and Africa-based academics. The Cambridge Centre of African Studies Series publishes work that emanates from this rich intellectual life. The series fosters dialogue across a broad range of disciplines in African studies and between scholars based in Africa and elsewhere.

Derek R. Peterson, ed.
Abolitionism and Imperialism in Britain, Africa, and the Atlantic

Harri Englund, ed.
Christianity and Public Culture in Africa

Devon Curtis and Gwinyayi A. Dzinesa, eds.
Peacebuilding, Power, and Politics in Africa

Ruth J. Prince and Rebecca Marsland, eds.
Making and Unmaking Public Health in Africa:
Ethnographic and Historical Perspectives

Making and Unmaking Public Health in Africa

Ethnographic and Historical Perspectives

Edited by Ruth J. Prince and Rebecca Marsland

Ohio University Press • *Athens*

Ohio University Press, Athens, Ohio 45701
ohioswallow.com
© 2014 by Ohio University Press
All rights reserved

To obtain permission to quote, reprint, or otherwise reproduce or distribute material
from Ohio University Press publications, please contact our rights and permissions
department at (740) 593-1154 or (740) 593-4536 (fax).

Printed in the United States of America
Ohio University Press books are printed on acid-free paper ⊗ ™

24 23 22 21 20 19 18 17 16 15 14   5 4 3 2 1

Library of Congress Cataloging-in-Publication Data

Making public health in Africa : ethnographic and historical perspectives / edited by Ruth J.
Prince and Rebecca Marsland.
    p. ; cm. — (Cambridge Centre of African Studies series)
Papers from a workshop held at the University of Cambridge's Centre of African Studies and
Department of Social Anthropology in June 2008.
Includes bibliographical references and index.
Summary: "Africa has emerged as a prime arena of global health interventions that focus
on particular diseases and health emergencies. These are framed increasingly in terms of
international concerns about security, human rights, and humanitarian crisis. This presents a stark
contrast to the 1960s and '70s, when many newly independent African governments pursued
the vision of public health "for all," of comprehensive health care services directed by the state
with support from foreign donors. These initiatives often failed, undermined by international
politics, structural adjustment, and neoliberal policies, and by African states themselves. Yet their
traces remain in contemporary expectations of and yearnings for a more robust public health.
This volume explores how medical professionals and patients, government officials, and ordinary
citizens approach questions of public health as they navigate contemporary landscapes of NGOs
and transnational projects, faltering state services, and expanding privatization. Its contributors
analyze the relations between the public and the private providers of public health, from the
state to new global biopolitical formations of political institutions, markets, human populations,
and health. Tensions and ambiguities animate these complex relationships, suggesting that
the question of what public health actually is in Africa cannot be taken for granted. Offering
historical and ethnographic analyses, the volume develops an anthropology of public health
in Africa. Contributors: P. Wenzel Geissler; Murray Last; Rebecca Marsland; Lotte Meinert;
Benson A. Mulemi; Ruth J. Prince; and Noémi Tousignant"—Provided by publisher.
    ISBN 978-0-8214-2057-7 (hardback : alk. paper) — ISBN 978-0-8214-2058-4 (pb : alk. paper) —
ISBN 978-0-8214-4466-5 (electronic)
    I. Prince, Ruth Jane, editor of compilation. II. Marsland, Rebecca, editor of compilation. III.
Series: Cambridge Centre of African Studies series.
    [DNLM: 1. Public Health—history—Africa South of the Sahara—Congresses. 2.
Anthropology, Cultural—Africa South of the Sahara—Congresses. 3. History, 20th Century—
Africa South of the Sahara—Congresses. 4. History, 21st Century—Africa South of the
Sahara—Congresses.
WA 11 HA12]
    RA552.A357
    362.10967—dc23
                                    2013030954

Contents

Contents

Acknowledgments

This volume is the result of a workshop held at the University of Cambridge's Centre of African Studies and Department of Social Anthropology in June 2008. The workshop was funded by the Economic and Social Research Council (ESRC) and the Centre of African Studies and hosted by Newnham College. The editors are especially grateful to the Cambridge Centre of African Studies Series editors, Derek Petersen, Harri Englund, and Christopher Warnes, and to Gillian Berchowitz at Ohio University Press for their intellectual support and encouragement. We would also like to thank colleagues who participated in the conference as speakers and discussants but whose contributions are not published here: Julie Livingston, Stacey Langwick, Hans-Jörg Dilger, and Steve Feierman.

Situating Health and the Public in Africa

Historical and Anthropological Perspectives

RUTH J. PRINCE

SINCE THE 1980S, MANY AFRICAN COUNTRIES HAVE WITNESSED THE decay of government-controlled health services and a corresponding proliferation of nongovernmental, transnational, private, and humanitarian organizations that target specific health-care needs, treat diseases, support service provision, or combine research with provision of health care—often through geographically and temporally limited projects. Since the turn of the twenty-first century, the language of health "emergencies" in Africa has gained increasing purchase in international concerns about security, conflict, and the spread of disease and is being linked to moral agendas and discourses of human rights. Africa has emerged as a prime arena of "global health" interventions focusing on the control of particular diseases. These high-profile interventions are reshaping social and political landscapes as well as infrastructures of health. Yet they exist alongside more mundane and persistent conditions and concerns. While global attention is focused on HIV activism and the terrain of antiretroviral provision, most African doctors, nurses, and health-care workers struggle with the day-to-day challenge of providing a reasonable standard of care in underresourced public health facilities.

This volume rethinks public health and what it means in Africa. The term public health implies the duty of government to provide for the health of its citizens, yet this situation has never been fully implemented on the continent. Attending to the legacies of earlier ameliorative drives to provide health care to national publics, to neoliberal structural adjustment, and to novel transnational interventions and biopolitical configurations, the volume assesses the uneven terrain of public health in Africa. It offers a critical analysis of widening global and national inequalities and the emptying out of the public as an inclusive terrain, as health-care provision is shifted towards the arena of the market and of nongovernmental and transnational organizations. At the same time, less visible engagements with the health of the public and with a public good open up new perspectives on the present and future. The book thus casts a critical eye on both the radical shifts in health-care provision and the less visible concerns and practices that connect the realm of "health" with that of the "public" (or publics) in Africa today. It presents ethnographic and historical perspectives on landscapes of what can be broadly termed "public health" in Africa, as well as on the regimes, relations, and tensions that animate them.

Contributors to the volume analyze the place of public health within emerging global "biopolitical" formations of political institutions, markets, human populations, and health, and explore how African professionals and citizens approach questions of responsibility for public health as they navigate contemporary landscapes of NGOs and transnational projects, faltering state services, and expanding privatization. The authors also attend to the broad range of moral and political practices that Africans have drawn upon to intervene on the health of a collective, practices that have a long history going back to the precolonial period. Individual chapters explore confrontations of official versions of public health with indigenous concerns about collective well-being in Tanzania; tensions between private and public spheres of responsibility for health and welfare in northern Nigeria; and attempts by pharmacists in Senegal to mediate public and private health sectors, state responsibilities, and citizenship. Other chapters follow how medical professionals, patients, "community-based organizations," and "volunteer" health workers navigate new regimes of HIV treatment in East Africa; negotiations of care for cancer patients in an underresourced public hospital ward; the struggles of people with diabetes within a disparate and uncoordinated landscape of health promotion, advice, and therapy in Uganda; and the interweaving of transnational medical research trials with health-care provision. Together, the chapters offer insights into widening global and national inequalities as well as present and future trajectories of public health in Africa.

The term *public health* conventionally refers to the duties of the modern state concerning the protection and care of the health of its citizens, through the application of modern, scientific medicine and rational administration—providing health-care services, preventive medicine, and environmental sanitation, as well as protective legislation concerning exposure to industrial, agricultural, or environmental hazards.[1] A vision of amelioration guides this drive toward public health, which applies biomedicine and bureaucratic procedures to state intervention and control, financed by national systems of taxation and health insurance. This vision, and the unity between "state" and "society" that it both assumes and strives for, was embodied most fully in the socialist and welfare regimes that were established in western European states during the mid-twentieth century.[2] It was exported to Africa in the halfhearted attempts of some colonial administrations in the 1940s to extend health and welfare services to broader segments of the population and was more enthusiastically pursued by some independent African governments in the "developmentalist" era of the 1960s and 1970s.[3] This vision of public health appears anachronistic when we consider contemporary landscapes of health-care provision, whether in Africa or in Europe. Yet it is one that should be taken seriously. The appeal of biomedicine to inclusive and expansive visions of progress and development and associated ideas about government responsibility, public service, and the public good are concepts that are now rarely associated with African states, yet they did play a part in the hopes and expectations many Africans had for development and for a national future.[4] In many countries after independence, especially those that appear in this book—Senegal and Nigeria in West Africa, and Uganda, Kenya, and Tanzania in East Africa—the extension of public health to an expectant citizenry became a nationalist project. It was pursued by governments and backed up by foreign aid and by the World Health Organization (WHO), and it had some success: hospitals and clinics were built in rural and urban centers; medical schools were set up; and primary health-care programs, vaccination and immunization campaigns, and maternal health services were extended. These visions were not, of course, shared across African countries (some of which were still fighting white supremacist regimes while others faced civil war, backed up by foreign political interference). They were also often tied to authoritarian and paternalistic regimes; they had to contend with, and were often deflected by, the very different concerns of what Rebecca Marsland in her chapter refers to as "indigenous" public health; and they were undermined by scarce resources. Still, their legacy is apparent today in the material and human infrastructure of government health services, even if much of this is currently in a state of disrepair and even ruin.[5]

The first objective of the book is to take these histories and legacies of biomedical modernization and associated public health initiatives seriously in our attention to how African publics—including medical professionals, scientists, government officials, staff of nongovernmental organizations (NGOs), community health workers, "volunteers," patients and their families, and clinical trial subjects—seek to provide or receive medical care. In doing so, we try to understand both why these initiatives often failed and how these actors navigate within contemporary landscapes of NGOs and transnational projects, faltering state services, and expanding privatization. The hospitals and clinics proudly built in the 1960s and 1970s today display peeling walls and leaking roofs, electricity and medical supplies are intermittent, and staff are overworked and often absent. The treatment of disease is always an uncertain task, but in the context of scarce resources, lack of diagnostic equipment, and poor working conditions, biomedical practice is often poor and may even be counterproductive. Lack of laboratory equipment to diagnose disease and the poor quality of existing equipment mean that medical professionals have to treat most diseases on a "best guess" basis.[6] In the face of this destruction and dysfunction, many of the doctors and nurses trained in African medical schools have migrated to work in countries of the Global North.[7] Others leave public medicine for private practice. Yet many continue with the struggle to diagnose disease and offer good care to the public under extremely difficult conditions, and many believe the state should take an active role in health-care provision.[8] Several of the chapters in this book observe the hopes and expectations that medical staff and patients initially bring to biomedical care and the afterlives of these hopes in the face of long-term illness and inequalities in access to treatment. Benson Mulemi, for example, shows how Kenyan doctors and nurses in a public hospital's cancer ward struggle to provide care to often very poor patients who arrive in a late stage of their illness, having been consistently misdiagnosed. Prince's chapter follows medical staff, volunteers, and patients attached to well-resourced, transnationally funded HIV clinics in the same country, while Susan Whyte explores the uncertain and diffuse landscape of diabetes treatment in Uganda.

A second objective of the book is to take a bearing on contemporary and past landscapes that connect health to—or disconnect health from—African publics. Despite the hopes placed in the developmentalist state, a national context in which public health is promoted by the government and extended to citizens on an equal basis has never really existed in Africa, either in the past or in the present. Moreover, conceptions of the public sphere, the public good, and the public itself are plural and cannot be taken for granted. There are three reasons for this.

First, health services have never been provided exclusively by the state. Colonial administrations began to attend to the health of African populations belatedly, and then only in limited ways.[9] Up to the Second World War, missionaries and private companies were more active providers of medical services, although rarely involved in extending them beyond a particular locality.[10] The attempts to extend public health provision by African governments after independence were undermined by global economic policies and political interests, lack of resources and political will, and large differences between urban and rural services, as well as by the burden of disease, and public health services remained patchy and inadequate. During the 1970s, as world economic recession impacted fragile national economies, modernization faltered and the vision of public health pursued by the developmentalist state was downscaled.[11] The 1980s saw a decisive shift away from developmentalist African states as aggressive neoliberal policies pushed by Western donors promoted privatization of health services and a dominant model of voluntary provision by humanitarian NGOs.[12]

Furthermore, the ideal vision of public health relies on a social contract between citizens and state and the existence of a state bureaucracy and civil service that serves the public interest, defined in this case in terms of biomedical health. As Murray Last argues in his chapter, both colonial and postcolonial government bureaucracies and political power may have only partially, if ever, functioned in this way, while Rebecca Marsland shows that district health officials' conceptions of public health and the public interest are not straightforwardly biomedical. Other "moral economies" relating to power, authority, the health of publics, and the relations between public and private interests operate as well.[13] Medical professionals, government officials, and patients must take into account these often-conflicting values and mores, and their own positions within them—shaped by past and present socioeconomic, class, education, religious, and ethnic differences—may be vastly different.[14]

Second, the association of biomedicine with colonial regimes of power and with national and global inequalities in the postcolonial era has undermined its promise as a means of amelioration. Biomedicine in colonial Africa was intimately tied to a repressive, coercive, and violent system of power and knowledge, which reached deep into African lives and identities.[15] Biomedicine's association with an externally imposed system of knowledge has continued to color encounters with health interventions in the postcolonial era. Suspicions and rumors about the nefarious intentions behind health interventions and medical professionals continue to circulate among African publics and have occasionally spilled out into resistance to public health campaigns.[16] This has not been confined to ordinary citizens or religious leaders. For example, in South Africa, former president Thabo Mbeki, together with other politicians and government officials, ignited fierce national and international disputes when he challenged the scientific consensus regarding antiretroviral treatment for HIV-positive people, evoking "dissident science" and the superiority of herbal and "indigenous" medicine.[17] Such suspicions of biomedical progress do not only speak truth to experiences of colonial and postcolonial domination. They also rest on experiences of scientific failure, as biomedicine often operates without adequate resources and in situations of deep uncertainty, in which mistakes are easily made. In her analysis of parents' resistance to polio vaccination in northern Nigeria, for example, Elisha Renne argues that mass immunization disrupted established patterns of immunity and led to the increased exposure of children to wild poliovirus, which fuelled fears of vaccination.[18]

Third, Africans have long been used to taking matters of health into their own hands. As the chapters in this book show, ordinary people are not passive recipients of health interventions. They have their own views on public health and their own concerns. These may include expectations of government action in relation to modern, formal public health, but responsibility for health and well-being has never rested in the hands of government or other biomedical authorities, and a thriving medical pluralism attests to the resonance of ideas about health and healing other than the biomedical. Biomedicine has had to coexist with these other epistemologies and practices, which locate health and therapy in arenas beyond the biological body, outside the clinic and the hospital and among nonbiomedical authorities. Given that biomedical practice has often been uncertain, inadequate, and sometimes counterproductive, its superiority over these other medical practices and forms of healing is fragile. Colonial governments recognized and feared the authority and power underlying indigenous forms of public health and therapeutic practices; the latter were labeled as antimodern and were repressed, sometimes violently. Yet they persisted and continue to shape conceptions of health, well-being, healing, and harm. In her chapter, Rebecca Marsland attends to the divergence in rural Tanzania between "indigenous" public health and district officials' visions of public health; she shows that although people cannot ignore government interventions, they can bend such interventions to fit their concerns.

Recent scholarship argues that a new form of "biopolitics" has emerged during the past two decades and is taking shape globally amid the shifting relations between political institutions, global markets, human populations, and health.[19] While Michel Foucault located biopolitics in the relations between the state and its populations, contemporary interventions into "life itself"—as the narrowly defined sphere of the vital processes of biological life—are driven by the market, specifically, the pharmaceutical industry and its pursuit of "biocapital."[20] As a result, health care is increasingly bifurcated: those who can afford it are offered the chance to "optimize" their health through advanced biomedical technology, produced through market investment, while the rest are left with a minimal form of care directed at their "bare life" and organized through voluntary and humanitarian interventions.[21] This zoning of health care reflects wider political and economic shifts in the relations between states, markets, and citizens as transnationalism and globalization create novel spatial and temporal forms of government: zones of "exception," a reconfiguration of sovereignty and belonging, and the fragmentation of national publics into smaller collectives gathered around specific needs.[22] While the example of AIDS activism and the new collectives forming around "rights to health" suggest that this situation does not necessarily prevent collective action and the pursuit of public goods, it is also true that the notion of "public" is heavily curtailed. As Nikolas Rose argues, "the idea of 'society' as a single, if heterogeneous, domain with the national culture, a national population, [and] a national destiny, coextensive with a national territory and the powers of a national political government, has entered a crisis."[23]

Between the vision—if not the reality—of the "developmental" past and this picture of a deeply fragmented present and uncertain but dystopian future, where does African public health lie? In the past two decades, attempts to build national health-care systems, patchy and fragmented as they were, have been replaced by humanitarian interventions and vertical disease programs with narrowly technical, targeted services—by projects that pursue "bare survival" rather than a vision of comprehensive care. The past decade has witnessed a narrowing of public health to target biologically defined (for example, HIV-positive) populations rather than a national public and citizenry. As such interventions focus more on the containment of diseases defined as "health emergencies" than on public health as a developmental goal, visions of public health have retreated further from the "health for all" goals of the 1960s and 1970s pursued by many African governments together with the World Health Organization. This increasingly transnational sphere of health provision has also created further shifts in the role of the state in relation to NGOs, in relations between public and private health services, and in imaginations of public health. While the displacement of the state and reduction of national sovereignty have not been confined to Africa, it has become a site par excellence of the "intermediary power formations"—the unstable and seemingly diffuse hybrids of public and private, state and nonstate, and national and transnational—that embody contemporary government.[24] Many African states, never strong in terms of trade relations with former colonial powers, foreign capital, or accountability to their citizens, have been particularly weakened in this move away from the modernist and nationalist project. Transnational and nongovernmental organizations often bypass national ministries of health and state institutions, leaving the state a weak role as "coordinator." Africa's marginality in what James Ferguson calls the "shadows" of the global political and economic system has left it open to a high degree of foreign intervention—to what Thandika Mkandawire calls a "reckless experimentation with African institutions."[25] Some scholars argue that this marginality and "crisis" have enabled African terrains to become sites of "experimentation" by external agents.[26]

This situation—and the claims made about it—calls for closer investigation. African states never formed taken-for-granted rational bureaucratic institutions but were always partial, in a process of being made (and unmade); moreover, they have always operated in an international field and have made use of external connections and relationships to pursue their own interests.[27] Health and the pursuit of treatment have also often escaped biopolitical framings in Africa, and citizenship has not been reduced to the "biological" or "therapeutic" domain, as has been claimed,[28] but remains, as Noémi Tousignant shows in her chapter, a complex field of negotiation and action. While people may make use of current opportunities to pursue livelihoods and careers, visions of a public good are not absent; they suffuse popular culture, public discussion, and national debates.

These tensions and the ambiguities that animate the relations between health and African publics suggest that the question of what public health actually *is* in Africa, whether today or in the past, cannot be taken for granted. An ethnographic and historical focus on the meanings and configurations of "public health" in Africa is therefore both timely and important. To locate and understand present and past forms of public health, we need to grasp the *particular* historical relations between political authorities, individuals, and collectives, as well as the often *plural* concepts of a "public" and practices of "public" health that exist. What has "public health" meant in particular African countries, at particular times? Did it ever exist, and if so, in which forms? Was there ever a narrative of "public" health, conceived of as the responsibility of the state to its citizens, and if so, what has become of it in a situation in which health interventions are funded and organized to a large extent by nonstate and extranational institutions? Which forms of responsibility, civic commitments, and collectives animate these new configurations of health care and intervention? What role do African states play in this? And what are the implications for African health—for the experiences of patients and the provision of services, as well as for notions of the public good and the responsibility of government? These questions provide a framework for this book. We use them to investigate the multiple relations between "health" and "the public" rather than assuming that there is a "system" of "public health."

The book explores, then, the regimes and relations, the interests and concerns, and the contradictions and negotiations that motivate, animate, or undermine the nebulous realm of public health in Africa. It asks who is taking care of whom, on what terms, and with which social, political, economic, and personal consequences.[29] It shows how those acting in relation to public health must contend with different historical legacies, conflicting interests, and uncertain futures. Offering insights from research in Nigeria, Senegal, Kenya, Uganda, and Tanzania, the contributing chapters examine the concerns and tensions that animate health-care provision and public health projects. The chapters explore various landscapes in which health is connected to—or disconnected from—various publics and follow the trajectories, motivations, expectations, and hopes of the actors that move within them. Thus, they explore how pharmacists, scientists and science workers, government officials, doctors, NGO staff, community health workers, and volunteers, as well as patients and laypeople, seek treatment or provide care, negotiate careers and seek livelihoods, and pursue their visions of development. Our analyses move between different levels of scale (the global, national, local, and individual), between public and private spaces, and between lives and technologies, medicines and bodies, organizations and individuals, and policies and practices, as well as between past and present. Some chapters attend to the hopes that Africans invest into biomedicine and health services and their visions of the public good in relation to health. Others point to the evacuation of the public as a national collective and the fragile status of the public good in the sphere of health, and trace the contours of new landscapes of health—"archipelagos," to adopt Geissler's term—that zoom in on particular groups and circumscribed publics or appeal to growing socioeconomic distinctions in an expanding market of privatized care. Several chapters point to a new "projectification" of health care and explore its implications. Others attend to older historical relations between health and the public or to "indigenous" forms of public health, which interact with formal health-care interventions in surprising ways. Together, they point to tensions between different versions of "public health" and open up debates about the very relevance of the term. In their exploration of the polyvalence of this landscape, the chapters offer an anthropology of public health in Africa.[30]

Within history and anthropology there is a rich literature on the coercive nature of the colonial campaigns against epidemic disease, the imperialist and racist visions that infused medical interventions, and the unequal power relations that continue to define biomedical intervention in Africa.[31] These analyses of repression and resistance are important, but they do not necessarily define the experience of Africans with public health and biomedicine.[32] Many Africans also appreciated scientific medicine and the opportunities it offered for curing disease. Scholars have paid much less attention to the hopes for health and the visions of national development and societal progress that many Africans associated with biomedicine and the pursuit of public health, especially in the years around independence but also since then. Even during the colonial period, biomedical interventions were not experienced solely as repressive; mission clinics and urban health centers were flooded with patients hoping to be cured, and Africans were eager to practice such medicine themselves.[33] In the years leading up to independence, biomedical services and public health campaigns offered people a vision of progress, and newly independent governments pushed the extension of public health services as a tool of "development." This drive for development by the state was fragmented, internally divisive, and contradictory and was quickly undermined by African governments themselves as well as by international interference. Yet it did provide a narrative of progress in independent Africa.[34] In the face of the destruction and fragmentation of public health systems by neoliberal policies and the massive privatization that has opened up health to market forces, including transnational business, on a new scale, these visions of the public good associated with public health appear as important objects of anthropological attention.

This book, then, offers various angles onto the differentiated forms of public health—or forms that relate to public health—that have emerged in recent years on the African continent. We pay attention not only to the new and old forms of power, and the violence, exclusions, and inequalities that are present within these formations, but also to the ways actors circumnavigate them, act upon them, and bend them to local interests and concerns. We use the frame of public health to interrogate visions of the public, the public good, and the public sphere that undergird particular interventions and to scrutinize the uneven and unstable relations between public and private health care and between public and private, government and nongovernmental organizations. We also examine the ways in which public health activities produce and interact with particular spheres of intervention—such as the domestic, the community, the market, lifestyle, behavior, the individual subject, and individual responsibility for health. Throughout, we point to historical legacies and present trajectories.

From Ritual and Healing to Biomedicine and Globalization

A rich historical and anthropological literature shows us that health and healing are at the heart of the socio-moral, political, and cosmological order in African societies past and present. Edward Evans-Pritchard's classic study of Azande witchcraft showed that Zande witchcraft beliefs and practices were at the center of societal order and notions of personhood. He argued that they formed a logical system of thought and practice, but he retained his faith in the ultimate truth of his scientific worldview and its superiority over what were, according to this perspective, cultural beliefs. His work is a reflection of his position as a colonial anthropologist, tasked with explaining African society to a bewildered colonial administration that was faced with the "otherness" of vastly different epistemological and ontological practices. Yet this cultural and political position on "science" versus "culture" has continued to shape anthropological analysis and to inform postcolonial governance and interventions into health and healing. Even though many anthropologists suspended their disbelief in the realities of African cosmologies and entered into different life worlds, the realm of scientific medicine was not treated with the same degree of symmetry.

From the 1950s to the 1970s, anthropologists' analyses of ritual and healing in African societies produced powerful insights into the rich cosmological worlds of African peoples and into the experience of illness, health, and therapy. Working in 1950s and 1960s Zambia, for example, Victor Turner explored the relations between symbols and experience and the transformative effect of ritual, laying the grounds for later anthropological treatments that related ritual practice to power, historical agency, and resistance to colonial hegemony.[35] In 1960s and 1970s Zaire, John Janzen explored the social organization of healing and the importance of "therapy management groups," that is, associations of family, neighbors, and friends that decide treatment pathways and manage the body of the patient.[36] By following case studies of illness and misfortune, he showed that people sought therapy within a landscape of medical pluralism, trying out both biomedical services and other forms of healing and approaching both therapeutic systems with caution, as medicine was understood to have the capacity to harm as well as heal. Janzen argued that the colonial suppression of healers and healing and accompanying shifts in the political and social landscapes of therapy had deeply influenced the therapeutic practices he observed. A growing body of historical research on how indigenous forms of healing were increasingly circumscribed by colonial power, administration, law, and medicine supported Janzen's views.[37]

These evocative studies of ritual and healing in Africa influenced subsequent work on cultural histories and colonialism, and they shaped a new subdiscipline, medical anthropology, which took seriously experiences of illness and therapeutic practices outside of scientific medicine.[38] Despite the recognition of medical pluralism, however, these and subsequent studies in Africa gave more attention to vernacular forms of healing than to the practice of biomedicine itself. This is strange, given that by the mid-twentieth century, particularly the anthropologists associated with the Rhodes-Livingstone Institute had already taken a keen interest in processes of colonialism, race relations, labor migration, and industrialization. Perhaps this blind spot was due to the fact that biomedical services were patchy and African encounters with them were more limited than with other colonial interventions, or perhaps it was because at the time anthropologists could not treat modern biomedicine with the same degree of cultural relativism. It was science, thus universal and outside the interests of the anthropology of the time.

In the 1980s and 1990s, however, anthropologists began to take a fresh look at the colonial encounter.[39] Influenced by Marshall Sahlins's work on Fijian histories, Jean and John Comaroff argued that dominant colonial, capitalist, and Christian practices and ideologies entered into extended interaction with African practices, producing "something altogether new."[40] This historical anthropology of colonialism opened up the study of colonial medicine as a system of power and knowledge and of contradictory practices.[41] Historians and anthropologists began to approach biomedicine as a "cultural system."[42] Influenced by Michel Foucault and Frantz Fanon, Megan Vaughan and Jean Comaroff scrutinized biomedicine as a system of knowledge and power that was imbued with racial and colonial stereotypes, objectifying Africans and Africa.[43] In her work on "blood stealing" rumors, Luise White points to the fears and suspicions, the ambivalence and the violence that suffused African experiences of colonial medicine, while Nancy Rose Hunt's account of the encounters between medical missionaries and Congolese in Belgian Congo offers a nuanced reading of the translations and misunderstandings as well as the violence of the exchanges that took place around biomedical practice.[44] Such studies underline that biomedicine cannot be considered predictable, coherent, or monolithic.

Medical anthropologists also began to turn their attention to biomedicine, offering acute analyses of the disconnects between biomedical disease and the patient's experience of illness, the political economy of health under capitalism, and the effects of globalization and neoliberal policies on the health of the poor.[45] Within Africa, however, ethnographic study until recently focused mainly on the informal sectors in which people accessed biomedical practice rather than on medical encounters within clinics and hospitals.[46] For example, Susan Whyte, Sjaak van der Geest, and Anita Hardon explored lay use of pharmaceuticals and the social histories of medicines as they circulated in the "informal" sector.[47] In revealing the mobilities of medicine, both within and beyond Africa, this work laid the grounds for more recent ethnographies of biomedicine and globalization. A new anthropology of biomedicine has taken shape,[48] which brings into focus new ethnographic sites. These include policy making, government bureaucracies, transnational NGOs such as World Vision and Médecins sans frontières (MSF), clinical research trials, drug donation projects, vaccination campaigns, and antiretroviral treatment programs—and the "assemblages" of transnational politics, ethics, science, technology, and expertise that support them.[49] Anthropologists have also turned to more mundane arenas of medical practices, such as hospitals, clinics, and medical colleges, the privatization of care, and its globalization.[50] Rather than engendering the inevitable transformation of "local" social and cultural forms by "universal" ones, globalization is recognized here as an unpredictable process that brings different trajectories, histories, and interests into friction as "universals" are engaged and made to work.[51] At the same time, neoliberal globalization has accentuated political and economic inequalities, particularly in Africa, where resources and technologies have leaped into bounded enclaves, benefiting an exclusive set of interests, often extractive and exploitative ones.[52] The anthropology of biomedicine has been inspired by recent ethnographies of development, which shift critique away from the hegemonic interests underlying development discourse to consider the practice of policy itself, the unexpected directions that development projects take, and ways different actors position themselves in relation to it.[53] These perspectives challenge the built-in bias of health interventions and development projects toward representing success rather than failures, and remind us of histories of dystopias.[54] Yet they also recognize that there may be, to use Julie Livingston's term, "productive misunderstandings," which enable public health interventions to encompass the multiple interests of actors involved.[55]

Social scientists argue that the present "neoliberal" order, with its particular imaginaries of society and the state, has narrowed the responsibility of health down to the individual while relating this individual—through his or her particular disease—to an increasingly transnational sphere of governance and privatized health. National sovereignty is pared away in this process, as state institutions are to a large extent bypassed or given a weak role. Such characterizations contain much truth yet also simplify a more complex reality. They lay bare political and economic exclusion, domination, and inequality, yet in privileging a narrative of biopolitical domination, they obscure other possibilities that may lie within the present.[56] The high-profile "global" regimes shaping health-care provision such as transnational HIV treatment programs are important objects of anthropological analysis. Yet they highlight only one arena shaping what has become of public health on the continent and overshadow the more mundane practices, policies, and struggles that form its less visible side. We must be careful not to privilege the agency of the global and overlook how local interests, actors, sensibilities, and social forms are often what anchor externally planned interventions in a meaningful way. Furthermore, Africa is not merely a recipient of humanitarian and development interventions; it is also a site of a thriving private therapeutic sector that builds on longer histories of mobility and encounters between different therapeutic traditions and health experts.[57] Public health care and interventions in Africa share the medical space not only with a vast variety of nonbiomedical therapies and traditions but also with increasing numbers of private hospitals and medical insurances, which offer biomedical treatment to the better-off middle classes, some of whom also go abroad for private medical care or fertility treatment.[58]

Such perspectives underline that the relations between health and the public in Africa encompass multiple interests, socioeconomic forms, and trajectories and that we cannot approach them through a singular object of study. These approaches inform the ethnographies of public health that we offer in this book. We show that public health cannot be taken for granted; it does not form a predictable space of intervention but is currently an open and even experimental arena, the future trajectories of which remain unclear.

Locating Health, Healing, and the Public in Africa

Steven Feierman's work on the "invisible histories" that surround biomedicine and colonialism reveals that present formations of health and the public have been shaped by longer histories, ideologies, and practices.[59] The encounter of these arenas in the colonial era with biomedicine involved violence and repression. These histories allow us to better understand contemporary encounters between health interventions and African publics.

In precolonial Africa (and up to the present day), health was understood to extend beyond the boundaries of the body and to be intimately tied to matters of production and reproduction, prosperity, and power.[60]

Interventions into health and well-being were directed not exclusively at bodies but also at the fertility of the land and livestock and relations with others, living and dead, while bodily health itself was conceived as part of wider relations. Given that such relations were always fraught and fragile, therapeutic power was considered highly ambivalent, as it could be directed to harm as well as to heal. Historians of Africa describe these forms of power, knowledge, and intervention that were concerned with the vitality and health of the collective as a kind of "public health."[61] Control over healing was at the heart of political power, albeit in different and often highly contested ways.[62] Chiefs were invested with power over the land, its fertility, and its vitality through their persons, their use of medicines, and their control over ritual and through their authority over healers and spirit mediums, rainmaking, and witchcraft. They could use this power to cleanse the land and persons of pollution but also to hold back growth and fertility. Yet healing was multifaceted. There was no one source of authority; chiefly power was not absolute, and chiefs were dependent on their people. If they were unable or unwilling to respond to misfortune, they would be deposed. Healers were not always intimate with those in political power; they could undermine such power or destabilize it.[63]

Through the introduction of Christianity, the suppression of uprisings, the killing and exile of chiefs and kings as well as healers and prophets, the reorganization of political economy, and the imposition of alien systems of authority and law, colonialism repressed and ruptured these forms of power and knowledge.[64] In the process, healing became severed from the political order. By the time anthropologists began observing rituals of healing and describing them in the 1930s and 1940s, many forms of public healing had gone underground or were forced to operate within a more circumscribed, private sphere.[65] Chiefs often became co-opted by colonial authorities as headmen; they lost their ritual authority but gained a position in the colonial order.[66] Meanwhile, colonial authorities began to intervene in matters of public health, such as disease epidemics and famines. At the same time, they tried to confine the realm of "African healing" to that of timeless, archaic tradition and sought to render healers' practices illegal.[67] The introduction of antiwitchcraft laws and the grouping of all practices regarded by the colonial authorities as "irrational" or "occult" into the category of witchcraft added to the confusion.[68] Christian missions reinforced these attitudes toward the realm of healing more intimately and intensely, as they demonized the African past, introducing polarities between "traditional" and "modern" and placing practices concerned with healing in the realm of the (archaic) past.[69] In their push for "development" and modernization, postcolonial governments largely took on colonial attitudes toward indigenous healing—at least officially—and labeled the realm of nonscientific medicine and healing practices as irrational and antimodern.[70] In the name of development or "scientific socialism," they continued to push popular concerns with the health of the public, and its location in practices pertaining to the growth and vitality of land and people, into the realm of custom, tradition, witchcraft, and the occult.

Even while public healing and public ritual were suppressed, however, "indigenous" understandings of health and healing did not disappear. The social, political, and economic tensions of the colonial era led to a rise in witchcraft accusations and the proliferation of witchcraft eradication movements and new forms of healing. The emergence of Christian healing and the persistence of ritual specialists and healers point to concerns about a broad realm of growth and vitality anchored not only within the body but also in the social, moral, and spiritual order. These concerns are still resonant today, even while they are deeply contested.[71] By contrast, biomedical practice attends to a circumscribed arena, that of the biological body. These issues are explored in the first section of this book. The chapters by Murray Last on northern Nigeria and Rebecca Marsland on contemporary Tanzania argue that colonial biomedicine and postcolonial attempts to intervene in public health share a tense space with other ideas and practices around health and healing, which engage with public morality.

Health, Development, and the Colonial State in Africa

While the particular interventions into health taken by different colonial governments in Africa—French, Portuguese, Belgian, and British—are diverse, until the 1920s colonial authorities confined their activities to providing health services to settler populations and combating epidemics of infectious and tropical disease that threatened pools of native labor and thus economic productivity.[72] Early disease campaigns focusing on sleeping sickness, plague, and smallpox were often coercive and violent and left a deep mark on African consciousness.[73] Curative services were mostly left to missionaries—although some medical care was provided to urban employees.[74] Colonial administrations gave African health more attention after the First World War but were mostly concerned with the reproduction of a healthy labor force, as the greater exposure to disease and poor nutrition of populations under colonial rule became apparent in high mortality and low birth rates. In the late 1920s and in the 1930s, some progressive voices called for improvement in socioeconomic conditions and for a focus on "African welfare," but the lack of political will meant that few of these initiatives were sustained.[75]

In the 1940s, the development of vaccinations and antibiotics and the increasing agitation of colonized peoples for better living standards and for political participation led to efforts, in the British and French colonies at least, to extend some health-care services and medical technologies to broader populations.[76] In the British colonies, postwar "development" and "welfare" acts were introduced, driven in part by self-interest but also by more progressive, if paternalistic, ideas about colonial trusteeship, in which government planning and investment would promote economic and social progress.[77] Interventions to improve living conditions and promote development remained half-hearted, patchy, and unfinished, however, and mostly focused on the most politically vocal groups, such as urban wage laborers, in the hope of diverting them from political protest.[78] This proved counterproductive to colonial rule, as "development" became a concept around which colonized peoples could formulate political and economic demands, while continued repression increased resistance to imperial power.[79]

The Developmentalist State in Africa

Frederick Cooper argues that "no word captures the hopes and ambitions of Africa's leaders, its educated populations, and many of its farmers and workers in the post-war decades better than 'development.'"[80] However, development in general, and public health in particular, was crisscrossed by contradictory impulses and experiences, as repression and violence coexisted with attempts at melioration across the colonial and postcolonial eras.[81]

From the 1950s to the 1970s, in the years up to and after independence, the vision of government planning and government investment as the key to economic and social progress had immense appeal both within and beyond Africa.[82] Despite different political approaches to economic development (for example, capitalism in Kenya and Senegal, socialism in Tanzania and Zambia), there was broad consensus that economic growth was to be complemented and driven by improving the education and health of citizens—and in the first two decades after independence, health, education, and social protectionism became a central part of the nation-building project and a central demand by the public of their government.[83] At the same time, development was located firmly in the international sphere and often undermined by cold war interests. Former colonial powers jostled with the United States and the Soviet Union to maintain trade and aid relationships with African states, setting up national "development agencies," which, together with the international organizations created in the 1940s under the Bretton-Woods Agreement, provided technical expertise as well as financial resources. This did not happen across Africa: South Africa, Mozambique, Namibia, and Rhodesia were still under colonial rule, while many newly independent states experienced further violence, even civil war. Still, development was a promise that captured the imagination of the African public.[84]

From the 1950s to the early 1970s, development through state planning had some success, even though its results were uneven. Growth rates in the 1960s and 1970s were mixed but largely positive. Urban economies expanded, as did agricultural exports and some industrial production.[85] The fruits of economic growth were unevenly distributed, disproportionately benefiting the elites, but between the 1950s and 1970s, life expectancy grew and mortality rates fell in many countries—the result of improved maternal and infant care services, the control of epidemics, the elimination of smallpox in 1950s, and the extension of immunization—while literacy rates also improved.[86] Some of the newly independent African states tried to address the imbalance of health services concentrated in urban areas, and there are indicators of widening access to health services and to education.[87]

Many Africans now look back on this era as one of optimism in the ability of the nation-state to deliver development.[88] Yet many states continued to be politically and economically subordinate to former colonial powers and to the international development regime, with its privileging of Western knowledge and technical expertise and belief in the "trickle-down" benefits of modernization projects.[89] At the same time, many postcolonial states continued to practice divisive and unequal forms of governance, inherited partly from their colonial predecessors.[90] Emerging elites rode roughshod over local knowledge and expertise, which contributed to the failure of many development projects. The period also saw the entrenchment of clientalism and political authoritarianism and the suppression of dissent by regimes that were often supported by the West.[91] As the rhetoric of participation in national development was replaced by policies of coercion and control, confidence in the nationalist project was "deeply undermined."[92] Recent scholarship on the rhetoric and realities of "development," "citizenship," "participation," and other postindependence nationalist projects further breaks up the vision of coherent wholes.[93] Still, critiques of the developmental state should not assume that developmentalism has disappeared without a trace; it was never a monolithic category, and for many Africans the project of national development is still one worth striving for.[94] Noémi Tousignant takes up these debates in her chapter on how Senegalese pharmacists have positioned themselves in relation to the state and its responsibility for public health.

The period of the developmentalist state was short-lived.[95] The dependence of many African economies on agricultural or mineral exports meant that the oil shocks and world economic recession of the early 1970s had immediate effects on economic growth. "Whereas in the decade before 1976, GNP per capital from Sub-Saharan Africa as a whole grew nearly 20 percent, in the next decade it fell 20 percent, and as of 1996 was only a little ahead of 1966."[96] If the 1960s was a period of "developmental authoritarianism," by the late 1970s "only the authoritarianism was left, for rarely was the state actually delivering on its developmental promises."[97] State leaders could no longer pass out resources to clients, leading to a highly unstable situation and giving rise to numerous coups and regional conflicts (exacerbated by cold war tensions) and to disillusionment and an increasing lack of faith in the state itself.[98] Governments were forced to borrow from Western institutions at high rates of interest. Growing debt and stalling economic growth began to reverse social and economic improvements; education systems declined, and there was a growing lack of medical facilities and supplies.[99]

The postcolonial period also saw the development of the field of "international health," led by the World Health Organization (which provided technical expertise to African governments) and funded by Northern governments through their development agencies. Health measures and advances were varied. Population control became a focus of intervention beginning in the 1960s, pushed by donors such as the U.S. Agency for International Development (USAID) and pursued by African governments, often through coercive measures. The World

Health Organization's successful eradication of smallpox in 1979 was a breakthrough for its role in overseeing and coordinating primary health campaigns. Overall, disease-eradication programs were favored until the 1970s, when growing disillusionment with "top-down" approaches led to calls for international and national efforts to focus on primary health care and the "grassroots"—captured in the World Health Organization's 1978 call for "Health for all by the year 2000" at its Alma Ata conference.[100] This was part of a broader critique of top-down, "one-size-fits-all" development in the face of the failure of large-scale modernization projects, and a turn toward small-scale projects, popular participation, and sustainable technology—in countries such as Kenya and Tanzania, it resonated with earlier calls for *harambee* ("pulling together") and *kujitegemea* ("self-reliance") in the name of national development.[101] The Alma Ata declaration called for strengthening health-care infrastructures, health worker training, redistribution of health resources to rural areas, and building on existing "community" strengths such as traditional midwives.[102] It emphasized preventive health care through a focus on immunization, reproductive health, contraception, sanitation, and the promotion of "safe motherhood." Based on successful models of health development in the socialist and communist world, it encouraged "community participation" as the means through which public health efforts would be responsive to local needs—"it was cheap, effective socialized health care."[103]

However, the Alma Ata vision of primary health care was also short-lived. Criticized for being overly ambitious and even expensive, it was disrupted by continuing economic recession in the 1980s, in addition to the rise of neoliberalism, market ideologies, and structural adjustment policies—and by new epidemiological challenges, foremost among them the appearance of HIV/AIDS. It was replaced, in the 1980s, by "selective primary health care," which focused on a few cheap and effective interventions requiring little investment in infrastructure—such as oral rehydration therapy for diarrheal disease in children and growth-monitoring, breast-feeding, and immunization programs.[104] During the 1980s, many national health-care systems were dismantled, and "the terms of Alma Ata, never fully implemented, were simply overtaken and made irrelevant by . . . global processes."[105] As neoliberal policies became dominant, health interventions became narrowly focused on promoting individual responsibility for health, rather than attempting to tackle the broader socioeconomic and political conditions underlying ill health.[106]

The 1980s: Neoliberalism, Structural Adjustment, and NGOs

The 1980s was a period of economic decline in Africa, engendered by increased oil prices and world economic recession, fluctuations in export prices, and governments' growing debt. At the same time, authoritarian governments became increasingly repressive (many of them, such as those in the Congo and Cameroon, were put in place and supported by Western powers). Faced with downward-spiraling revenues, African governments applied for financial loans to the International Monetary Fund (IMF) and World Bank, which imposed stringent conditions, known as "structural adjustment," forcing them to cut down expenditures and scale back development objectives. IMF economists considered Africa's economic crisis to be caused by misjudged economic policies but also, above all, by what they saw as "bloated" state institutions and corruption ("rent-seeking" behavior). While this diagnosis contained some truth, the solution imposed—drastically cutting state resources for health and education and cutting back finances for the civil service, including teachers and health workers—is now widely accepted to have done little to reduce corruption, while having devastating effects on health and education provision, on the morale of civil servants, and on living standards, as formal sector wages fell, while more and more people were forced to find a living in the informal economy.[107] The collapse of primary health care services and the decimation of public health systems pushed people to seek treatment outside the formal sector, in informal pharmaceutical markets and within the diverse arena of "traditional" medicine.[108] National pharmaceutical industries collapsed, too: "By 1990," argues Kristin Petersen, "the domestic production of pharmaceuticals ceased almost entirely not only in Nigeria but throughout Africa; most pharmaceutical and medical supply industries were pushed into bankruptcy."[109] This further opened up African markets to the global pharmaceutical industry. It reflected a widespread "dispossession" of local manufacturing and small-scale enterprise by neoliberal policies across the globe.[110]

The story of 1980s neoliberalism in Africa and beyond (and its consequences for power relations between national, transnational, and global scales) is by now well-known.[111] The 1970s economic crises led to the dismantling of the Bretton-Woods system of fixed exchange rates and controls on capital and to the encouragement of speculative financial movements. The New Right, led by the United States and the United Kingdom, endorsed neoclassical economic theories advocating growth through opening up markets and reducing the role of the state.[112] Liberal theories in which the state and citizens are conceived as separate and antagonistic entities replaced social democratic ideas of the duties and relationships between them. Neoclassical economics came to dominate powerful international institutions such as the World Bank and International Monetary Fund (IMF), which "shifted their focus from economic specialization within a national framework to specialization in a world economy; thus, for the Bank, development became 'participation in the world market.'"[113] Health markets were opened up to transnational corporate entitles, leaving national governments with little control over prices and supplies of medicines and equipment.[114] At the same time, responsibility for health development in African countries increasingly shifted out of the hands of ministries of health and into a globalized policy environment, dominated by the World Bank and IMF.[115]

The World Bank's 1981 *Berg Report* made the case for structural adjustment and the minimalist role of the state, while the 1991 World Bank Development Report, titled *The Challenge of Development*, signaled the final break from state-led development approaches: the role of the government was to be confined to providing a legal and regulatory framework within which markets could operate, that is, to being a "night-watchman."[116] The 1993 World Bank Development Report (titled *Investing in Health*) observed that direct government provision of health care is inefficient. Governments should provide a "minimum package" of health services, which World Bank experts believed would ensure equal access to basic health services, leaving all other services to be covered by medical insurance or shifted to the private sector.[117]

The degree to which governments and citizens accepted the neoliberal ideology of reduced state expenditure and bureaucracy varied—Kenya adopted it with less resistance than did Tanzania or Zambia.[118] However, African governments applied structural adjustment policies through the 1980s while development policies became driven by the neoliberal agenda—termed the "New Policy Agenda."[119] This focused on a "rollback" of the state, the encouragement of private-sector health services, and an increased flow of external aid to nongovernmental organizations rather than to governments.[120] It involved not only the cutting back of state expenditure but also experimentation with new social forms in health service delivery. Characteristic public health interventions of the time were the Bamako Initiative—a form of "cost sharing" that involved the introduction of "community pharmacies," for which the community had to pay, and "social marketing" initiatives, for example, marketing condoms as a response to the HIV/AIDS epidemic.[121] Cost sharing was supposed to make individuals more responsible for their consumption of health services, and in the 1980s and 1990s the ideology of the patient as a "consumer" who should exercise "choice" (reflected in the use of the term *client*) became dominant.[122]

There is ample evidence that privatization of previously public services gathered pace and that this occurred within a fundamental shift in the ideology of public health. However, this overlays a complex intertwining of public and private health care from the colonial period on, particularly in African nations that followed a capitalist model of development.[123] The shift away from state health provision is indisputable, yet an association of the pre-1980s with public health and the post-1980s with private health is too simple. As Noémi Tousignant's chapter in this volume underlines, since independence in Senegal, pharmacists have mediated and moved between public and private sectors, appealing to state responsibility for public health care while taking advantage of the state's support for private enterprise. This story could be told elsewhere, particularly in countries, such as Kenya, that followed a capitalist model of development. John Iliffe documents how the Kenyan government encouraged the commercial sale of medicines and of medical expertise; only a minority of Kenya's doctors, even before the 1980s, were in public medicine, and those who were supplemented their state incomes with private practice.[124] The prominence of NGOs or "private voluntary groups" in the provision of health care in African countries also has a long history, as already noted.[125] Their increased role does not necessarily cancel out the state; many health workers are still employed by the state, and clinics and hospitals are run by it, but public health institutions are crisscrossed with "public-private partnerships" and nongovernmental projects. "Demarcation between the public and private sectors is blurred and there are transfers of control, funds and personnel not only from the state to the voluntary sector but also in the reverse direction. Links between the voluntary sector and the state are becoming more—not less—important for service provision: 'straddling' between the public and voluntary sectors is a key feature of privatization."[126]

Nongovernmental Governance?

NGOs became popular vehicles for the implementation of official donor aid objectives at a time of dissatisfaction with state-led development and a search for alternatives. They were endorsed by both sides of the political spectrum, as the Left was frustrated with corruption and political repression in some African states and with "top-down" development. Supporting nongovernmental organizations thus became a strategy to build up "civil society," framed again by the liberal idea, dominant in the United States, of state versus citizens.[127] NGOs were also regarded as more transparent, less weighed down by bureaucracy and corruption, more efficient, and closer to "the grassroots"—hence, better able to deliver the promises of "bottom-up" development.[128] Because of their humanitarian or mission roots, NGOs were also regarded by those on the Left as better advocates for the world's poor than were aid bureaucracies of donor countries or international institutions such as the United Nations. Meanwhile, the political Right regarded the voluntary sector as a cheaper and more efficient alternative; the small size of NGOs gave them a supposed "comparative advantage."[129]

The 1980s and 1990s experienced an "NGO revolution" in many African nations[130]—such that by the mid-1990s, collaboration with NGOs was an established feature of international development. International NGOs have become household names in many African countries.[131] Major bilateral and multilateral actors in international health, including USAID and the World Bank, increasingly channeled aid to the health sector in poor countries through NGOs, producing an "unruly mélange" of international donors and NGOs.[132] Meanwhile, the number of development NGOs in the global North rose from 1,600 in 1980 to between 3,000 and 5,000 in 1993, many of them funded partly by Northern governments.[133] The largest NGOs have budgets larger than the gross domestic product of some African nations.[134] A significant proportion of the NGOs operating in East Africa are American evangelical Christian groups, which registered as NGOs to receive USAID funding,[135] underlining the growing prominence of faith-based organizations in development projects and in providing health services, particularly those directed at HIV/AIDS.[136]

While the focus on civil society and NGOs has contributed to political democratization, in the field of health provision it is generally accepted to have led to poorly regulated, often parallel and competing "projectification" of health care—a focus on isolated islands of intervention rather than national development.[137] There is a large literature on the NGO phenomenon and the largely negative consequences of this model of development, including lack of aid coordination, fragmentation and decline in quality of health services, and increasing inequality.[138]

For example, in East Africa, AIDS interventions aim at getting people to "own" development projects, drawing on a language of "stakeholders" and community "participation." Yet NGOs and "community-based organizations" end up responding more to pressures from above—from donor funding cycles and bureaucracies—than to interests from below, creating an externally orientated and highly dependent health sector.[139] In Mozambique during the late 1990s, the multiplicity of organizations working on health projects and providing health services were found to "duplicate programme support, create parallel projects, pull health services workers away from routine duties and disrupt planning procedures" and to reinforce "a two-tiered provision of services that siphons off resources and personnel from a poorly funded public system, further undermining morale, commitment and organizational capacity."[140] NGO projects pay higher salaries, drawing professionals out of the state system both permanently and on a daily or weekly basis (as they attend training "workshops" run by NGOs and supplemented by generous allowances). State actors are reduced to "coordinators," but they have little incentive in trying to control NGO projects, as these bring in much-needed income and resources.

Across East and southern Africa, then, the turn toward NGOs has increased donor power to direct agendas, weakened state authority, and created a poorly regulated "NGO-isation of society."[141] Moreover, the very qualities that give NGOs a supposed "comparative advantage" limit their effectiveness at promoting societal development. Developmental problems are vast and cannot be tackled by islands of intervention targeting specific populations. Operating short-term and discrete projects, NGOs do not have the reach of state institutions.[142] As NGOs are given an increasingly prominent role, the unit of development is no longer society but the "community": "Some fortunate individuals and communities may experience an improvement in their living standards and quality of life as the result of NGO interventions but the rest of society around them remains stagnant and impoverished."[143] The process of development is, by definition, fragmented, with no provision of universal services and no attempt at equity. As NGO projects, directed at meeting survival needs, replace a vision of development (however fragmented it actually was) as broad-based, equitable economic growth and improvement in living standards, two models of development are produced: "survival of sorts in Africa, and progress for the rest of the world."[144] Despite their avowedly nonpolitical and humanitarian stance, NGOs are political actors whose presence and activities have reconfigured the politics of health provision, development, and ultimately statehood and citizenship.[145] Although old hierarchies have not disappeared—the state is by no means absent, or simply "failing," despite Afro-pessimistic diagnoses—there has been a fundamental rescaling of power.[146]

There is ample evidence that the turn toward NGOs and "civil society" organizations has had detrimental effects. But what of the argument that state institutions were inefficient, corrupt, and unable to deliver development? Alan Fowler argues that the "comparative advantage" of NGOs was deliberately constructed, lying in their ability to mobilize resources.[147] Thandika Mkandawire argues that the neoliberal view of state inefficiency became a "self-perpetuating reality" and, moreover, that it rested on a misinterpretation of the policies behind the East Asian "tiger" economies' successes.[148] From the early 1990s on, as African countries' economic performance continued to decline while social and health indicators worsened, structural adjustment was reappraised. Recognizing that the tiger economies were in fact dependent on strong states governing markets and ensuring national self-interest, the World Bank has moved toward a more positive view of the role that the state can play in development. It now urges combining financial rigor with a return to basic priorities—health, education, and quality of government.[149] But this return of the state, argues Mkandawire, has focused on issues such as technical competence and "capacity" rather than dealing with the low morale and poor pay of government employees.[150] Governance, which began as a concern for accountability, has become "entirely about accounting," a "depoliticized quest for technocratic governance" underlying what he sees as an "ideological vacuum" in which African elites pursue their self-interest, with no sense of the public good.[151] Mkandawire's analysis, however, does not analyze terms such as *accountability* and *good governance*, nor does it raise the important questions of what a "public good" is, who defines it, and how it is acted upon.[152] Several chapters in the book take up these questions surrounding the role of the state and provocatively address issues of the "public" and the public good in relation to public health.

From Public Health to Global Health?

The twenty-first century has seen major shifts concerning how health problems in Africa are conceptualized and in the international responses to them—a shift, some argue, from public health to "global health."[153]

Political scientists define global health normatively as the field of policy and intervention addressing problems of health that "circumvent, undermine, or are oblivious to the territorial boundaries of states, and thus lie beyond the capacity of states to address effectively through state institutions alone."[154] The turn toward global health has taken shape in an ideological framework dominated on the one hand by "emergency," "crisis," and concerns about "global security" and on the other by humanitarianism, both of which have proven powerful forces for mobilizing resources and action.[155] It occurs within a globalized landscape of science and pharmaceutical research, in which there is a dense interpenetration of public and private interests. In the past fifteen years, an increasing number of transnational and nongovernmental organizations compete to provide health services and target disease—from development agencies to private philanthropic groups, transnational NGOs, well-endowed Northern universities (which conduct research and provide health care), and pharmaceutical companies—whose scientists, researchers, policy makers, and academics belong to a powerful "global health elite." Below, I sketch out this new landscape of global health and consider whether the global health orthodoxy oversees a further seeping of power away from African states and their citizens into the nonnational and transnational arena.

The African AIDS epidemic appeared in the 1980s and quickly gathered force. It reached epidemic proportions first in Uganda, moving across East Africa and then to southern Africa.[156] Its effects—during a time of economic crisis and of huge cuts in health budgets—were catastrophic. Most governments did not face up to the problem, with the exception of Uganda, which mobilized a "multisectorial" approach, setting up a National AIDS Control Council and encouraging donor agencies, NGOs, and church-based and grassroots efforts (often by women who were faced with the burden of care).[157] A few other countries, notably, Botswana and Senegal, made early attempts to address AIDS through public education and blood surveillance. Senegal, like much of West Africa, was spared a devastating epidemic, partly for biological reasons, while Botswana's following of expert advice, which at that time linked HIV/AIDS to "risky" behavior, proved irrelevant for much of the population, and HIV prevalence soared.[158]

The AIDS epidemic focused international attention. Beginning in the mid-1980s, the World Health Organization worked with governments to set up national AIDS control councils, introduce national surveillance and blood screening, and oversee preventative efforts.[159] Yet prevention was for many years modeled on ideas of individual responsibility and focused on "risk groups" rather than the socioeconomic conditions that render people vulnerable to HIV infection.[160] Meanwhile, despite the known extent of the epidemic, external funding for health interventions in Africa declined during the 1990s, and African governments had to deal with the surge in morbidity by themselves. Grappling with structural adjustment, they had few resources to mobilize: clinics and hospitals were overwhelmed and doctors and nurses faced appalling conditions, while patients and their families had to sell off assets to pay for medicines and hospital care.[161] Only a tiny proportion of patients could access the new antiretroviral therapies—those who were wealthy or managed to enroll themselves in research programs (or, more rarely, HIV activist networks).[162] The majority sought treatment for opportunistic infections, from which they eventually died.

Beginning in the year 2000, this situation began to change. After effective antiretroviral medicines became available (in 1994), HIV activists pushed the lack of access to treatment in the Global South into a moral issue, forcing the suffering of AIDS patients—and the associated role of global markets, pharmaceutical companies, and governments, together with questions of ethics and responsibility—onto the global health agenda.[163] In 2001 in South Africa, a coalition of HIV activists, international and local NGOs, and the South African government successfully used "right of access" arguments to pressure pharmaceutical companies to lower prices.[164] Earlier, the South African "Treatment Action Campaign" group had, together with MSF, successfully taken the government to court for its refusal to authorize the purchase of generic nivirapine for the prevention of mother-to-child transmission of HIV. These cases drew attention to the vastly unequal resources and inadequate care available to African citizens and to the positive role that NGOs and activist groups could play in publicizing such inequalities. Funding for interventions into HIV/AIDS and, to a much lesser extent, tuberculosis and malaria in Africa increased hugely in the 2000s, with the introduction of the Global Fund to Fight AIDS, Tuberculosis and Malaria in 2001 and the President's Emergency Plan for AIDS Relief (PEPFAR, set up by George W. Bush) in 2003. Together with Northern donors, the World Bank and private philanthropic groups, they channel funds to a mélange of governmental and nongovernmental organizations that are involved in antiretroviral treatment (ART) programs.[165] The deployment of power through the new global funds and interventions is enormous; according to Vinh-Kim Nguyen, in some African countries, PEPFAR and the Global Fund together have at their disposal funds exceeding the entire national health budget.[166] Like NGO-led development, these interventions focus on geographical enclaves, particular populations, and "hot spots" of disease. Although they operate within a language of "partnership" between Northern and Southern institutions, they have been criticized for draining resources and professional expertise away from government health systems, undermining their sustainability.[167]

A body of anthropological scholarship has emerged in response to the AIDS epidemic. This can be divided into pre-ART and post-ART ethnography.[168] Initially, anthropologists examined the disjuncture between public health and prevention messages and local concerns around AIDS, including religious engagements with the epidemic and the attempts of African citizens to make sense of it and to cope with illness and death.[169] Once ART was introduced, attention shifted to the "global assemblages" connected to HIV treatment: the movements of medicines, resources, and expertise, as well as global HIV scripts such as the "confessional technologies" that developed around positive living, new forms of "biosociality," and activism.[170] Steve Robbins, writing from South Africa, argues that these new languages and alliances form a novel political force with effects outside of AIDS activism, producing "empowered citizens" aware of their rights and entitlements.[171] Aside from these pockets of activism in South Africa, however, the apparatus of ART programs in Africa has been accompanied by little political agitation, let alone transformative politics. Instead, ART programs tend to reduce health outcomes among people struggling to survive amid the ravages of structural adjustment to individual responsibility for "adherence" to medical regimens.[172] Ethnographic work from both West and East Africa shows that grassroots activity around HIV/AIDS is marked more often by patronage networks than by political activism; most PLWHAs (people living with HIV/AIDS), as they are now referred to, are struggling to survive in the informal economy, and they are more concerned with accessing resources made available by NGOs than with agitating for their rights in relation to the state.[173] At the same time, ART programs represent a shift away from national sovereignty to the global scale, leaving populations dependent on external aid and depleting resources and expertise from other health-care services.[174]

Some argue that the current structuring of AIDS treatments and the humanitarian economy allow African states to continue to pursue their own modes of accumulation—which means channeling resources to political and economic elites, while leaving the rest to survive in the informal economy or to struggle for charitable handouts.[175]

In summary, although the provision of free ART is a vast improvement over the neglect of the past, the structures in which it is organized produce an impoverished sphere of public health in which specific populations receive specific treatments, while other pressing health issues, the socioeconomic inequalities producing ill health, and the challenges facing national health-care systems are inadequately addressed. Rather than being tied to a developmentalist vision of a national public health system, visions of health are further reduced to survival needs, and public health-care provision is reduced to a technology-driven humanitarian intervention.

Still, HIV/AIDS interventions have introduced new languages of rights and entitlements into national and global arenas, and they have been incredibly productive—of new networks, new identities, and new associations and forms of belonging. They have also intersected with government health services and sites, rather than bypassing them completely. In this book, the chapters by Lotte Meinert, Hannah Brown, and Ruth Prince offer perspectives on AIDS interventions that move away from metanarratives of "biopower" to explore how new therapeutic regimes and governmental practices overlay and interact with existing relations, associations, and connections. Rather than being victims of therapeutic domination, those on the receiving end of such interventions use them to explore new opportunities and pursue their own interests.

The prominence of ART programs as a paradigm of public health in many African countries points toward a new political economy of pharmaceuticals shaping the contours and imaginations of public health—a "pharmaceuticalization of public health," as João Biehl puts it. The focus of public health interventions on problems that can be solved through biomedical and technological intervention was a feature of international health efforts throughout the twentieth century, driven by scientific progress and the desire to solve problems quickly and "efficiently."[176] Progressive moves toward the promotion of health through socioeconomic reform that were discussed and occasionally implemented during the 1920s–40s were quickly supplanted by disease control through the magic bullet of medicine.[177] This technical orientation has only become stronger in recent years. It is supported by the dominance, across wide domains of policy and intervention, of an "audit culture," which evaluates the success of vertical disease programs in terms of numbers of drugs dispensed or numbers of people receiving pharmaceutical treatment, rather than in relation to longer-term health outcomes. Commenting on charitable drug donation programs by pharmaceutical companies to African "communities," Ari Samsky argues, "We no longer talk about health, really, we talk about disease, but when we talk about disease we're really talking about treatment, and even when we elaborate treatment philosophies and techniques we're really talking about a drug."[178]

The pharmaceutical paradigm of health is also driven by an ever more powerful global pharmaceutical industry, its pursuit of "biocapital," and associated intellectual property regimes.[179] Even public health initiatives such as PEPFAR are intimately tied to the North American and global pharmaceutical industry: for the first five years of the program (2003–8), PEPFAR was licensed to purchase only U.S.-patented drugs; it shifted to cheaper generics manufactured in India and Brazil only after vociferous criticism.[180] The subservience of public health to global capital and the drive for profit on a transnational scale is not confined to Africa, of course. We see this in the current privatization of national health systems in Europe such as the National Health Service in the United Kingdom. Meanwhile, in Brazil and Mexico, the state encourages profit-motivated pharmaceutical companies to cater to a citizenship that is regarded as a "therapeutic market," leading to an increasing interpenetration of public with private sectors.[181]

In many African countries, competing kinds of drug markets characterize the production and distribution of pharmaceuticals. Although some countries, such as Nigeria, developed a strong generic drug manufacturing industry, this was decimated by structural adjustment policies in the 1980s, which made the costs of production too high.[182] Meanwhile, African governments are under intense pressure to conform to the World Trade Organization's TRIP (Trade Related Intellectual Property) Agreement, which gives proprietary (U.S. and European) pharmaceutical companies exclusive twenty-year rights on their drug patents. This is undercut, however, by a thriving informal market in pharmaceuticals—in which the production and sale of counterfeit drugs overshadows the formal sector of licensed pharmacies. In Nigeria, not only private doctors but also public hospitals and clinics prefer to buy their drugs from these informal markets; these "out-compete" both U.S. proprietary drugs and

Nigerian generics but at a great cost to the safety of the populations consuming these poor-quality medicines.[183] National and international attempts to ensure better regulation of quality in the name of public health are a drop in the ocean in the face of these illegal pharmaceutical markets.[184] Meanwhile, it is difficult for qualified pharmacists to make a living in a country flooded by cheap counterfeit drugs. In her chapter, Noémi Tousignant shows how, in appealing to the state to take more control over the quality of the medicines available, Senegalese pharmacists struggle to make a space for their professional commercial practice (and livelihood) in the face of the flourishing informal market and to ensure the protection of the public from poor-quality and unsafe medication.

The interpenetration of private and public interests in the name of public health and global philanthropy is reflected in the new orthodoxy of "public-private partnerships" (or PPPs) as a paradigm of global health intervention, and indeed of governance.[185] The term *PPPs* refers to the transnational partnerships between private philanthropic groups, NGOs, charities, and governments, which together pursue health or humanitarian interventions, such as organizing malaria control or conducting publicly funded research into HIV treatment. Public-private partnerships also frame the charitable donations of drugs by pharmaceutical companies, which work with African governments to target communities exposed to "neglected tropical diseases" in the name of "corporate social responsibility."[186] The use of the term *partnership* in both global health and development interventions is a self-conscious move away from paternalist regimes of international development, yet it conceals the continuing, even deepening, inequality between Northern and Southern institutions and, in doing so, may reinforce the discourse of Western "donor(s)" and African "recipients."[187] These unequal power relations have become more embarrassing than they were in the colonial era, but rather than confronting them, the response is to look away, to clothe inequality in a language of equality and deflect it through the language of technical intervention.[188] P. Wenzel Geissler argues that the power inequalities of both past and present are not simply overlooked by the rhetoric of "partnership" (or, in the humanitarian domain, by that of "saving lives" and "numbers on treatment"); rather, this entails an active state of "not-knowing."[189]

Global health interventions targeting HIV/AIDS and other vertical disease programs also pay lip service to another orthodoxy of development practice: "community participation," or getting a community to "own" intervention projects—whether HIV/AIDS prevention, malaria control, or drug donation programs. Yet rarely are people in "the community" the ones who decide what kind of health intervention they receive, and if they are asked, they often have different opinions of what they find most useful: "We are very thankful for this unique chance, because we are selected from the district," a hamlet chairperson told Samsky in reply to his questions about drug donations for river blindness, but she went on to suggest that a primary health-care clinic would be even more useful.[190] Elisha Renne argues that in refusing to let their children get the polio vaccine, parents in northern Nigeria were showing "their disapproval of their own government's support for international health programs while failing to provide local primary health care" or to address child health problems that they considered to be more serious.[191]

As in other regions of the world where populations are poorly protected by their governments, African countries have also become sites for clinical trials by pharmaceutical companies. Some notorious clinical trials conducted by pharmaceutical companies—for example, Pfizer's trial of Trovan in Nigeria in 1996, which resulted in the deaths of children and a court case—draw attention to the "ethical variability" characterizing such profit-motivated research.[192] Although the majority of medical research in Africa is public health research, conducted through collaborations between public institutions from the Global North, such as universities and government research groups (for example, the UK's Medical Research Council and the U.S. Centers for Disease Control and Prevention), and African state institutions, often parastatals—and it is motivated not by profit but by the desire to improve health outcomes in Africa[193]—such research sites are still structured by inequality. Geissler's chapter in this volume is based on a long-term ethnography of a "trial community"—the scientists, researchers, fieldworkers, and trial participants who gather around publicly funded clinical trials in Kenya. It explores the implications of the architecture of research "zones" for landscapes of public health in East Africa.

Futures?

Can we find ways of thinking creatively about the progressive policies (and not only the reactionary dangers) of this new terrain of transnational organization of funds, energies and affects? Can we imagine new "arts of government"?[194]

This discussion of historical trajectories and recent developments underlines that, far from the scenario imagined by modernization theories of the 1950s, the space of public health as a relation between the state, biomedicine, government, and citizenship has, in most African countries, never developed in a predictable fashion—just as the global movement of science, modern government, and economic progress has not transpired as earlier historians of science imagined. The present situation is even less clear. Unlike an earlier era in which health interventions were framed by grand narratives of modernization and by a broad consensus in state-led development, the only strong political ideology of the day pushes, from the Right, for minimal state intervention, for private enterprise and individual responsibility for health. Meanwhile, the Left calls weakly for grassroots and community development. Public health measures are concerned with the containment of disease—pushed by a language of emergency and crisis—rather than tied to a language of social transformation and society-wide progress.[195] The transnational space in which public health concerns are formulated promotes disparate, not very well coordinated, interventions. Meanwhile, the privatization and marketization of health care has reached new dimensions, in Africa and across the world. The present situation thus involves emerging, unstable, and contingent assemblages and a multiplicity of actors and collectives, which narrow the space of public health to disease control and targeted interventions, leaving the rest of health care to the private sector. The 1990s and 2000s also saw the emergence of new forms of health activism, the global circulation of human rights and humanitarian discourses, new networks, and new forms of politics, which, while allowing states to divest themselves of responsibilities at one level, create new obligations at another level. Thus, there are openings as well as closures. This situation calls for ethnographic scrutiny—for us to bring ethnographic tools and anthropological methods to bear on the question of what public health is, who makes it, and with what consequences.

The volume offered here, through its attention to policies and practices and their effects on the ground, will help take our thinking about the present and future relations between public health, biomedicine, and social progress further and in new directions. While this book does not offer solutions, it offers close readings of actual practices and formations—which speak of power, inequality and dispossession, pain, frustration, and disillusionment but also of solidarities and common concerns. It underlines the fact that public health in Africa is pluralistic and polyvalent. This situation can be considered as an opportunity to look at the present as a starting point for possible futures, to move away from deterministic visions of neoliberalism and transnationalism in order to appreciate present opportunities and to develop a vision of possible ways forward toward the progressive goal of public health—a citizenry with equitable access to public health care, protected by a more accountable state. The authors of this volume reject singular descriptions of the present to offer analyses of the heterogeneous regimes and relations, the policies and interests, tensions and contradictions that produce, negotiate, or undermine the health of the public in Africa.

Overview of the Chapters

The chapters are grouped into three sections. The first section, "Whose Public Health?" unpacks the concept of public health, holding up to scrutiny the question of what public health is, whose interests define it, the relations between the public and private sphere of health, and conceptions of the public sphere, the public good, and the public itself as an imagined collective.

Drawing on historical and ethnographic research and his long engagement with Nigeria, the first chapter, by Murray Last, embeds what he argues is an absence of "public" health in northern Nigeria within a discussion of imaginations of and relations between "public" and "private" in the wider region—which have been shaped by class and ethnic relations, by Islam, and by British colonialism, as well as by the policies of the postcolonial Nigerian state. His chapter lends historical texture to received visions of "failing" or "absent" states by pointing to the historical, cultural, and political trajectories that shape relations between the Nigerian state and its public.

Rebecca Marsland likewise explores the tensions between different versions of public health, this time in present-day Tanzania. Here, district health officials have attempted to legislate against "misleading traditions," mostly concerned with funeral practices, which they present as threats to the public health order. However, these funeral practices speak to an indigenous realm of public health that is concerned with maintaining the social-moral order. She argues that public health in Tanzania has never constituted a straightforward concern with "citizens." Government officials' attempts to control public health draw upon other imaginations of publics—as crowds and populations—that are interwoven with class, regional, and ethnic prejudices, as well as with techniques of government. Some populations were considered less as citizens and more as crowds to be controlled.

Both Last and Marsland embed their discussion of governmental imaginations of public health in broader histories; they show how district health statecraft coexists with an "indigenous public health" concerned with the well-being of the social collective and explore how it overlays older ways of conceiving political power and responsibility. Colonial and postcolonial forms of public health coexist with, and must often contend with, other practices concerned with well-being—although the relation of these older practices to governmental forms of public health may seem obscure, irrelevant, or even, as Marsland shows, antagonistic.

Moving to Senegal, Noémi Tousignant's chapter suggests that state-directed attempts to improve public health and access to services have, since independence, encompassed efforts to develop the private sector, through the privatization of pharmacies. Pharmacists' private practice, together with the development of the public's pharmaceutical consumption, was promoted in this context as an engine of national development and economic growth. In the wake of structural adjustment policies, pharmacists have become concerned with the lack of regulation over pharmaceuticals and have begun to call for the state to take a stronger role in monitoring, controlling, and assessing the quality of medicines. In doing so, they see themselves as both protecting their profession and providing a better service to the public.

The chapters by Tousignant and Last encourage a rethinking of divisions between "public" and "private" in the incorporation of people into wider collectives and in related visions of social responsibility and the public "good." While Tousignant's chapter underlines how African professionals draw upon both older developmentalist narratives and neoliberal concerns in their quests to "develop" their country and attend to the public "good" as well as to their professional careers, Last suggests that in northern Nigeria, the public good, outside of personal relationships, has never carried much weight.

The second section, "Regimes and Relations of Care," asks who is taking care of whom, on what terms, and with what social and personal consequences. The chapters by Lotte Meinert and Hannah Brown look into the intimate spaces of public health care and the personal lives and motivations of patients and caregivers within the "public" system. Through case studies of HIV/AIDS interventions in Uganda and Kenya, respectively, they examine conceptualizations of "community" and the "domestic," as well as "care" and "patient-responsibilization." They offer insights into contemporary arts of government that characterize public health formations beyond AIDS care but also show how the targets of interventions use them to create unexpected connections and opportunities.

Lotte Meinert moves away from metanarratives of biopower to offer a subtle reading of the interaction of ART programs in Uganda with individual lives and the environments in which they live. Meinert follows the case of "Anna" as she falls sick, seeks care, is incorporated into an HIV treatment program, and then finds that the regimes of care it imposes upon her chafe against her desires and hopes for the future, as she moves beyond simply keeping alive. Here, Meinert builds on her ongoing work with Susan Whyte and colleagues in Uganda, which follows the first generation of people on ART in Uganda.[196]

Hannah Brown shows that recent home-based care interventions in Kenya are layered upon older histories of governmental interventions, which targeted particular public and private spheres—such as the "domestic" and the "community"—for "development." Focusing on a women's grassroots group that provides home-based care, she shows how rural women appropriate these interventions for their own ends as they strive to bring development into their locality and to benefit from it.

The third chapter in this section, by Benson Mulemi, describes the struggle to treat cancer in Kenya's largest public oncology ward. He highlights the concerns of doctors, nurses, and patients and their families as they seek to provide or access care in the absence of adequate medicines as well as diagnostic technologies—and the limited resources they have to draw upon. He shows the tensions that develop around diagnosis and prognosis, between hospital staff and patients and their families, as cancer upsets and challenges expectations of biomedical technology and hospital provision of care. He also follows how patients, sometimes with the help of nurses, experiment with the wide range of alternative therapies and discourses about health promotion and prevention that are currently crowding into the medical marketplace.

The final section, "Emerging Landscapes of Public Health," explores new geographies of disease, health-care provision, and medical research, which overlap and are layered upon one another, appearing as transient and unstable. The chapters in this section show how these landscapes animate particular collectives, lifestyles, and aspirations for the future but at the same time heighten socioeconomic and political inequalities.

Like Mulemi, Susan Reynolds Whyte draws attention to a disease that has been much less visible to funders and governments but is increasingly intruding upon people's lives—in this case, diabetes. Like cancer, diabetes has been ignored in recent concerns with global health, and the landscape of diabetes in Uganda provides a stark contrast to that of global health interventions focused on HIV/AIDS. Knowledge of the condition and the search for ways of managing it and for therapeutic intervention are left to individual initiative, piecemeal NGO projects, and the marketization of health promotion and care. The chapter draws attention to the gaping holes in public health provision and the flourishing market in private health care in places such as Uganda and explores how these intersect with the socioeconomic relations and conditions that underlie diabetes in Uganda. Whyte points out that the focus on individual "lifestyles" in diabetes management—on diet and exercise and the proliferation of private and expensive dietary and medical supplements—overlooks the more challenging burden of "life conditions," as well as the relation of diabetes to pathologies of stress that seem to be increasingly affecting both the poor and the middle classes.

The chapters by Ruth Prince and P. Wenzel Geissler explore the landscapes that global health interventions and medical research activities produce as they pour resources, expertise, and globally circulating regimes of knowledge into an East African city, superimposing a layer of global connectivity on a crumbling public health infrastructure.

Focusing on the city of Kisumu in Kenya, Prince follows the frictions that arise as globalized health resources, discourses, technologies, and expertise—embodied in the new HIV clinics and time-limited projects—intersect with local economies and livelihoods and with aspirations and imaginations for "development," in a city marked by poverty and inequality. Following how various actors—health professionals, patients of HIV clinics, and "volunteer" health workers—navigate these spaces, the chapter explores the gaps left behind and opened up by global health interventions, as they touch only particular nodes and operate within circumscribed locations. While these gaps are supposed to be filled by "self-help" and "community-based" initiatives, this move merely deflects responsibility for a more robust public health onto the poor and onto unsustainable structures. The chapter draws attention to the insecurity and vulnerability of those who seek health, livelihoods, and futures in this unstable landscape of global health.

In the final chapter, Geissler explores a trend that is becoming increasingly evident in African public health—the interpenetration of scientific medical research work with health-care provision. He examines how scientific research work operates spaces of inclusion and exclusion, reflecting and extending the targeted interventions and archipelago pattern that have become typical of public health projects. He looks at the "in-between" lives and movements of "science workers," those involved in medical research projects, and calls for an ethnography of the spatial forms, the geographies of connection and disconnection, and the movements and circulations that contemporary public health research produces and extends in Africa.

Notes

1. Examining the history of the modern European state, the historian George Rosen argued that the application of biomedicine (modern scientific medical knowledge and practice) to the building of a modern society was coterminous with the development of the modern state and a modern citizenry or public; see George Rosen, *A History of Public Health: Expanded Edition* (Baltimore, MD: John Hopkins University Press, 1993). See also Dorothy Porter, ed., *The History of Public Health and the Modern State*, Welcome Institute Series in the History of Medicine (Amsterdam: Editions Rodopi, 1994).

2. Dorothy Porter, introduction to Porter, *History of Public Health*, 1–44; Didier Fassin and Jean-Pierre Dozon, eds., *Critique de la santé publique: Une approche anthropologique* (Paris: Editions Balland, 2001).

3. Thandika Mkandawire, "Thinking about Developmental States in Africa," *Cambridge Journal of Economics* 25, no. 3 (2001): 289–314; Frederick Cooper, *Africa since 1940: The Past of the Present* (Cambridge: Cambridge University Press, 2002); Joanna Lewis, *Empire State-Building: War and Welfare in Kenya, 1925–52* (Oxford: James Currey, 2000); Helen Tilley, *Africa as a Living Laboratory: Empire, Development and the Problem of Scientific Knowledge, 1870–1950* (Chicago: University of Chicago Press, 2011); Pauline Kusiak, "Instrumentalized Rationality, Cross-Cultural Mediators, and Civil Epistemologies of Late Colonialism," *Social Studies of Science* 20, no. 10 (2010): 1–32.

4. Ann Beck, *A History of the British Medical Administration of East Africa, 1900–1950* (Cambridge, MA: Harvard University Press, 1970); John Iliffe, *East African Doctors: A History of the Modern Profession* (Cambridge: Cambridge University Press, 1998); James Ferguson, *Expectations of Modernity: Myths and Meanings of Urban Life on the Zambian Copperbelt* (Berkeley: University of California Press, 1999).

5. Adeline Masquelier, "Behind the Dispensary's Prosperous Façade: Imagining the State in Rural Niger," *Public Culture* 13, no. 2 (2001): 267–91; Annettee Nakimuli, "What Are the Main Causes of Maternal Morality in Africa?" and Godfrey Mbaruku, "Health Systems' Policy towards Reducing Maternal and Neonatal Deaths" (papers presented at the conference "Maternal Mortality in Africa," 2–3 July 2012, Cambridge, UK).

6. Iruka N. Okeke, *Divining without Seeds: The Case for Strengthening Laboratory Medicine in Africa* (New York: Cornell University Press, 2011).

7. Kenneth Sherr et al., "Brain Drain and Health Worker Distortions in Mozambique," *PLoS One* 7, no. 4 (2012), www.ncbi.nlm.nih.gov/pmc/articles/PMC3338796/.

8. Claire L. Wendland, *A Heart for the Matter: Journeys through an African Medical School* (Chicago: University of Chicago Press, 2010); Karen Booth, *Local Women, Global Science: Fighting AIDS in Kenya* (Bloomington: Indiana University Press, 2004); Steven Feierman, "When Physicians Meet: Local Medical Knowledge and Global Public Goods," in *Evidence, Ethos and Experiment: The Anthropology and History of Medical Research in Africa*, ed. P. Wenzel Geissler and Catherine Molyneux, 171–96 (New York: Berghahn Books, 2011).

9. E.g., Randall Packard, *White Plague, Black Labour: Tuberculosis and the Political Economy of Health and Disease in South Africa* (Berkeley: University of California Press, 1989); Megan Vaughan, *Curing Their Ills: Colonial Power and African Illness* (Stanford: Stanford University Press, 1992).

10. Terence Ranger, "Godly Medicine: The Ambiguities of Medical Mission in Southeastern Tanzania, 1900–1945," in *The Social Basis of Health and Healing in Africa*, ed. Steven Feierman and John M. Janzen, 256–82 (Berkeley: University of California Press, 1992); Nancy Rose Hunt, "'Le Bébé en Brousse': European Women, African Birth Spacing, and Colonial Intervention in Breast Feeding in the Belgian Congo," in *Tensions of Empire: Colonial Cultures in a Bourgeois World*, ed. Frederick Cooper and Ann Laura Stoler, 287–321 (Berkeley: University of California Press, 1997); Lyn Schumaker, "Slimes and Death-Dealing Dambos: Water, Industry and the Garden City on Zambia's Copperbelt," *Journal of Southern African Studies* 34, no. 4 (2008): 823–40.

11. Cooper, *Africa since 1940*.

12. Meredeth Turshen, *Privatizing Health Services in Africa* (New Brunswick, NJ: Rutgers University Press, 1999); Sheelagh Stewart, "Happy Ever After in the Marketplace: Non-government Organisations and Uncivil Society," *Review of African Political Economy* 24, no. 71 (1997): 11–34; M. R. Reich, "Reshaping the State from Above, from Within, from Below: Implications for Public Health," *Social Science and Medicine* 54, no. 11 (2002): 1669–75.

13. Jean-Pierre Olivier de Sardan, "A Moral Economy of Corruption in Africa," *Journal of Modern African Studies* 37, no. 1 (1995): 25–52.

14. Mahmood Mamdani, *Citizen and Subject: Contemporary Africa and the Legacy of Late Colonialism* (Princeton: Princeton University Press, 1996).

15. E.g., Vaughan, *Curing Their Ills*; Frantz Fanon, *Black Skin, White Masks* (New York: Grove, 1967); Luise White, *Speaking with Vampires: Rumor and History in Colonial Africa* (Berkeley: University of California Press, 2000).

16. James Fairhead, Melissa Leach, and Mary Small, "Where Techno-Science Meets Poverty: Medical Research and the Economy of Blood in the Gambia, West Africa," *Social Science and Medicine* 63, no. 4 (2006): 1109–20; P. Wenzel Geissler, "Kachinja Are Coming! Encounters around Medical Research Work in a Kenyan Village," *Africa* 75, no. 2 (2005): 174–202; Melissa Graboyes, "Fines, Orders, Fear . . . and Consent? Medical Research in East Africa, c. 1950s," *Developing World Bioethics* 10, no. 1 (2010): 34–41; Adeline Masquelier, "Public Health or Public Threat: Polio Eradication Campaigns, Islamic Revival and the Materialization of State Power in Niger," in *Medicine, Mobility and Power in Global Africa: Transnational Health and Healing*, ed. Hansjörg Dilger, Abdulaye Kane, and Stacey Langwick, 213–40 (Bloomington: University of Indiana Press, 2012).

17. Didier Fassin, *When Bodies Remember: Experiences and Politics of AIDS in South Africa* (Berkeley: University of California Press, 2007).

18. Elisha P. Renne, *The Politics of Polio in Northern Nigeria* (Bloomington: Indiana University Press, 2010).

19. Paul Rabinow and Nikolas Rose, "Biopower Today," *BioSocieties* 1 (2006): 195–217; Nikolas Rose, *The Politics of Life Itself: Biomedicine, Power, and Subjectivity in the Twenty-First Century* (Princeton: Princeton University Press, 2007).

20. Kaushik Sunder Rajan, *Biocapital: The Constitution of Postgenomic Life* (Durham, NC: Duke University Press, 2006).

21. Rebecca Marsland and Ruth J. Prince, "What Is Life Worth? Biomedical Intervention, Survival and the Politics of Life," *Medical Anthropology Quarterly* 24, no. 4 (2012): 453–69; Didier Fassin, "Another Politics of Life Is Possible," *Theory, Culture and Society* 26, no. 5 (2009): 44–60.

22. E.g., Aihwa Ong, *Neoliberalism as Exception: Mutations in Citizenship and Sovereignty* (Durham, NC: Duke University Press, 2006).

23. Nikolas Rose, "The Politics of Life Itself," *Theory, Culture and Society* 18, no. 6 (2001): 5.

24. João Biehl, "Pharmaceuticalization: AIDS Treatment and Global Health Politics," *Anthropological Quarterly* 80, no. 4 (2007): 1083–1126; Saskia Sassen, "Globalization or Denationalization?" *Review of International Political Economy* 10, no. 1 (2003): 1–22; Janet Roitman, *Fiscal Disobedience: An Anthropology of Economic Regulation in Central Africa* (Princeton: Princeton University Press, 2005).

25. Mkandawire, "Thinking about Developmental States," 307n2; James Ferguson, *Global Shadows: Africa in the Neoliberal World Order* (Durham, NC: Duke University Press, 2006).

26. Richard Rottenburg, "Social and Public Experiments and New Figurations of Science and Politics in Postcolonial Africa," *Postcolonial Studies* 12, no. 4 (2009): 423–40; Vinh-Kim Nguyen, "Government by Exception: Enrolment and Experimentality in Mass HIV Treatment Programs in Africa," *Social Theory and Health* 7, no. 3 (2009): 196–218.

27. Jean-François Bayart, "Africa in the World: A History of Extraversion," *African Affairs* 99 (2000): 239. See also Thomas Blom Hansen and Finn Stepputat, eds., *States of Imagination: Ethnographic Explorations of the Postcolonial State* (Durham, NC: Duke University Press, 2001).

28. Nikolas Rose and Carlos Novas, "Biological Citizenship," in *Global Assemblages: Technology, Politics, and Ethics as Anthropological Problems*, ed. Aihwa Ong and Stephen J. Collier, 439–63 (Malden, MA: Blackwell, 2005).

29. I am grateful to one of the reviewers for offering this formulation.

30. Melissa Parker and Ian Harper, "The Anthropology of Public Health," *Journal of Biosocial Science* 38, no. 1 (2006): 1–5.

31. E.g., Packard, *White Plague, Black Labour*; Vaughan, *Curing Their Ills*; Maryinez Lyons, *The Colonial Disease: A Social History of Sleeping Sickness in Northern Zaire, 1900–1940* (Cambridge: Cambridge University Press, 1992); Nancy Rose Hunt, *A Colonial Lexicon: Of Birth Ritual, Medicalization, and Mobility in the Congo* (Durham, NC: Duke University Press, 1999); Renne, *Politics of Polio*.

32. Maureen Malowany, "Unfinished Agendas: Writing the History of Medicine of Sub-Saharan Africa," *African Affairs* 99 (2000): 325–49.

33. Vaughan, *Curing Their Ills*; Hunt, *Colonial Lexicon*; Walima T. Kalusa, "Language, Medical Auxiliaries, and the Re-interpretation of Missionary Medicine in Colonial Mwinilunga, Zambia, 1922–51," *Journal of Eastern African Studies* 1, no. 1 (2007): 57–78.

34. Ferguson, *Expectations of Modernity*.

35. Victor Turner, *The Forest of Symbols: Aspects of Ndembu Ritual* (Ithaca, NY: Cornell University Press, 1967); Turner, *The Ritual Process: Structure and Anti-structure* (Chicago: Aldine Publishing, 1969).

36. John M. Janzen, *The Quest for Therapy: Medical Pluralism in Lower Zaire* (Berkeley: University of California Press, 1978).

37. Steven Feierman, "Colonizers, Scholars, and the Creation of Invisible Histories," in *Beyond the Cultural Turn: New Directions in the Study of Society and Culture*, ed. Victoria Bonnell and Lynn Hunt, 182–216 (Berkeley: University of California Press, 1999).

38. Classics include Harriet Ngubane, *Body and Mind in Zulu Medicine* (London: Academic Press, 1977); Murray Last, "The Importance of Knowing about Not Knowing: Observations from Hausaland," in Feierman and Janzen, *Social Basis of Health and Healing in Africa*, 393–407; Robert Pool, *Dialogue and the Interpretation of Illness: Conversations in a Cameroon Village* (Oxford: Berg, 1994); Susan R. Whyte, *Questioning Misfortune: The Pragmatics of Uncertainty in Eastern Uganda* (Cambridge: Cambridge University Press, 1997); Jean Comaroff, *Body of Power, Spirit of Resistance* (Chicago: University of Chicago Press, 1985).

39. Marshall Sahlins, *Islands of History* (Chicago: University of Chicago Press, 1987); John L. Comaroff and Jean Comaroff, *Ethnography and the Historical Imagination* (Boulder, CO: Westview Press, 1992); John L. Comaroff and Jean Comaroff, *Of Revelation and Revolution*, vol. 2, *The Dialectics of Modernity on a South African Frontier* (Chicago: University of Chicago Press, 1997).

40. Feierman, "Colonizers, Scholars," 185.

41. E.g., Packard, *White Plague, Black Labour*; Vaughan, *Curing Their Ills*; Philip Curtin, "Medical Knowledge and Urban Planning in Colonial Tropical Africa," in Feierman and Janzen, *Social Basis of Health and Healing in Africa*, 235–55; Shula Marks, "What Is Colonial about Colonial Medicine? And What Happened to Imperialism and Health?" *Social History of Medicine* 10, no. 2 (1997): 205–19; Michael Worboys, "The Colonial World as Mission and Mandate: Leprosy and Empire, 1900–1940," *Osiris Nature and Empire: Science and the Colonial Enterprise*, 2nd series, vol. 15 (2000): 190–206; Hunt, *Colonial Lexicon*; Julie Livingston, *Debility and the Modern Imagination in Botswana* (Bloomington: Indiana University Press, 2005).

42. Jean Comaroff, "The Diseased Heart of Africa: Medicine, Colonialism, and the Black Body," in *Knowledge, Power, and Practice: The Anthropology of Medicine and Everyday Life*, ed. Shirley Lindenbaum and Margaret Lock, 305–27 (Berkeley: University of California Press, 1993).

43. Vaughan, *Curing Their Ills*; Comaroff, "Diseased Heart of Africa."

44. White, *Speaking with Vampires*; Hunt, *Colonial Lexicon*.

45. E.g., Paul Farmer, *AIDS and Accusation: Haiti and the Geography of Blame* (Berkeley: University of California Press, 1992); Farmer, *Infections and Inequalities: The Modern Plagues* (Berkeley: University of California Press, 1999); Hans A. Baer, Merrill Singer, and Ida Susser, *Medical Anthropology and the World System: A Critical Perspective* (Westport, CT: Bergin and Garvey, 1997). The work of Arthur Kleinman and Bryan Good developed medical anthropology as a subdiscipline that gave equal attention to biomedicine.

46. Exceptions include Carol MacCormack, "Health Care and the Concept of Legitimacy in Sierra Leone," in Feierman and Janzen, *Social Basis of Health and Healing in Africa*, 426–36.

47. Susan Reynolds Whyte, "The Power of Medicines in East Africa," in *The Context of Medicines in Developing Countries: Studies in Pharmaceutical Anthropology*, ed. Sjaak van der Geest and Susan R. Whyte, 217–33 (Dordrecht: Kluwer, 1988); Sjaak van der Geest, Susan R. Whyte, and Anita Hardon, "The Anthropology of Pharmaceuticals: A Biographical Approach," *Annual Review of Anthropology* 25 (1996): 153–78.

48. See Margaret Lock and Vinh-Kim Nguyen, *The Anthropology of Biomedicine* (Oxford: Blackwell, 2010). The literature is too vast to give it justice here, but notable contributions include Sarah Franklin and Margaret Lock, *Remaking Life and Death: Towards an Anthropology of the Biosciences* (Santa Fe, NM: School of American Research Press; Oxford: James Currey, 2003); João Biehl, *Will to Live: AIDS Therapies and the Politics of Survival* (Princeton: Princeton University Press, 2007); Adriana Petryna, Andrew Lakoff, and Arthur Kleinman, eds., *Global Pharmaceuticals: Ethics, Markets, Practices* (Durham, NC: Duke University Press, 2006); Margaret Lock, *Twice Dead: Organ Transplants* (Berkeley: University of California Press, 2007); Annemarie Mol, *The Body Multiple* (Durham, NC: Duke University Press, 2005); Rose, *Politics of Life Itself.*

49. E.g., Peter Redfield, "Doctors, Borders, and Life in Crisis," *Cultural Anthropology* 20, no. 3 (2005): 328–61; Erica Bornstein and Peter Redfield, eds., *Forces of Compassion: Humanitarianism between Ethics and Politics* (Santa Fe, NM: School for Advanced Research Press, 2011); Ari Samsky, "Scientific Sovereignty: How International Drug Donation Programmes Reshape Health, Disease and the State," *Cultural Anthropology* 27, no. 2 (2012): 310–32; Johanna Crane, "Adverse Events and Placebo Effects: African Scientists, HIV, and Ethics in the 'Global Health Sciences,'" *Social Studies of Science* 40, no. 6 (2010): 843–70; Fairhead, Leach, and Small, "Where Techno-Science Meets Poverty"; P. Wenzel Geissler and Catherine Molyneux, eds., *Evidence, Ethos and Experiment: The Anthropology and History of Medical Research in Africa* (New York: Berghahn Books, 2011); Vinh-Kim Nguyen, *The Republic of Therapy: Triage and Sovereignty in West Africa's Time of AIDS* (Durham, NC: Duke University Press, 2011); Jean Comaroff, "Beyond Bare Life: AIDS, (Bio)politics, and the Neoliberal Order," *Public Culture* 19, no. 1 (2007): 197–219; Ong and Collier, *Global Assemblages.*

50. Wendland, *Heart for the Matter;* Sjaak van der Geest and Kaja Finkler, "Hospital Ethnography: Special Issue," *Social Science and Medicine* 59, no. 10 (2004): 1995–2001; Hannah Brown, "Hospital Domestics: Care Work in a Kenyan Hospital," *Space and Culture* 15 (2012): 18–30; Anita Hardon and Hansjörg Dilger, "Global AIDS Medicines in East African Health Institutions," in "AIDS Treatment in East Africa," special issue, *Medical Anthropology* 30, no. 2 (2011): 136–57.

51. Anna Lowenhaupt Tsing, *Friction: An Ethnography of Global Connection* (Princeton: Princeton University Press, 2005).

52. Ferguson, *Global Shadows.*

53. David Mosse, *Cultivating Development: An Ethnography of Aid Policy and Practice* (London: Pluto Press, 2005); Tom Yarrow, "Life/History: Personal Narratives of Development amongst NGO Workers and Activists in Ghana," *Africa* 78, no. 3 (2009): 334–58.

54. Guillaume Lachenal, "Le médecin qui voulut être roi: Médecine coloniale et utopie au Cameroun," *Annales HSS* 1 (January–February 2010): 121–56.

55. Julie Livingston, "Productive Misunderstandings and the Dynamism of Plural Medicine in Mid-Century Bechuanaland," *Journal of Southern African Studies* 33, no. 4 (2007): 801–10.

56. Tracy J. Luedke and Harry G. West, eds., *Borders and Healers: Brokering Therapeutic Resources in Southeast Africa* (Bloomington: Indiana University Press, 2005); Dilger, Kane, and Langwick, *Medicine, Mobility and Power.*

57. Angelika Wolf, "Health Security on the Move: Biobureaucracy, Solidarity and the Transfer of Health Insurance to Senegal," in Dilger, Kane, and Langwick, *Medicine, Mobility and Power,* 92–114; Viola Hürbst, "Assisted Reproductive Technologies in Mali and Togo: Circulating Knowledge, Mobile Technologies," in Dilger, Kane, and Langwick, *Medicine, Mobility and Power,* 162–89.

58. James Ferguson, "The Uses of Neoliberalism," *Antipode* 41, no. 1 (2009): 166–84, esp. 169.

59. Feierman, "Colonizers, Scholars"; Janzen, *Quest for Therapy.*

60. Steve Feierman, "Struggles for Control: The Social Roots of Health and Healing in Modern Africa," *African Studies Review* 28 (1985): 73–147; John M. Janzen, "Ideologies and Institutions in Pre-colonial Western Equatorial African Therapeutics," in Feierman and Janzen, *Social Basis of Health and Healing in Africa,* 195–211.

61. Gloria Waite, "Public Health in Pre-colonial East Africa," in Feierman and Janzen, *Social Basis of Health and Healing in Africa,* 212–33; Murray Last, "Understanding Health," in *Culture and Global Change,* ed. Tim Allen and Tracey Skelton, 72–86 (London: Routledge, 1999); Feierman, "Colonizers, Scholars"; Livingston, *Debility and the Modern Imagination,* 17.

62. Steve Feierman, "On Socially Composed Knowledge: Reconstructing a Shambaa Royal Ritual," in *In Search of a Nation: Histories of Authority and Dissidence in Tanzania,* ed. James L. Giblin and Gregory H. Maddox, 14–32 (Athens: Ohio University Press, 2005).

63. Ibid.

64. Janzen, *Quest for Therapy;* Feierman, "Colonizers, Scholars."

65. Janzen, *Quest for Therapy;* Feierman and Janzen, *Social Basis of Health and Healing in Africa;* Janzen, "Ideologies and Institutions."

66. Steve Feierman, *Peasant Intellectuals: Anthropology and History in Tanzania* (Madison: University of Wisconsin Press, 1990).

67. Feierman, "Struggles for Control."

68. Stacey A. Langwick, *Bodies, Politics and African Healing: The Matter of Maladies in Tanzania* (Bloomington: Indiana University Press, 2011), chap. 2; see also Tilley, *Africa as a Living Laboratory,* chap. 6.

69. Comaroff and Comaroff, *Dialectics of Modernity;* Birgit Meyer, *Translating the Devil: Religion and Modernity among the Ewe in Ghana* (Edinburgh: Edinburgh University Press, 1999); P. Wenzel Geissler and Ruth J. Prince, *The Land Is Dying: Contingency, Creativity and Conflict in Western Kenya* (New York: Berghahn Books, 2010).

70. Langwick, *Bodies, Politics and African Healing;* Harry West, *Kupilikula: Governance and the Invisible Realm in Mozambique* (Chicago: University of Chicago Press, 2005).

71. Geissler and Prince, *Land Is Dying.*

72. Lyons, *Colonial Disease.*

73. Vaughan, *Curing Their Ills;* Fanon, *Black Skin, White Masks;* White, *Speaking with Vampires;* Achille Mbembe, "Provisional Notes on the Postcolony," *Africa* 62, no. 1 (1992): 3–37; Fassin, *When Bodies Remember.*

74. Hunt, "Le Bébé en Brousse"; Worboys, "Colonial World"; Schumaker, "Slimes and Death-Dealing Dambos."

75. Shula Marks and Neil Andersson, "Industrialization, Rural Health and the 1944 National Health Services Commission in South Africa," in Feierman and Janzen, *Social Basis of Health and Healing in Africa,* 131–62; Lewis, *Empire State-Building;* Randall Packard, "Visions of Postwar Health and Development and Their Impact on Public Health Interventions in the Developing World," in *International Development and the Social Sciences: Essays on the History and Politics of Knowledge,* ed. Frederick Cooper and Randall Packard, 93–115 (Berkeley: University of California Press, 1997), esp. 95.

76. Packard, "Visions of Postwar Health"; Lewis, *Empire State-Building;* Tilley, *Africa as a Living Laboratory.*

77. Lewis, *Empire State-Building,* 79, 86, 105. This contrasted with Belgian and Portuguese colonies in Africa, as well as South Africa and Rhodesia, which gave little thought to the welfare of most Africans.

78. Cooper, *Africa since 1940*, 44, 85; Andrew Burton and Michael Jennings, "The Emperor's New Clothes? Continuities in Governance in Late Colonial and Early Postcolonial East Africa," *International Journal of African Historical Studies* 40, no. 1 (2007): 1–25.

79. Cooper, *Africa since 1940*.

80. Ibid., 91.

81. Tilley, *Africa as a Living Laboratory*.

82. Ibid., 86; Ferguson, *Expectations of Modernity;* Mkandawire, "Thinking about Developmental States"; Christophe Bonneuil, "Development as Experiment: Science and State Building in Late Colonial and Postcolonial Africa, 1930–1970," *Osiris* 15 (2000): 258–81.

83. Mkandawire, "Thinking about Developmental States"; Iliffe, *East African Doctors*.

84. Ferguson, *Expectations of Modernity;* Frederick Cooper and Randall Packard, introduction to Cooper and Packard, *International Development and the Social Sciences*, 10.

85. Ferguson, *Expectations of Modernity;* Cooper, *Africa since 1940*.

86. Cooper, *Africa since 1940*, 88; Iliffe, *East African Doctors*.

87. Mkandawire, "Thinking about Developmental States."

88. Ferguson, *Expectations of Modernity*.

89. James Ferguson, *The Anti-politics Machine* (Cambridge: Cambridge University Press, 1991); James C. Scott, *Seeing Like a State: How Certain Schemes to Improve the Human Condition Have Failed* (New Haven, CT: Yale University Press, 1998); Timothy Mitchell, *Rule of Experts: Egypt, Techno-Politics, Modernity* (Berkeley: University of California Press, 2002).

90. Mamdani, *Citizen and Subject;* Burton and Jennings, "Emperor's New Clothes."

91. African statecraft has since become characterized by "Afro-pessimistic" diagnoses, as a "politics of the belly"; see Jean-François Bayart, *The State in Africa: The Politics of the Belly* (London: Longman, 1993). See also Cooper, *Africa since 1940*, 88; Frederick Cooper, "The Dialectics of Decolonization: Nationalism and Labour Movements in Postwar French West Africa," in Cooper and Stoler, *Tensions of Empire*, 406–35.

92. Burton and Jennings, "Emperor's New Clothes," 24.

93. Priya Lal, "Self-Reliance and the State: The Multiple Meanings of Development in Early Post-colonial Tanzania," *Africa* 82, no. 2 (2012): 205–19; Rebecca Marsland, "Community Participation the Tanzania Way: Conceptual Contiguity or Power Struggle?" *Oxford Development Studies* 34, no. 1 (2006): 65–79.

94. Priya Lal, "Self-Reliance and the State," 213; Cooper and Packard, *International Development and the Social Sciences*; Tom Yarrow and Soumhya Venkatesan, "Anthropology and Development: Critical Framings," in *Differentiating Development: Beyond an Anthropology of Critique* (New York: Berghahn Books, 2012), 1–22.

95. Mkandawire, "Thinking about Developmental States."

96. Cooper, *Africa since 1940*, 107.

97. Ibid., 89.

98. See Achille Mbembe and Janet Roitman, "Figures of the Subject in Times of Crisis," *Public Culture* 7 (1995): 323–52.

99. Cooper, *Africa since 1940*, 115.

100. Packard, "Visions of Postwar Health"; Craig R. Janes, "Going Global in Century XXI: Medical Anthropology and the New Primary Health Care," *Human Organization* 63, no. 4 (2004): 457–71.

101. Robert Maxon, "The Kenyatta Era, 1963–78: Social and Cultural Changes," in *Decolonization and Independence in Kenya: 1940–93*, ed. Bethwell A. Ogot and W. R. Ochieng' (Athens: Ohio University Press, 1995), 137–38.

102. Janes, "Going Global."

103. Ibid., 458

104. Packard, "Visions of Postwar Health"; Janes, "Going Global," 458.

105. Janes, "Going Global," 458.

106. Vicente Navarro, "Neoliberalism and Its Consequences: The World Health Situation since Alma Ata," *Global Social Policy* 8 (2008): 152–55.

107. Thomas Bierschenk, "The Everyday Functioning of an African Public Service: Informalization, Privatization and Corruption in Benin's Legal System," *Journal of Legal Pluralism and Unofficial Law* 57 (2008): 101–39.

108. Sjaak van der Geest and Susan R. Whyte, eds., *The Context of Medicines in Developing Countries: Studies in Pharmaceutical Anthropology* (Dordrecht: Kluwer, 1988); Renne, *Politics of Polio.*

109. Kristin Petersen, "AIDS Policies for Markets and Warriors: Dispossession, Capital and Pharmaceuticals in Nigeria," in Dilger, Kane, and Langwick, *Medicine, Mobility and Power,* 153.

110. Julia Elyachar, *Markets of Dispossession: NGOs, Economic Development and the State in Egypt* (Durham, NC: Duke University Press, 2005); Janet Roitman, *Fiscal Disobedience: An Anthropology of Economic Regulation in Central Africa* (Princeton: Princeton University Press, 2005).

111. Ferguson, *Global Shadows;* James Ferguson and Akhil Gupta, "Spatializing States: Toward an Ethnography of Neoliberal Governmentality," *American Ethnologist* 29, no. 4 (2002): 981–1002; Sassen, "Globalization or Denationalization?"

112. David Harvey, *A Brief History of Neoliberalism* (Oxford: Oxford University Press, 2005).

113. Marc Edelman and Angelique Haugerud, "Introduction: The Anthropology of Development and Globalization," in *The Anthropology of Development and Globalization: From Classical Political Economy to Contemporary Neoliberalism,* ed. Marc Edelman and Angelique Haugerud (Malden, MA: Blackwell Publishing, 2005), 17.

114. Adriana Petryna and Arthur Kleinman, "The Pharmaceutical Nexus," in Petryna, Lakoff, and Kleinman, *Global Pharmaceuticals,* 1–32; João Biehl, "Pharmaceutical Governance," in Petryna, Lakoff, and Kleinman, *Global Pharmaceuticals,* 206–39.

115. Janes, "Going Global," 459.

116. Mkandawire, "Thinking about Developmental States," 292.

117. Janes, "Going Global"; World Bank Development Report 1993, *Investing in Health.*

118. Robert M. Maxon and Peter Ndege, "The Economics of Structural Adjustment," in *Decolonization and Independence in Kenya, 1940–93,* ed. Bethwell A. Ogot and William R. Ochieng', 151–86 (London: James Currey, 1995).

119. Peter Gibbon, "Structural Adjustment and Structural Change in Sub-Saharan Africa: Some Provisional Conclusions," *Development and Change* 27, no. 4 (1996): 751–84; Joseph K Kipkemboi Rono, "The Impact of Structural Adjustment Programmes on Kenyan Society," *Journal of Social Development in Africa* 17, no. 1 (2002): 81–98.

120. In Kenya, for example, the Ministry of Health's budget in 1995/6 was half that of 1980/1; see Julie Hearn, "The NGO-isation of Kenyan Society: USAID and the Restructuring of Health Care," *Review of African Political Economy* 25 (1998): 89–100, esp. 91.

121. James Pfeiffer, "Condoms and Social Marketing: Pentecostalism and Structural Adjustment in Mozambique," *Medical Anthropology Quarterly* 18, no. 1 (2004): 77–103; Helen Epstein, *The Invisible Cure: Africa, the West, and the Fight against AIDS* (New York: Farrar, Straus and Giroux, 2007).

122. Mol, *Logic of Care.*

123. Iliffe, *East African Doctors*.

124. Ibid.

125. However, colonial and postcolonial governments at that time controlled funds and channeled some of these into the mission medical sector. Since the 1990s, this process has been reversed: NGOs receive funds and invite government institutions to enter into "partnerships" or government employees to attend "capacity-building" seminars.

126. Joseph Semboja and Ole Therkildsen, eds., *Service Provision under Stress in East Africa: The State, NGOs and People's Organizations in Kenya, Tanzania and Uganda* (Copenhagen: Centre for Development Research; Nairobi: East African Educational Publishers, 1995).

127. Stewart, "Happy Ever After."

128. See Edelman and Haugerud, "Introduction."

129. Stewart, "Happy Ever After."

130. Julie Hearn, "The 'Invisible' NGO: US Evangelical Missions in Kenya," in "Christian and Islamic Non-governmental Organisations in Contemporary Africa," special issue, *Journal of Religion in Africa* 32, no. 1 (2002): 44.

131. E.g., Family Health International, Population Services International, Marie Stopes, Save the Children, MSF, Africare, Care, World Vision, Oxfam, Concern, Food for the Hungry International, Pathfinder, and Catholic Relief Services.

132. Kent Buse and Gill Walt, "An Unruly Melange? Coordinating External Resources to the Health Sector; A Review," *Social Science and Medicine* 45, no. 3 (1997): 449–62; James Pfeiffer, "International NGOs in the Mozambique Health Sector: The 'Velvet Glove' of Privatization," in *Unhealthy Health Policy: A Critical Anthropological Examination*, ed. Arachu Castro and Merrill Singer, 43–62 (Walnut Creek, CA: Altamira Press, 2004).

133. Hearn, "NGO-isation of Kenyan Society"; Hearn, "'Invisible' NGO," 44.

134. Hearn, "'Invisible' NGO," 45; Stewart, "Happy Ever After," 11.

135. During the 1990s, U.S. evangelical Christian groups formed a significant constituency for U.S. funding. Hearn, "NGO-isation of Kenya," 43; Hearn, "'Invisible' NGO," 33. See also Epstein, *Invisible Cure*.

136. Ruth J. Prince, with Rijk van Dijk and Philippe Denis, "Engaging Christianities: Negotiating HIV/AIDS, Health and Social Relations in East and Southern Africa," *Africa Today* 56, no. 1 (2009): v–xviii; Hansjörg Dilger, "Doing Better? Religion, the Virtue-Ethics of Development, and the Fragmentation of Health Politics in Tanzania," *Africa Today* 56, no. 1 (2009): 89–110.

137. Stephen N. Ndegwa, "Civil Society and Political Change in Africa: The Case of Non-governmental Organizations in Kenya," *International Journal of Comparative Sociology* 35, no. 1/2 (1994): 19–36.

138. Issa G. Shivji, *Silences in NGO Discourse: The Role and Future of NGOs in Africa* (Nairobi: Pambazuka Press / Fahamu Books, 2007).

139. Hearn, "NGO-isation of Kenya"; Reich, "Reshaping the State"; Jelke Boesten, Anna Mdee, and Frances Cleaver, "Service Delivery on the Cheap? Community-Based Workers in Development Interventions," *Development in Practice* 21, no. 1 (2011): 41–58; Jelke Boesten, "Navigating the AIDS Industry: Being Poor and Positive in Tanzania," *Development and Change* 42, no. 3 (2011): 781–803; Rebecca Marsland, "(Bio)sociality and HIV in Tanzania"; Ruth J. Prince, "HIV and the Moral Economy of Survival in an East African City," *Medical Anthropology Quarterly* 24, no. 4 (2012): 534–56.

140. James Pfeiffer, "International NGOs and Primary Health Care in Mozambique: The Need for a New Model of Collaboration," *Social Science and Medicine* 56 (2003): 726 and 737.

141. Hearn, "NGO-isation of Kenya."

142. E.g., Stewart, "Happy Ever After"; Pfeiffer, "International NGOs."

143. Hearn, "'Invisible' NGO," 99.

144. Ibid.

145. Michel Feher, "The Governed in Politics," in *Nongovernmental Politics*, ed. Michel Feher, 12–27 (New York: Zone Books, 2007); Didier Fassin, "Humanitarianism: A Nongovernmental Government," in Feher, *Nongovernmental Politics*, 149–60; William F. Fisher, "Doing Good? The Politics and Anti-politics of NGO Practices," *Annual Review of Anthropology* 27 (1997): 439–64.

146. Bayart, *State in Africa*; Patrick Chabal and Jean-Pascal Daloz, *Africa Works: Disorder as Political Instrument* (London: James Currey, 1999); Sassen, "Globalization or Denationalization?" 6; Bayart, "Africa in the World"; Ferguson, *Global Shadows*.

147. Quoted in Hearns, "NGO-isation of Kenya," 94.

148. Mkandawire, "Thinking about Developmental States."

149. Cooper, *Africa since 1940*.

150. Mkandawire, "Thinking about Developmental States," 291.

151. Ibid.

152. Olivier de Sardan, "Moral Economy of Corruption"; Laura Routley, "NGOs and the Formation of the Public: Grey Practices and Accountability," *African Affairs* 111, no. 442 (2012): 116–34.

153. Theodore M. Brown, Marcos Cueto, and Elizabeth Fee, "The World Health Organization and the Transition from 'International' to 'Global' Public Health," *American Journal of Public Health* 96, no. 1 (2006): 62–72; Vincanne Adams, Thomas E. Novotny, and Hannah Leslie, "Global Health Diplomacy," *Medical Anthropology* 27, no. 4 (2008): 315–23; Mark Nichter, *Global Health: Why Cultural Perceptions, Social Representations and Biopolitics Matter* (Tucson: University of Arizona Press, 2008); Craig R. Janes and Kitty Corbitt, "Anthropology and Global Health," *Annual Review of Anthropology* 38 (2009): 167–83; James Pfeiffer and Mark Nichter, "What Can Critical Medical Anthropology Contribute to Global Health?" *Medical Anthropological Quarterly* 22 (2008): 410–15; Joanna Crane, "Unequal Partners: AIDS, Academia and the Rise of Global Health," *Behemoth* 3 (2010): 78–98; Paul Farmer, *Pathologies of Power: Health, Human Rights and the New War on the Poor* (Berkeley: University of California Press, 2005).

154. K. Lee, S. Fustukian, and K. Buse, "An Introduction to Global Health Policy," in *Health Policy in a Globalizing World*, ed. S. H. Lee, K. Buse, and S. Fustukian (Cambridge: Cambridge University Press, 2002), 5 (quoted in Janes and Corbitt, "Anthropology and Global Health," 168).

155. Nikolas B. King, "Security, Disease, Commerce: Ideologies of Postcolonial Global Health," *Social Studies of Science* 32, no. 5/6 (2002): 763–89; Andrew Lakoff, "The Problem of Securing Health," in *Biosecurity Interventions: Global Health and Security in Question*, ed. Andrew Lakoff and Stephen J. Collier, 7–32 (New York: Columbia University Press, 2008); Didier Fassin and Maria Pandolfi, *Contemporary States of Emergency: The Politics of Military and Humanitarian Interventions* (New York: Zone Books, 2010); Peter Redfield and Erica Bornstein, eds., *Forces of Compassion: Humanitarianism between Ethics and Politics* (Santa Fe, NM: School for Advanced Research Press, 2011).

156. John Iliffe, *The African AIDS Epidemic: A History* (Oxford: James Currey, 2006).

157. Ibid.; Justin Parkhurst, "The Crisis of AIDS and the Politics of Response: The Case of Uganda," *International Relations* 15, no. 6 (2001): 69–87; Epstein, *Invisible Cure*.

158. Suzette Heald, "It's Never as Easy as ABC: Understandings of AIDS in Botswana," *International Journal of African AIDS Research* 1 (2002): 1–10.

159. Iliffe, *African AIDS Epidemic.*

160. Ibid.; Epstein, *Invisible Cure.*

161. Mary-Jo DelVecchio Good et al., "Clinical Realities and Moral Dilemmas: Contrasting Perspectives from Academic Medicine in Kenya, Tanzania, and America," *Daedalus* 128, no. 4 (1999): 167–96; Susan Whyte et al., "Treating AIDS: Dilemmas of Unequal Access in Uganda," in Petryna, Lakoff, and Kleinman, *Global Pharmaceuticals.* See also Geissler and Prince, "Purity Is Danger," in *Morality, Hope and Grief: Anthropologies of AIDS in Africa,* ed. Hansjörg Dilger and Ute Luig, 240–69 (New York: Berghahn Books, 2010).

162. Susan Reynolds Whyted, ed., *Second Chances: Surviving AIDS in Uganda* (Durham, NC: Duke University Press, forthcoming).

163. Biehl, *Will to Live;* Vinh-Kim Nguyen, "Antiretroviral Globalism, Biopolitics, and Therapeutic Citizenship," in Ong and Collier, *Global Assemblages,* 124–44.

164. Comaroff, "Beyond Bare Life" (2007); Fassin, *When Bodies Remember.* Highly active antiretroviral medicine (HAART) was created in 1994, and combination ART was made available to HIV-positive people in the North beginning in 1996.

165. Crane, "Unequal Partners"; Nguyen, "Government by Exception."

166. Nguyen, "Government by Exception."

167. Laurie Garret, "The Challenge of Global Health," *Foreign Affairs* 86, no. 1 (2007): 14–38; Wim Van Damme, Katharina Kober, and Guy Kegels, "Scaling Up Antiretroviral Treatment in Southern African Countries with Human Resource Shortage: How Will Health Systems Adapt?" *Social Science and Medicine* 66, no. 10 (2008): 2108–21; Crane, "Unequal Partners"; "What Has the Gates Foundation Done for Global Health?" editorial, *Lancet* 373 (2009): 1577.

168. Anita Hardon and Hansjörg Dilger, "Global AIDS Medicines in East African Health Institutions," in "AIDS Treatment in East Africa," special issue, *Medical Anthropology* 30, no. 2 (2011): 136–57.

169. E.g., Frederick Klaits, "The Widow in Blue: Blood and the Morality of Remembering in Botswana," *Africa* 75, no. 1 (2005): 46–62; Klaits, *Death in a Church of Life: Moral Passion in a Time of AIDS* (Berkeley: University of California Press, 2010); Prince, Denis, and van Dijk, introduction to "Engaging Christianities"; Dilger and Luig, *Morality, Hope and Grief;* Philip W. Setel, Milton Lewis, and Maryinez Lyons, eds., *Histories of Sexually Transmitted Diseases and HIV/AIDS in Sub-Saharan Africa* (London: Greenwood Press, 1999).

170. Ong and Collier, *Global Assemblages;* Nguyen, "Antiretroviral Globalism"; Comaroff, "Beyond Bare Life" (2007); Nancy Rose Hunt, "Condoms, Confessors, Conferences: Among AIDS Derivatives in Africa," *Journal of the International Institute* 4, no. 3 (1997): 15–17.

171. Steve Robbins, "'Long Live Zackie, Long Live': AIDS Activism, Science and Citizenship after Apartheid," *Journal of Southern African Studies* 30 (2004): 651–72; Steve Robbins, "Humanitarian Aid beyond 'Bare Survival': Social Movement Responses to Xenophobic Violence in South Africa," *American Ethnologist* 36, no. 4 (2009): 637–50. For Brazil, see Biehl, "Will to Live."

172. Ippolytos Kalofenos, "'All I Eat Is ARVs!' The Paradox of AIDS Treatment Interventions in Mozambique," *Medical Anthropology Quarterly* 24, no. 3 (2010): 363–80; Ruth J. Prince, "HIV and the Moral Economy of Survival."

173. Nguyen, *Republic of Therapy;* Nadine Beckmann and Janet Bujra, "The Politics of the Queue: The Politicisation of People Living with HIV/AIDS in Tanzania," *Development and Change* 41, no. 6 (2010): 1041–64; Rebecca Marsland, "(Bio)sociality and HIV in Tanzania."

174. Rottenburg, "Social and Public Experiments"; Nguyen, "Government by Exception."

175. Ruth J. Prince, "The Politics and Anti-politics of HIV Interventions in Kenya," in *Biomedicine and Governance in Africa*, ed. Paul Wenzel Geissler, Richard Rottenburg, and Julia Zenker, 97–116 (Bielefeld, Germany: Transcript Verlag, 2012).

176. Packard, "Visions of Postwar Health."

177. Marks and Andersson, "Industrialization, Rural Health"; see also Tilley, *Africa as a Living Laboratory*.

178. Samsky, "Scientific Sovereignty," 328.

179. Biehl, *Will to Live*, 10–11; see also Stefan Ecks, "Pharmaceutical Citizenship: Antidepressant Marketing and the Promise of Demarginalization in India," *Anthropology and Medicine* 12, no. 3 (2005): 239–54; Rajan, *Biocapital*; Melinda Cooper, *Life as Surplus: Biotechnology and Capitalism in the Neoliberal Era* (Seattle: University of Washington Press, 2008).

180. Nguyen, "Government by Exception."

181. Cori Hayden, "A Generic Solution? Pharmaceuticals and the Politics of the Similar in Mexico," *Current Anthropology* 48, no. 4 (2007): 475–95.

182. Petersen, "AIDS Policies."

183. Ibid.

184. Susan Whyte, Sjaak van der Geest, and Anita Hardon, eds., *Social Lives of Medicines* (Cambridge: Cambridge University Press, 2002).

185. Michael Reich, "Public-Private Partnerships for Public Health," *Nature Medicine* 6, no. 6 (2000): 617–20; Comaroff, "Beyond Bare Life" (2007); Ann Kelly, "The Progress of the Project: Scientific Traction in the Gambia," in *Differentiating Development: Beyond an Anthropology of Critique*, ed. Tom Yarrow and Soumhya Venkatesan, 65–83 (New York: Berghahn Books, 2012); Rene Gerrets, "International Health and the Proliferation of 'Partnerships': Unintended Boosts for State Institutions in Tanzania?" in *Para-states of Science: Ethnographic and Historical Perspectives on Life-Science, Government, and Public in Twenty-First-Century Africa*, ed. P. Wenzel Geissler (Durham, NC: Duke University Press, forthcoming).

186. Samsky, "Scientific Sovereignty."

187. Crane, "Unequal Partners"; P. Wenzel Geissler, "Studying Trial Communities: Anthropological and Historical Inquiries into Ethos, Politics and Economy of Medical Research in Africa," in Geissler and Molyneux, *Evidence, Ethos and Experiment*, 1–28.

188. P. Wenzel Geissler, "Public Secrets in Public Health: Knowing What Not to Know When Making Scientific Knowledge," *American Ethnologist* 40, no. 2 (2013): 13–34.

189. Ibid.

190. Samsky, "Scientific Sovereignty," 324.

191. Renne, *Politics of Polio*, 7.

192. Adriana Petryna, "Ethical Variability: Drug Development and Globalizing Clinical Trials," *American Ethnologist* 32 (2005): 183–97.

193. Fairhead, Leach, and Small, "Where Techno-Science Meets Poverty"; Crane, "Adverse Events and Placebo Effects"; Geissler, *Para-states of Science*.

194. Ferguson, "Uses of Neoliberalism," 169.

195. James Ferguson, "Formalities of Poverty: Thinking about Social Assistance in Neoliberal South Africa," *African Studies Review* 50, no. 2 (2007): 71–86; Eric Hobsbawm, "The Future of the State," *Development and Change* 27, no. 2 (1996): 267–78.

196. Lotte Meinert, Hanne O. Mogensen, and Jenipher Twebaze, "Tests for Life Chances: CD4 Miracles and Obstacles in Uganda," *Anthropology and Medicine* 16, no. 2 (2009): 195–209; Whyte et al., "Treating AIDS," 240–62.

PART ONE

Whose Public Health?

ONE

The Peculiarly Political Problem behind
Nigeria's Primary Health Care Provision

MURRAY LAST

THE TERM *PUBLIC HEALTH* PRESUPPOSES THE EXISTENCE OF A CENTRAL government or a local administration that puts a high priority on minimizing the incidence of "ill health" among its people by, for example, lessening the risk of epidemics through the provision of vaccinations as well as providing water, drainage, rubbish removal, and so forth—not to mention the maintenance of local, accessible clinics offering free primary health care to all. But what happens when there is *not* that priority for the public's health—when, for example, education is seen as much more worthwhile an investment? How does the public then manage its own "public health"? In this chapter I wish to suggest that northern Nigeria is an example in which governmental public health has largely lapsed in some if not all local government administrations (LGAs) despite a rhetoric of concern for health. Though there are, I believe, plausible reasons for this, at its root there is the problem of the politics underlying health provision—a problem that could be put right once the political will was there. If the first question is why did this problem ever arise, the second question must be how to solve it: is it primarily a problem of governance and bureaucratic malfunction—how does one get local health delivery to work efficiently?—or is it primarily political or even, at a deeper level, cultural?

But first, we need to understand the broader context. Northern Nigeria, where I have been working for the past fifty years, has changed its governance hugely since the country as a whole gained independence from Britain in 1961. The period 1966–67 was one of intense reform: two violent coups prompted a long process of change in the structures of government and local administration from a centralized, authoritarian system concerned with security and revenue raising (through local taxation) to today's decentralized polity of thirty-six states and 774 local government areas with a federal government at the new capital, Abuja. The other major change has been in revenue: the federal oil account at Abuja receives monthly payments from the major oil companies, and this revenue is then distributed according to a set formula to states, LGAs, and other institutions on the list. The sums thus regularly disbursed are enormous, more really than the three tiers of government are able (or willing) to use for development; much of the money is simply privatized, one way or another. But because the money has not been "earned" by anyone—nor has it come from citizens' paying taxes out of their earnings from hard work—there is, Nigerians tell me, a certain unreality to this flow of cash. "Development" as a discourse is still on the agenda, but personal consumption is more pressing: a degree of both is possible, given the quantity of cash on the table. Politics is a highly expensive occupation: everyone expects a politician to be very generous, and so people hassle their local politician day and night, weekday or weekend, in their search for a job, a contract, a handout, or help in a crisis. For a politician to be successful he has to be a successful patron, with all the trappings of success (and therefore power) on display. At root, then, even LGA councillors, but especially the LGA chairman, have to be full-time politicians, at least for the maximum number of terms in office they are allowed (for the chairman, that is eight years). Everyone labels the system as corrupt—and certainly personal enrichment occurs on a major scale—but in many instances it is also a system of redistribution. One governor needed four million naira (about thirty thousand U.S. dollars) each weekend for handouts, and when a first lady needed a similar sum for a brief trip to her own place, a civil servant on a Friday afternoon had to drive around the capital looking for the sum required—in cash, of course. This, then, is the context in which this chapter on local health services is set: above the ordinary farmer or trader and his family out in the countryside or somewhere deep in a megacity "slum" is this elite with access to a scale of wealth that is extraordinary in the local context. What is striking is how the two milieux do not clash: they pass each other by in peace. But there is an element of resentment in the farmer on the roadside and an element of unease inside the new, air-conditioned Honda Accord speeding by; my friends in Abuja say they half expect to die in their beds—murdered, by their servants.

Almost all my field data relate to the Hausa-speaking peoples, both Muslim and non-Muslim (*Maguzawa*), with whom I have lived as a long-term guest in their houses. They have been part of Islamic states whose recorded histories go back at least five hundred years. Nigeria was part of the British Empire from 1903 to 1960, and the administrative system set up by the British in the emirates of northern Nigeria has become known as "indirect rule": modeled on British practice in India, it enabled the emirs to head a "native authority" staffed by local officials, all under the eye of a small British-staffed office. Each native authority ran in its emirate its own *shari'a* judiciary, a police force, and a prison, as well as collecting taxes from all adults. As a reaction to this rather oppressive regime, the reforms promoting decentralization of government were initially popular.

This chapter looks at the fate of the primary health services under this new decentralized system of government. Underlying my argument is the assumption that Nigeria's system of administration is still a work in progress. Everyone knows it needs reform, and many a commission over the years has made recommendations (often accepted by the government), but the central dilemma is implementation of such reforms. Reforms do not simply "happen" as and when government orders them: someone has not only to enforce implementation but also to ensure that those newly empowered by the reforms comply with both the letter of the law and its spirit. But the very act of decentralization has removed legitimacy from any single institution that might have ensured that the system worked as it was meant to: in short, you can break the rules and get away with it. It may cost you something, but the risk is small compared to the rewards of getting away with the "loot." Nigeria thus offers most of its citizens enormous freedoms to do as they will—there is now no colonial-style authority enforcing its will and ensuring that its policies are carried out to the letter; no system of close surveillance controls the population.

My focus here is more on how ordinary people I have known over the years at the grassroots level of northern Nigerian society respond to the problems of health, both personal and public. There is a cultural dimension, as well as a political one, underlying people's broad reactions to the lack of coherent health services from the state. Cultures change, of course, but "common sense" is remarkably persistent, and this is important if only because it is so often unspoken or unrecorded.

Decentralizing the Administration: Or Why Every Politician Wants a Local Government of His Own

We need initially to recognize how fashionable it has been for foreign agencies and donors to promote, even to insist upon, decentralization— politically in the name of furthering democracy, medico-managerially in the name of prioritizing primary health care.[1] Yet sometimes these calls for decentralization also echoed the internal politics of the state, especially when separatism was in the air, as it was in Nigeria during the 1960s and 1970s or in Mali in the 1990s: minority groups needed to be co-opted into the state, and this could be done, it was thought, by giving them their own local governments complete with their own budgets.[2] The policy assumed that local politicians could, or would soon learn to, organize and maintain whatever was primary—primary education, primary health care—and not just such basic primary services as local markets, sanitation, and the registration of births and deaths. Another assumption was that newly fashionable "one-line" budgets (block grants made out to a single top official) could still be accounted for at the local level, no matter how huge they were—thanks to oil rents—and that any financial malpractice could be checked both by the democratic process and by transparency or, failing that, that corruption could be deterred by an economic and financial crimes commission given real teeth by central government.

If these were indeed the assumptions that policy makers in the late 1970s had at the time the policy was formulated, they soon proved overly optimistic. Horror stories quickly circulated: one colleague told me how his friend, a local government chairman, used to collect the local government's monthly allocation of cash from the bank and take it home, where he and some of his friends would sit on the floor and divide it up; my colleague was once offered a wad of naira notes. However, for items such as health and education there was formally a "joint state and local government account" in which the relevant local government funds were kept; the state's governor had access to it (again on a "one-line budget" system), as did the LGA chairman. Local government chairmen had little option but to comply, as the state's governor (and his party) had usually ensured that his nominees were "elected" as local government chairmen. Even more disturbing is that some state governors have often behaved no better than local government chairmen: the "joint account" only increased the amount of funds to which the governor had access, though he might have to share some of them with his House of Assembly.

Nigeria has thus devolved or delegated many functions of government, first by creating new states and then (since 1976, when the main reforms were to start) by establishing local government administrations, both to lessen tensions during and after the "Biafran" civil war and to manage more acceptably, if not better, the distribution of the burgeoning oil wealth that began to be massive in the 1970s. Over the years, local demands have since brought about a huge increase in the number of local government administrations; it pays to get one, though these are agreed to by the central government only after hard campaigning. Despite several attempts to get the system to work well, the politics of local governments, with its intense competitiveness, has only increased local conflict while failing to deliver the allocated services. The democratic "bonus" has also been strikingly absent. Though the early horror stories about the stealing by those running the LGAs are, it seems, no longer so true, the LGAs' provision of primary health services is strikingly poor.

Local Government Authorities: Or Why Do Large Health Budgets Seem to Have So Little to Show for Them?

Unlike most developing countries, Nigeria has followed supposedly "best policy" and decentralized its primary health care along with local government. Constitutionally, responsibility for "participating" in the provision of primary health care lies with 774 local government authorities, over whom there is effectively no budgetary oversight (though some state governors do indeed control the LGA chairmen). Finance should not be a problem: it comes directly from the federal government's ample oil revenues. The problem lies in that monies allocated to health services do not always reach those meant to utilize them. The buildings are there (if not always well maintained), but staff are sometimes not paid for months at a time (and so are often absent from work), medicines are not in the clinics, and the necessary medical equipment and sometimes bedding and even beds are nowhere to be seen. Nor, of course, are well-paid "ghost workers." The key issue is not the giving out of huge contracts to build or repair various health facilities: the problem lies with the recurrent expenditures on salaries, drug stocks, and repair and maintenance of equipment. Building is easy, and opening a grand new clinic is a good photo opportunity: the hard part is manning and running the necessary services consistently, day by day, year-in and year-out—that requires good, honest budgetary management. If that is not possible locally, then who should take charge of the health services? There seems to be widespread reluctance to hand over still more power to the states' governors by ceding them control over the entire public health budget. And a return to old-style central control from Abuja would be controversial and perhaps not feasible now: a careful, recent study of the running of centralized vaccination programs, especially against polio, suggests that control from the center is no longer a viable option.[3] Nigeria is too large (both in population and in distances to be covered) and too complex culturally to be run really effectively by a centralized civil service. So much has already been devolved down to the states and their LGAs that the central administration is dependent on them; not even commercial operations under contract can, it seems, deliver the services required.

Clearly, some LGAs are more honestly run than others, but overall the result is that patients and their kin resort to the private sector, not only for medicines but also for hospital care. The boom in private hospitals and specialist clinics, even in small towns, is evidence of this: they may look ramshackle but are no worse than the LGA facilities—at least the staff are there. However, the governments of the thirty-six states have the responsibility for hospitals, while the federal government runs the university teaching hospitals and the National Hospital as well as crucial agencies such as the National Agency for Food and Drug Administration and Control (NAFDAC), which tries to eliminate "fake" drugs from the marketplace. So why is there not more public outrage over the failure of the politicians who run the LGAs to provide what they are constitutionally allocated to do?

Admittedly, the fact that local voters pay no taxes, now that the government is so rich in oil revenues, means that those they elect are not seen as misusing the taxpayers' hard-earned money when the local councillors "steal" the health budget's cash. Demands for proper primary health care do not seem to be a major issue at election time. Schools and roads, by contrast, are on the agenda, though given the amount of election rigging, the failures of the LGA scarcely affect the result. But there is another serious political problem with LGAs today:

who are their "public"? The debate lies in their right to issue "certifi-cates of indigeneity" to whomever they please—but, more important, to *deny* a certificate to anyone (or any group) who displeases them.[4] Your family may have lived in a town for a hundred years—indeed, helped to develop it—but this will not necessarily guarantee you a certificate of indigeneity, and without such a certificate you and your children cannot access local schools, scholarships, local jobs, or welfare benefits (in an emergency, though, you will not be turned away from a hospi-tal, I was told, but some did not rule out the possibility of that). As a Nigerian citizen, then, you can literally be "stateless"—with no state or LGA willing to grant you rights as an "indigene." You still have the constitutional right to vote, but that will make little difference to your local status or get you contracts. You are effectively not a member of the Nigerian "public." This is a new development that is generating much anger and resentment; not religious difference but indigeneity thus lies at the heart of local political conflict. At root, only indigenes are likely to win office in their LGA, and with that office they have access to the huge wealth that is allocated to the LGA's coffers each month. Competition to control the certificates that ensure classification as an indigene is obviously fierce, since by it you can exclude all kinds of categories of rivals: any group that has moved for work or trade (and maybe has become rich and potentially powerful) can find themselves reduced politically to nonentities in the local context.

One might have thought the federal government could have reined in the excesses of the LGA system, but no political party feels they can risk the wrath of their LGAs, since the LGA is what effectively controls the votes (or at least the polling booths and the paperwork returning the voting figures). Obasanjo had serious plans in 2005 to reform the LGAs, but they fell through along with his project to get a third term in office. Only a strong military regime might have the nerve, immediately after it had seized power, to cancel the consti-tutional rights given to LGAs and thus depend on people's evident discontent to outweigh any self-interested mayhem the local politi-cians might try to mobilize. For the LGAs will not willingly forgo their access to the local health budget, seeing what a large part it can play in the politicians' personal incomes. In short, I do not foresee any immediate change in the way the "public" is deprived of government-sourced "public health" and primary health care on any scale com-mensurate with the funds available.

On the Origins of the Concept of "Public" in Northern Nigeria: Or Why Are the Attitudes toward the Government's Health Programs So Ambivalent?

I want here to offer some historical and "cultural" data on deep-rural people's experience of modern, government-driven health care, if only to show, first, how the ordinary people I lived with for two years (and have revisited every year for the past forty years) might not be so worried by the lack of a "public health" that they would take the risk of public protest and, second, why the local politicians of the LGA apparently feel no guilt over pocketing money meant for health.

"Domestic Religion"—or Who Actually Uses Primary Health Care Where I Lived?

By *deep-rural* I mean people off the main roads and a hundred miles or more away from the major conurbations, and by *people* I mean women and adolescents as well as men, since I would argue strongly for a distinction between, first, "domestic" religion (the practices done privately within the house that are designed to maintain the well-being of that house and to keep at bay the various kinds of "evil" that can bring about illness, women being crucial to the performance of these practices) and, second, "public" religion (which in most of northern Nigeria is Islam and performed most commonly by men, often collectively).[5] Because the vast majority of illness within the house is experienced by children and their mothers, domestic religion is an essential part of everyday therapy. Public health and primary health care can be seen, then, as an adjunct of domestic religion and its therapeutic program to prevent illness. Therefore, women's views, however implicit, of public health are crucial to our understanding of public health and the way it is or is not taken up in everyday life. Yet often, visiting researchers, in my experience, hear from their interviewees only the conventional, "public" account of health care. I can show how in practice the contents of a discussion on health are geared to be appropriate to the enquirer—my first eight-month experience of fieldwork while living in one farmstead was, it turned out, confined to "the conventional." By happenstance, however, one of my host's wives, in a break during hoeing her field, decided to tell me about the parallel understanding, current in the house, of their health problems, problems that included anxieties about the possible effects of spirits, witches, and sorcery on my neighbors in the farmstead, children and adults alike. There was a layer of therapy—as well as an "ethno-anatomy," an "ethno-physiology"—that I had had no knowledge of, indeed, no right to know about: it was private (but *not* secret). (The kind of public, entrepreneurial witch finding that occurs elsewhere in Africa is absent in northern Nigeria: youths might drive out a "witch" from their farmstead, yet whether a person was or was not a real "witch" remained an open question, though one not readily discussed. Much is simply not spoken about; reticence, if not silence, is admired—yet it is also a source of others' anxiety.)

The Absence of the "Public" in the Precolonial Polity

In the precolonial period (pre-1903), the traditional authorities' concern over "public health" was focused less on health at the family level than on the well-being of the "land" on a spiritual plane. Ultimate responsibility for an epidemic (such as meningitis or cholera) was laid at the door of the emir and his various officials in the countryside: their implicit role was to ensure that their territory was "clean" spiritually (which might mean morally, too)—hence, failure of the community to be properly Muslim could result not only in droughts but also in other communal disasters (such as a famine or an epidemic—perhaps even colonial invasion). The local definition of an epidemic was when those who do not "normally" die start dying in large numbers—namely, young adult men and women, for because babies and the elderly are always dying, the many deaths among them, especially at specific seasons of the year, do not constitute an "epidemic." There were officials (such as *muhtasib* and *lumo*) concerned with the maintenance of the streets and the market, but their role, along with a *Qadi* or two, was to ensure public order rather than public health. Justice, as a core element of Islamic government, itself provides the public with a kind of social "health."

In the early nineteenth century there was an attempt to Islamicize local therapies and replace non-Muslim healers (such as *boka* and *maye*) with medically minded *ʿulamaʾ*; texts spelled out the appropriate prayers for a variety of ills. Classical Arabic medical handbooks were in limited circulation, but often the plants and minerals mentioned in them were not available in northern Nigeria or the appropriate translation/equivalence was not known. In practice, traditional healers survived into the colonial period simply because there were no alternative sources of treatment, no official institutions for Islamic medicine. The new *jihadi* authorities in the nineteenth century did not set up hospitals or asylums:

no *maristan* was ever established, in part because even institutions that elsewhere attract the support of a *waqf* (a charitable bequest such as for schools or libraries) were left to individuals. Welfare was in the hands of the big houses: even today, food for the poor in the early evening is put out in dishes outside the doors of great houses, and people can eat freely there on their way back from the mosque. In theory, the palace had the means (and the stores) to support anyone seriously in need, but I have known a house to send out food nightly to some two hundred people in need (I was sometimes a beneficiary), using grain given by others.

More important, perhaps, the notion of "public" (as distinct from the notion of *jama'a*, the community of Muslims) was ignored, though undoubtedly the ruling scholarly elites who founded the Sokoto caliphate knew the concept of "nonpersonal property" or waqf (they were competent lawyers, after all!). For example, mosques, "palaces," and even prisons precolonially were private property, not "public" in terms of control or construction, though they may have been managed by a specific official. Even the water supply (in the form of wells) was private property; but because everyone had a right in theory to draw water, if necessary, from even a well inside a house, wells were often dug in a house's front courtyard or in the corner of a field where access would not prove a problem. In the cities, there were no public fountains, let alone a public washbasin for bathing or laundry. Similarly, "police," such as there were, were the private staff of officials or followers from a big house, and armies were raised for a specific campaign from personal retainers (including one's slaves) and fellow townsmen—there was not a "national" army, even when invasion threatened. Similarly, judges were in a sense personal appointees—in a huge emirate such as Kano, there were only three or four of them, one in the marketplace and the others attached to certain major rulers as legal assistants: justice (and the resolving of domestic conflicts) came from rulers, not from judges. Justice was personal and done in the house, not in a "public" court. Not until the British colonial regime (1903–60) was a formal "public" dimension instituted, with specific departments of the new "native authorities" responsible in the manner of a British bureaucracy: new courts with judges, a formal uniformed police, and a prison, as well as a hospital and doctor and so forth.[6] Even the palace became an "official" residence and not the ruling family's personal house—it was "public" property. Similarly, "corruption," if defined as diverting public goods into private hands, became a new offence once so much that had once been personal was reclassified as "public goods." Furthermore, this new offence was taken very seriously by the new British officials overseeing their colonial system.

I think the only truly public space was (and is) the marketplace, often sited just out of the village or town (on the west) or in some liminal spot (such as the banks of the river that divides Kano city into two distinct parts—so distinct that people preferred not to cross into the other side). The "market" has a life of its own—the "market" (as a mob) can, with impunity, lynch a thief; no one will be charged with murder. The marketplace was the site for executions, either beheading with the sword or skewering alive on a stake; the bodies were left there. It is still a place to hide in by day or sleep by night. But more generally, the marketplace is where named individuals can become an anonymous mass, a "public": where public spectacles are witnessed, where public announcements are made.

I am, then, suggesting that Muslim northern Nigeria precolonially was unlike, say, Egypt or the Maghreb. It did not have a "public" dimension in the way those states did; instead, the leading big houses or families provided all that was needed, especially in their own sections (*ungwoyi*) of the city. The needy "public," such as it was, attached themselves to one or another of these houses, though the begging blind would usually form a village of their own. Visitors en masse, such as the porters and drivers for the caravans, had separate settlements of their own on the edge of town; there, things could be done (such as gambling, drinking, sex for hire) that shari'a law in the city would have stopped. (A further, practical reason was that city gates, for security's sake built with a dogleg passageway, rarely had space enough for a loaded camel to pass through; hence, merchants preferred to lodge outside rather than load and unload within the city walls.) What concerned—and controlled— most people were more often personal ties than anything institutional. The British colonial regime, then, imposed on the community an extra institutional layer—not just themselves as "indirect rulers" but also a public, bureaucratic domain. Bureaucracy, the domain of "the public," was thus a *colonial* institution—alien and Christian—that had no place in Hausa political or cultural life. With the colonial rulers gone, why continue to give bureaucracy the same importance as the officious colonialists had?

Rulers, whatever their stripe, are responsible for the broad well-being of those they rule. In this context, then, it seemed fitting locally that the early years of colonial rule, when Muslim lands were being ruled for the first time by alien Christians, should also witness other disasters—especially a severe famine and major epidemics such as Spanish influenza. Though the new government was to blame, primarily it was Allah who was punishing His people both by imposing on them these strange non-Muslims and by inflicting, a little later, a series of new, lethal illnesses (such as flu after World War I and cerebrospinal meningitis circa 1924). People's response to these crises was to improve their practice of Islam, to join reformed Sufi brotherhoods (such as the Tijaniyya and the Mahdiyya), and, more keenly than ever, to send their children to Qur'anic schools—in the firm belief that they would please Allah enough for Him to remove again the Christians whom He had brought. Many, however, decided to move away instead of waiting for Him to act—to go east to Mecca to await the Mahdi there. The exodus was huge, but the hardships endured were so great that many finally decided to settle in the Sudan, never making it to Mecca. Theirs was not, of course, a "public" decision: large extended families came together and met to discuss who among them should emigrate east and who should stay behind to manage the properties and herds and care for those too elderly to travel. Again, it was at the level of the family that decisions were taken and provision made. Though the Amir al-mu'minin, after his defeat at Sokoto in March 1903, also made his way eastward, it made matters worse if the masses went with him—water and food were desperately short at that time. Emigration (*hijra*) was not "public policy."

"Subsistence Health"

For their part, the British in the face of these famines and epidemics in northern Nigeria were primarily concerned with ensuring the health of themselves and their Nigerian military and police forces. Medical services, as so often occurs, were initially linked to military, not civilian (let alone "native" or the public's), needs. With so much concern among Muslims about the legitimacy of accepting non-Muslim "rulers" (however few and inconspicuous the non-Muslims may have been), in their forts the colonial British needed, if only for their own sense of security, a force that was never too ill to fight in an emergency. Many of the early British officials were chosen because they were ex-army men (often with experience of fighting Boers in South Africa); hence, a concern for military health was habitual. Only in Zaria did the new British regime allow a missionary to stay in a Muslim city, and he eventually opened a medical station (at Babban Dodo); his success, however, in converting some Muslim "princes" to Christianity caused such alarm that he was ordered by the colonial authorities to move his station south out of the city and into a new separate settlement (Wusasa). Otherwise, the barracks (*bariki*) north of the city across the river were the main site of what early colonial medicine there was. Indeed, *bariki* became synonymous with a certain style of non-Muslim life that was usually also seen as disreputable. Medicine, then, started in surroundings that for Hausa were culturally low-class and off-limits; it was a service primarily for "others." The rank and file of the military who fought for the Christian British were drawn from peoples ("martial races," of course) whom the Muslim Hausa both despised and feared: "[S]ome even filed their teeth like cannibals," said an early colonial note, referring especially to local Dakarawa recruits.

Nonetheless, from their bases in the new mixed-race settlements, pioneer traders such as John Holt imported patent remedies (such as *pengo*, or "pain-go"), quinine, and soap to sell over the counter in their "go-downs" along the "beach" (as the main trading streets in the colonial cantonments were called even in dry Sokoto and hilly Jos). In time, specially iodized salt was imported to limit the incidence of goiter, but petty traders, especially from the Christian south of Nigeria, penetrated deep into the countryside on their bicycles selling medicines alongside hurricane lamps, matches, candles, soap, and ordinary salt (as well as cigarettes at a penny or less a stick). These traders are the ones who introduced "Western" medicines into deep-rural communities, just as did soldiers and police on their return home to villages. In this context, any government service promoting primary health care or public health was irrelevant to people's understanding.

The British colonial government, being short of cash (and concerned about its ability to collect taxes), therefore had a policy of "subsistence health" not dissimilar to the notion of "subsistence agriculture." Health was left to ordinary people to continue their ordinary therapies. In the Muslim emirates of northern Nigeria, the colonial policy was that Christian missionaries should not be allowed to set up mission stations (apart from some leprosy stations in the 1930s), so that all schools and hospitals/dispensaries were effectively run by the "native authorities," the powerful administrations staffed by local emirate officials under "indirect" British supervision. These schools and medical facilities were staffed often by Christians (whether Nigerian or foreign), with the result that "medicine" has become one of the occupations primarily identified with Christianity, despite the presence of some Muslims as teachers, nurses, and (later) doctors. But missionaries, people told me, were apt to exact an unpleasant price: as you waited for hours in a long queue to be seen in the hospital or dispensary, you were subjected to endless preaching in an attempt to have you convert to Christianity. People went there for treatment, not for a diatribe against "pagan" beliefs (which I would include in "domestic" therapy) and pressure to join a church. Mission schools were similarly hard on non-Christian boys; the pressure did sometimes result in conversion, but in the long term it also won them an education—and they could always leave Christianity later. In short, altruism among whites was in short supply; you had to know their price. Yet at the same time, people recognized genuine selflessness among whites when they met it and warmly remember it still.

The Move toward Active "Public Health"—and People's Suspicions of It

The colonial government by the 1950s (in the run-up toward independence) had initiated a more public health–oriented policy that saw teams of sanitary inspectors (*duba gari*, in Hausa) who could enter everyone's house (since one of the team was always a woman): each week, people tidied their compounds carefully before the inspectors came. In the countryside, district officers on tour would check (and report on) the sanitary conditions of farmsteads and their environs, including the removal of thorny plants (such as *kashin yawo*) that were regarded as a health hazard; they would also supervise the refurbishment of improved wells with concrete tops. Sleeping-sickness surveys of the general population were instituted (beginning in the late 1940s), and people with swollen neck glands were compulsorily taken to a camp for treatment. This turned into an exploitative process, as beautiful women and girls were clearly the majority of the ones identified as having swollen glands and therefore taken away. It took money to save your wife or daughter from this official abduction—I watched the process happen even in the early 1970s. It is important to remember how oppressive were government officials of all kinds then. With no oil revenue to finance their wants, officials from the towns would come out to the village head's house on a weekly basis with some new scheme to make the farmers pay. In short, government was synonymous with extortion—even a supposed celebration such as a *durbar* was an excuse to take away the most beautiful of the local farmers' daughters, to the despair if not fury of their families. Hence, the notion that the government might have the "public good" in mind, even in matters of health, was repeatedly proved false. I saw it happen myself; it was not hidden.

But the practice was established well before my time. There had already developed a very real suspicion that medical services from the government were *not* beneficial, at least not for the ordinary person. This suspicion dates back to early colonial days when "whites" (or, rather, "reds," as Europeans were classified) were considered as being possibly a kind of fish or manatee that came out of the ocean: the dye of their clothes did not run, they needed constant water (showers, baths), they could not really walk (they had to have shoes and socks and were carried about in hammocks), and they liked to build dams and create lakes (which they visited for picnics, and some even dived in and swam—maybe they were doing nefarious things underwater). Their liking for ice and cold water at dusk was a significant proof of their essential witchiness.[7] It was typical of people's doubts about whites' work as doctors that the spirit-possession (*bori*) depiction of a doctor was of man sitting with a stethoscope around his neck and the house's most beautiful small girl beside him—the stethoscope he used to suck blood from her.

These notions may seem absurd now (certainly old-fashioned and stale), but even during my two years in a farmstead as recently as 1970–72 I found that some of my co-residents thought they might possibly be true of me. The local "cottage hospital," an outlying unit of the university's teaching hospital, was similarly a focus of suspicion, especially as patients often died there (having been taken in as a last resort) and their bodies might be subject to a postmortem after which not all the body parts were always replaced, and the returned body, under its winding sheet, might have its chest stuffed with paper—but wiser relatives usually did not look before burial. In short, there was a rumor that hospitals were a kind of "power-station" where whites extracted the crucial body parts of blacks so that otherwise ineffectual whites could exert their improbable power over the local black population and its age-old political authorities. Hospital medicine was, in their eyes, a kind of magic, a magic that at its core is harmful: X-rays and other techniques of seeing inside a person were the attributes of witches. After a while, however, a witch might become sated and use his powers for good, not evil, at which point he could be a useful friend. To some in the farmstead I was such an ex-witch, but I was only told some eight months after my arrival in the farmstead that they knew I had witchly powers: at the time, I was apparently in a battle to the death with another witch in the farmstead. To my chagrin at the time, my hosts quite expected him to win and me to die or flee. Given some of these suspicions (remember, they are not "beliefs," nor are they "facts," yet they just might turn out to be true), entry inside the high barbed-wire fence of a government hospital was seen as a potentially risky business; people went to have their pains and blockages relieved—*not* to have their lives "saved," since Allah alone determined the moment they would die. So people took patients in by their own choice; it was they who decided (and took the risk), and the decision was certainly not at the behest of a government official.

Today's "Private Health": Or How Has Child Mortality Decreased So Much Today?

When I lived in a deep-rural farmstead circa 1970–72, the child mortality rate was approximately 50 percent. Of the 131 children I knew there, 66 died and 65 remained alive. Today, nearly forty years on, when I visit the farmstead's graveyard (as I do each year), I can count at most 4 children's graves dug during the previous year, yet the farmstead now has nearly five times more children alive—up from 60 to about 300—than it had forty years ago (for the first time, not one child died in the year 2009–10). It is an astonishing change, with, of course, huge implications for land and jobs, both of which are in such short supply that most of the young men have gone to the cities to find work; they return to the farmstead only to see and support their wives and children financially. The population of the wider village area has grown from 1,500 taxpayers in 1954 to over 75,000 residents in 2007, but only since the 1980s or later has "maternal and child health" (MCH) been transformed. One needs to remember that traditional medicine (what I call "ethno-pediatrics") has never been very successful in managing the acute infections that kill babies and young children—or, indeed, in saving their mothers from catastrophic pregnancies and childbirth. MCH, with its drugs and potential surgery, offers women what was not available before: though there are traditional remedies, for example, for peripartal heart failure (such as the plant *daita*), the necessary dosages cannot be calculated— so sometimes it worked, sometimes it did not.

Although there are local MCH clinics and surgical facilities in the state government- and university-run hospitals, the major change in the local "therapeutic culture" has come about through local youths becoming interested in biomedicine—partly through wanting to trade in medicines in the marketplace, where you have to be able to explain to customers what each item for sale is meant to do for them; even in urban chemist stalls, young boys are often the ones who explain the medicines that their fathers or uncles are selling. In the farmstead I stay in, two or three youths have gone into biomedicine as their career, not as doctors but as community or theatre nurses. The result is that in the farmstead they put up drips, administer injections, and care for their sick relatives. And they are competent: one neighbor, an elderly HIV-positive woman, they kept alive for a year by using various drugs to fend off the opportunistic infections she picked up in her farmstead. Their newly learned expertise rubs off not just on their wives but also on the mothers in the farmstead and neighboring houses more generally. Mosquito nets, which no one (except me) had in the farmstead in 1970, are now appreciated, even if not all use them—you have to buy them, and they are not impregnated; but a young bride might well expect to find one ready for her in her bridal chamber alongside a nice bed and armchair. No electric light or running water will greet her, however—even if the wires and pipes are there (as they might be in a roadside village), the government has yet to provide power and water. (Wires and pipes, like roads, involve profitable work for both private contractors and those awarding the contracts, whereas keeping power and water flowing does not.)

These developments depend on "private" initiative, "private" medicine, and "private" facilities (even the wells are usually personally dug by hand). The young men get formal jobs in privately owned clinics (usually belonging to a doctor with a government practice in a state-run hospital). In one case, as a theatre nurse, a youth I know learned how to do operations and on occasions had to instruct the surgeon on what to do and what not to do; the newly appointed "surgeon" turned out to be wholly untrained (and lethal) though licensed by government—you can buy your qualifications and practice (if you are bold enough and/or persuasive enough to blame God rather than your lack of skill when your patient dies). People are aware that some who offer medicine may be poseurs: for example, one "dispenser" in a local village specialized in injecting his own homemade fluids into the eye, often with dire results. The youths I know have usually been trained in state-run schools for community health, but many also learn from each other; books are rarely an adequate source, as villagers' command of written English is poor and textbooks have not been translated into Hausa (which can, anyway, be hard to read). The government system, then, does run after a fashion, and there are dedicated young Nigerians providing health care at the grass roots. I would suggest, however, that people's self-motivated health-care system, not the government's public health program, is primarily what has brought about the marked change in morbidity and mortality in the deep-rural countryside.

One exception remains to be noted, however. Guinea worm, which was a devastating plague on farmers, their wives, and especially their children, has been eradicated. It was a government program funded and supported by overseas governments, but it was carried out systematically and has worked. It was not, I admit, a product of LGAs, but it was public health in the conventional sense, and it has transformed lives. Similarly, our village head is serious, working for his people much as his father did for some fifty years before him. He has ensured that polio vaccine was administered but admits it was imperfectly done (you cannot force people to take it). Despite the much-publicized controversy over its safety and the suspicions that it was designed to make Muslim girls infertile, he has seen it administered to cooperative villagers (some have had over twenty doses) to appear to fill a quota, while everyone else in the village's administrative area seems to have been left alone. People know about the value of vaccines, especially the all-important measles vaccine, without which infant mortality rose each April and May, but one major campaign I witnessed (against measles) never reached the women and children who sought it, because the vaccine needed to be kept chilled and the cold boxes given for storage were "privatized" (that is, stolen) and the vaccine spoiled. In any case, the vaccinating team members were reluctant to leave the main, tarred road, and did not stay long—they were gone before women could get to them with their children. The sense of "service" to the individual is strong, but altruistic service to a general "public" seems rare.

Conclusions? Or Why It May Not Matter to People if the Situation Does Not Change Soon

Without major political change at the center of the federal government, the LGAs are unlikely to reform themselves spontaneously or seriously to offer primary health care *to all*. Certainly, some state governors do better than others, and in time maybe more governors will emulate them, but the creation of local government was a political solution to a pressing political problem at a time when political discontent at the local level was getting fierce: the profits from oil had to be better and more widely distributed, and decentralization was the answer chosen. There is little enthusiasm for increasing even further the powers of state governors over the LGAs—decentralization is not about further enriching those at the state's capital. Local money, even if misspent or invested far outside the LGA's area, is still potentially more accessible to ordinary people living in the locality.

The comparison of primary health with primary education—both are the constitutional responsibility of LGAs—is indicative of the way health has never had the same priority as education, for two simple reasons: first, "modern" education is necessary for one's children to acquire if they are not to be condemned to a farming future precisely at a time when there will not be enough farmland for them to live off; and second, modern education can be supplied only by schools with educated teachers. Unlike health care, which you can access in a variety of ways, education is strictly controlled through certificates: you must get your certificate somehow, and your competence as an educated man or woman must show in daily life and work if you are to get and keep a job. Hence, when in the 1990s there was a crisis in the schools on account of the teachers never being paid by the LGAs, there was so strong a row over schools' closure that the federal government had to step in and subtract the teachers' salaries from the block grant to the LGAs and ensure that teachers were paid. Schooling mattered in a way health does not. That emphasis goes back a long way: we know that school budgets in twentieth-century Africa were conventionally up to four times the size of health budgets, and people seem to share this priority for their children to be educated. Indeed, once children have reached school age, the worst period of child mortality is over, so schooling is the best investment for the future of both them and their parents.

By contrast, as an adult (with long-developed immunity and resistance), you can get by with minimal health care provided by all kinds of people: in an emergency, admittedly, you may have to be taken (at great risk and possibly great cost) to a hospital or clinic. But ultimately, whether you live or die depends on Allah, not on the doctor. People see "public health" as giving jobs and power currently to a set of individuals whose primary concern is not "the public" but themselves: primarily, they are their own "public," promoting their own (financial) "health." Serious suspicion about colonial intentions with medicine has given way to cynicism about government's claims to altruism and service: the end result is much the same—do not waste time campaigning for health services, for it is better to ensure your family's health with well-chosen carers you can trust. Were local government ever to provide public health and primary health care, that would be a bonus; meanwhile, we must care for ourselves, they say.

Notes

1. E.g., the "Bamako Initiative" of 1987, organized by WHO and UNICEF and taken up by African health ministers, focused on the decentralization of maternal and child health and the provision of primary health care. Immunization and guinea-worm eradication were also on the agenda.

2. On Mali, see Jennifer Seely, "A Political Analysis of Decentralisation: Co-opting the Tuareg Threat in Mali," *Journal of Modern African Studies* 39, no. 3 (2001): 499–524.

3. Elisha Renne, *The Politics of Polio in Northern Nigeria* (Bloomington: Indiana University Press, 2010).

4. On "indigeneity," see Human Rights Watch, *"They Do Not Own This Place": Government Discrimination against "Non-indigenes" in Nigeria* (New York: Human Rights Watch, 2006). The distinction between indigenes to a specific place and "settlers" goes back to precolonial times but was reinforced during colonial rule and further reinforced with the 1970s increase in LGAs. Since about 2002 in Jos it has become deeply contentious.

5. Domestic religion involves the cult of spirits (*iskoki, aljanu*) and perhaps the use of various "magic" charms, as well as a range of special prayers to Allah. It is quite elaborate, I am told, and kept secret (or at least private), even from one's husband or wife. Such practices are not, of course, confined to the countryside; my urban colleagues have told me (and shown me) what is being done in their households, but it is not something one normally discusses. Domestic medicines, then, are a very different matter: they include common plants, foods, and, today, pills specially given as tonics to strengthen or ease the sickly.

6. Government doctors in this new system were more than medical: in an emergency and in the absence of the Resident, a doctor would take over command of the province.

7. The crucial substance that witches (unlike ordinary people) are believed to have in their stomachs is ice—traditionally, a piece of hail, which was the only known occurrence of ice in Hausaland. Thus, the introduction by "whites" of refrigerator-made ice cubes made them objects of suspicion. Normal people are warm inside.

TWO

Who Are the "Public" in Public Health?

Debating Crowds, Populations, and Publics in Tanzania

REBECCA MARSLAND

IN 2002, NEW BYLAWS WERE APPROVED IN KYELA DISTRICT IN southwestern Tanzania to legislate against what were described as "misleading traditions" (*mila potovu*) of the Nyakyusa. These "misleading traditions" include matters relating to inheritance, mourning, funerals, and a range of different customs loosely grouped under the heading "Cleanliness, Care, and Improvement of the Environment." Anyone caught following these traditions can be fined ten thousand shillings (equivalent to a month's income for many farmers during most of the year) or receive six months in jail.

Kyela, located in the floodplains of the north shore of Lake Nyasa, is a bustling and economically prosperous district in Tanzania. The Nyakyusa who dominate the district farm rice, cocoa, bananas, and palm oil and engage in trade over the border with Malawi and farther afield on the road to Dar es Salaam. To the north of Kyela are the equally prosperous highlands of Rungwe District, also mainly inhabited by Nyakyusa. The fieldwork on which this chapter is based took place from 2000 to 2002, in six weeks in 2007, and in a final four months in 2009, mainly in a village close to the lakeshore. It also draws on the monographs and unpublished field notes of Monica and Godfrey Wilson, who worked in the area in the 1930s.

In this chapter, I ask how we can account for these bylaws as a public health intervention, and thus my analysis is framed in terms of an anthropology *of* public health, as opposed to an anthropology *in* public health.[1] The *of* requires that anthropologists put public health under the ethnographic lens, whereas the *in* compels us to offer a service, such as cultural broker, to public health. Part of this ethnographic understanding of public health includes a clarification of what the "public" in public health means to public health workers, in this case in Tanzania. I therefore examine how the bylaws against "misleading traditions" offer an insight into how public health officials imagine a "public" in Kyela; for them, a public as a critical rational debating group does not exist. Instead, they imagine something akin to a crowd or population, which are quite different things.[2] The bylaws are an intervention to create the "right" kind of population, and they do this by distinguishing "good" traditions from "bad."[3]

There is, however, a second layer to consider. Public health is made not only by public health professionals but also by those who use or choose not to use their services. Therefore, I ask how the people in Kyela who practice the "misleading traditions" construe the field of public health and their role in it. In doing so, I examine the relationship between historical forms of indigenous public health and what have come to be known as challenging attitudes toward authority in the district, for the "public" have taken control of one aspect of indigenous public health for themselves. A deeper understanding reveals that the bylaws operate "between" these two "kinds" of public health. The bylaws reflect the view of official public health that indigenous public health is a threat to public health in its own right—it is unruly and dangerous and represents an informal alternative to state-authorized forms of authority. The bylaws can be construed as an attempt by external authorities to close down debate about areas of moral uncertainty, which have been debated intensively in Bunyakusa at least since Monica and Godfrey Wilson were working in the region in the 1930s.

Debating Funerals

Over the past ten years, there has been an upsurge of interest in funerals in African countries. This reflects the high frequency of funerals—when I was in Kyela, I would usually encounter at least one each week. Sometimes there were three funerals in one day. This can partly be attributed to the AIDS epidemic but is also a consequence of increased mortality rates caused by the rise of infectious diseases, changes to health-care provision, and economic insecurity. In Kyela, these deaths were also associated with "tradition."

Funerals combine a bewildering number of contentious issues. They are significant primarily because they mark loss, and with that comes all the complicated emotions of grief, anger, sorrow, and fear, as people mourn and try to make sense of what are often premature deaths. This often results in disputes about the cause of death and can lead to accusations of neglect or witchcraft. Funerals consolidate identity, both of the dead and of the living, and bring people together to carry out the work of relatedness and reestablish bonds of connection.[4] They are also a major context in which tensions of obligation between urban elites and villagers are played out.[5] Funerals necessitate great expenditure, which can get people into debt or lead people to spend money that some would argue could be better used to improve living standards or health care.[6] Conflict about the use of gifts contributed to the bereaved family by relatives and friends, the misuse of money donated for funeral expenses, and the failure of the bereaved family to provide sufficient refreshments for visiting mourners is common. Such disputes about reciprocal gift giving can be dangerous because they predispose people to ill feeling and jealousy, sentiments that can urge people toward indulging in witchcraft. Deborah Durham has described this as the "double-edge of sociality."[7] Governments, churches, and chiefs in some places have addressed these matters with initiatives to regulate funeral celebrations, often aiming to cut down ostentation and cost.[8] However, I have not yet come across regulations like those in Kyela, which construe funerals as a public health hazard or seek to control the acts of witchcraft that can result from the jealousy and ill feeling that are often generated at funeral sites.

In Kyela, as in other parts of Africa, funerals are thus significant and contentious. This is nothing new. They make up a central component of Godfrey and Monica Wilson's two monographs on ritual, both of which go into detailed symbolic analysis of rituals of death and mourning.[9] The Wilsons' field notes from the 1930s contain numerous examples of disputes over these rituals, provoked by missionary influence, education, and exposure to other ways of life as Nyakyusa men traveled farther afield during the colonial period.[10]

Today, Nyakyusa funerals remain major events. When somebody dies, the body must be returned "home" to the place of his or her father's lineage or, in the case of married women, to the place of her husband's father's lineage. On the day of the burial, hundreds of relatives, friends, and the entire village gather at the deceased person's "home." Men and women congregate in separate spaces, the women sitting on the ground on mats or banana leaves around the side or the back of the house, and the men at the front, seated on chairs, usually arranged in a circle. The assembled mourners are given refreshments—*kande* (a stew made of beans and maize) and sweet black tea. As newcomers arrive, singly or as long lines of women carrying *ipijilo* (food such as bananas, rice, and beer) in distinctive blackened baskets on their heads, they give condolences first to the men in a manner determined by the visitors' sex: men shake hands; women kneel at a respectful distance. The newcomers then go to the assembled women, where they must work their way through the seated masses to the key mourners, who are often in the center of closely gathered bodies, where on their knees and weeping they offer their hands, saying, *"Ndaga ndaga"* (sorry, sorry), setting off a new wave of wailing. Gifts of money, sheets, or cloth are given to both male and female mourners by their friends and relatives. Comfort is offered by women singing hymns and songs of mourning to each other, in addition to entertainment in the form of a church choir or *ngoma* (drum) performance. The atmosphere is a heady mixture of grief, noise, gossip, and hilarity.

Young men from the village work together to dig the grave. When it is time for the burial, everybody gets up and heads to the graveside, where the main mourners are seated and everybody else crowds around. The coffin is lowered in. There are speeches by religious leaders and senior relatives, and the village chairperson takes the opportunity to remind everyone of the bylaws pertaining to funeral procedures. Afterward, the young men fill in the grave with earth, accompanied by the singing of those assembled. Once this is over, most people file off home, but the main relatives, friends, and neighbors remain. If the burial is of a married woman, then one of her brothers will "carry the funeral" *(kubeba kilio)* to her father's home—where her father awaits the accompanying mourners, further refreshments are distributed, and gifts are given.

The mourning is not over at this stage. Women and a few men remain at the funeral site for days or weeks to help cook and to comfort their bereaved relative or friend. During this time, the "owner" of the funeral (the senior man in the household) must foot the often-considerable bill to provide food, soft drinks, and beer for these visitors. If the house is not big enough, the women will sleep outside on mats. In 2000–2002 they did so without mosquito nets (women would show me the bites on their arms as evidence of their suffering at the funeral), but the new bylaws ensured that by 2009 mosquito nets were tied up under trees. Women used to be "afraid" to sleep under a mosquito net at a funeral, because it would appear as if they were "showing off," sleeping in comfort while their friends suffered, and so they feared they might be bewitched in reprisal. Mourning also requires that a bereaved woman does not wash, wear shoes, or change her clothes, and the ground is not swept. Nothing is cleaned until the day of *ukujola imindu* (sweeping up the rubbish), when the wives of the dead person's brothers come to sweep the ground and are given doughnuts, soft drinks, and cash for their work. Then, after a final wail, the bereaved can wash and put on clean clothes. The mourners' hair used to be shaved *(kunyoa nywele)*, but these days, because young women like their hair to be long, a small lock is snipped off as a gesture to the custom. In the past it could take months for this stage to be reached, and old women complained to me that they would be infested with lice. Now, because of the bylaws, this period should take no longer than three days, although it may in practice be a matter of weeks.

The bylaws are mainly concerned with the "misleading traditions" described above that take place at funerals, although they also refer to other matters, such as feasts cooked for the inheritance ritual, when an estranged wife returns to her husband or after a dispute, on the birth of a new baby, or to apologize for failing to follow any of these "misleading traditions." In addition, they cover other traditions, such as the obligation for sons to build a brick house for their father before they build one for themselves, an obligation that leaves many young families living in houses constructed from bamboo and plastered with mud. They also deal with the mistreatment of widows.

I first learned of these bylaws in a National Malaria Control Programme (NMCP) document, which stated that as the result of a community exercise in Kyela District, some traditions had been identified as "hinder[ing] the community interventions against malaria" and that bylaws against these "traditional beliefs" had been passed to prevent their continued practice.[11] Not until 2009 did I discover that the bylaws had never been approved by the national government; throughout the period of my research, government officers in the district believed that they had been and were acting accordingly. A key figure who pushed for these bylaws was the district medical officer (DMO). When I met him, he had recently returned from studying for his MPH at the University of Leeds, where he had written his dissertation on the relationship between Nyakyusa tradition and the spread of disease. I discussed the bylaws with different government health workers in the district, all of whom framed them unambiguously in terms of public health. The traditions they targeted were deemed to be unhygienic and therefore to encourage the spread of infectious disease: malaria, cholera and other waterborne diseases, meningitis, and sexually transmitted infections, including HIV.

That the bylaws are also concerned with witchcraft as a problem for public health could only be partially acknowledged by members of the medical profession. The DMO explained to me in 2002 that belief in witchcraft has a "psychological" effect, which causes people to seek treatment outside of the biomedical health services, for example, from traditional healers. As a Nyakyusa man from Rungwe District, he recognized that people are under pressure to conform to "tradition" at funerals and other occasions. Even his own wife would be expected not to sleep under a mosquito net when mourning, to go barefoot and not change her clothes, and to bring considerable gifts of food and money at times when relationships are being mended or renegotiated. But it took the Society for Traditional Healers to explain to me that these "traditions" can be enforced by a kind of community witchcraft known in Kinyakyusa as *imbepo sya bandu*.[12] Outlawing such "traditions" would free people from the pressure to conform to what are often difficult or expensive obligations and restrictions on behavior. Subsequently, I found in conversation after conversation with acquaintances in the village where I lived, and in interviews, that the bylaws had widely been interpreted as a means to control imbepo sya bandu, which was widely perceived to have grown out of control.

That funerals attract witches is not a new concern. Conversations recorded by Godfrey Wilson during his fieldwork in the 1930s reveal that witches were thought to kill people so that they could eat meat at funerals (in the days when cattle were killed for funeral feasts).[13] The hunger of witches for meat is a theme that is familiar to Africanists and has led contemporary debates to focus on how witchcraft as the epitome of greed and jealousy is deployed as a critical discourse on the moral corruption of modernity and the inequalities brought about by global capitalism.[14] In contrast, the bylaws in Kyela illustrate how witchcraft is experienced as very real,[15] and its prevalence is taken as evidence for the widely held view that tradition has become morally corrupt.[16]

The bylaws thus address an amalgam of public health concerns. From the point of the view of the state, these are hygiene, the spread of infectious disease, and delays in consulting biomedical practitioners because of irrational beliefs in witchcraft. From the point of view of an indigenous public health, they address a kind of witchcraft that is either considered to be a necessary curb on antisocial behavior, when people do not conform to "traditional" norms, or is considered to have gone too far, reflecting the greed and jealousy of witches.

This double function of the bylaws can be traced to the consultative procedure that was followed by the district government. The DMO and other senior district-level officials first drafted the bylaws and then circulated them to ward and village committees. As a result, many more "misleading traditions" were added in. This public consultation exercise revealed critical thinking on the part of these committees, who saw tradition as threatening public health as they defined it. District officials were unable to acknowledge openly this critique, however, because it would require entering into the logic of witchcraft, a logic that is not officially sanctioned.[17]

Public Health without a Public?

How can we understand these bylaws in the context of public health in Tanzania, and what do they tell us about how public health authorities view the citizenry? One problem that continually troubled me during fieldwork was the tendency of many who occupy positions of public authority in Tanzania to view "ordinary people" as superstitious, backward, and uneducated. They are, in the words of Charles L. Briggs and Clara Mantini-Briggs, "unsanitary subjects."[18] This stance can be attributed to the centrality that development holds in the postcolonial Tanzanian state. The successors to the British colonial administration might have repudiated many aspects of colonial rule, but one attitude they shared was the view that rural people were irrational, superstitious, backward, lazy, and drunken.[19] This is why I decided to ask myself whether public health authorities recognize the existence of a "public," in Jürgen Habermas's sense of citizens who engage in "rational-critical debate" about themselves and shape the field in which public authorities operate, while bringing to account, through publicity, those in power.[20] Below I argue that such a public does exist but that public health authorities do not see it—instead, they see crowds and populations.

In anthropology, thinking about publics has tended to focus on the distinction between public and private. Feminists have critiqued the power relationships that create a gendered hierarchy between public and private.[21] This is one possible line of inquiry, if we are to ask questions of public health and its publics. For example, the private sphere of intimate and domestic practices is invaded by public health interventions about safe sex or mosquito nets. This government over the everyday labor that keep us alive illustrates how "the life process itself . . . has been channelled into the public realm."[22] Power is chan-neled through our will to live and is manifest in bodily disciplines such as "techniques of the self" in which we internalize the advice of public health authorities.[23] However, these techniques hinge on a body that is managed by the "self" and not by others. In an African context, it is often "others"—family, friends, neighbors—who manage bodies. They determine the choice of therapy and provide the context through which publicly sanctioned moralities of the body are understood (pertaining to sexuality, bodily comportment, and sickness caused by antisocial or im-moral behavior).[24] This does not mean, however, that power in African countries is not dependent on matters of sheer survival or public health. On the contrary, political authority once depended on indigenous forms of public health that ensured that life circulates within the "country."

If public health were to have a public, it might be one that reflects rationally and critically about survival and the activities its members undertake to keep themselves alive. It might also reflect critically on the work of public health authorities. Bruno Latour claims that "matters of fact" are commonly used by those in authority to close down debate.[25] Those (like rural Tanzanians) who are skeptical of "facts" are seen to be irrational. It would be more democratic, he argues, if we could step away from facts and recognize that they are often produced by interested par-ties. He recommends that we return debate and dispute to the political arena and take an interest in "matters of concern": those complex issues that cannot easily be explained by facts. We would all benefit if "the public adopts problems that no one else is taking care of."[26]

Returning to the bylaws, I argue that from the point of view of public health authorities, funerals raise "matters of fact": they are indis-putably unhygienic and lead to the spread of infectious disease, even if the authorities offer no empirical evidence as proof of these facts. From the point of view of the public of public health, however, funerals raise "matters of concern." The responsibility to mourn properly and with consideration toward others vies with the considerable discomfort involved and is contradicted by health education messages. The obliga-tion to bring gifts to the bereaved, and for the bereaved to offer food and drink in return, consolidates social relations on the one hand and raises the risk of witchcraft on the other.

It is important, of course, to acknowledge that my starting point for thinking about publics stems from concepts rooted in the Western history of thought. The conditions in which a public might emerge in Africa are necessarily going to be different, but that does not mean to say that the notion is irrelevant. As Michael Warner suggests, the notion of a public has "gone traveling"; it is a concept that is widely understood in many different contexts.[27] Certainly, the activity of critical debate is one that is most familiar to Africans. Habermas's notion of the public hinged on a particular socioeconomic moment in history—in which capitalism brought together members of the bourgeoisie as equals, and which was mediated by literacy and print media. Print media is not freely accessible to many in an African context, but as Karin Barber makes clear, print was useful to "convene" new publics but not necessary for them to emerge.[28] There are other spaces, such as funerals, markets, and drinking "clubs," where people assemble and debate. In a context in which witchcraft is a "matter of concern," the rationality of public debate might also be contested. In their discussion of funerals in Botswana, Deborah Durham and Frederick Klaits prefer to talk about a "public *space* of funerals" instead of a public sphere, which brings people together through shared sentiment instead of rational debate,[29] and certainly this applies to the public who assemble at funerals in Kyela. Yet there is also rational debate about the sentiments of greed and jealousy at funerals—a debate that operates within the logic of witchcraft but is also critical of the use of it as social sanction and of the social norms it seeks to maintain.

Crowds

Historically, crowds have been thought of as irrational and dangerous and as a pathological and criminal form of social gathering. Crowds are contrasted to publics, whose "advantages . . . are to be found in replacing custom by mode, tradition by innovation."[30] The historian George Rudé instead considers crowds as a form of populist political movement.[31] The bylaws in Kyela criminalize the kind of "traditional" crowd that gathers to mourn or to feast. Crowds are unruly mobs who take action, but not on the basis of reason. They prefer tradition and custom to progress and science.

In Kyela, public health officials and other public authorities imagine that local people constitute a crowd and not a public. In particular, crowds of women at funerals do not behave "reasonably" from a public health point of view. Mourning compels them to give up their personal hygiene and go without shoes and clean clothes. They do not comb their hair, and they sit in a litter of banana leaves instead of on mats. For fear that they will be bewitched, they do not sleep under mosquito nets, putting themselves and young children at risk of malaria. Public health officers informed me that people at funerals will defecate in the surrounding area (leading to diarrheal diseases, including cholera); the sheer number of people in close proximity encourages the spread of skin diseases and meningitis; and the custom for female friends and relatives to stay overnight and sleep at the home of the deceased provides an opportunity for them to meet lovers under cover of night while they are away from their husbands, thus spreading HIV and other sexually transmitted infections. The bylaws paint a picture of funeral crowds as irrational masses of unhygienic bodies.

Crowds have also been said to be heedless of authority. People in Kyela have long been construed as "noncompliant." Indeed, when I first arrived in Mbeya (the regional capital), several people took it upon themselves to dissuade me from doing my fieldwork in Kyela at all. According to them, the Nyakyusa in Kyela were uncooperative, did "not want development," and were drunken, promiscuous, and belligerent, and in addition the land is hot, muddy, and malarious. My advisors suggested I would be much better off studying the Nyakyusa in the cooler hills of Rungwe, where people are said to be better educated, live in brick houses, and are good Christians. This also happens to be the home of the DMO who initiated the bylaws in Kyela.

Ever since "outsiders" have begun to attempt to govern the part of the world where the Nyakyusa live, there has been a tension between government and what government officials see as their noncompliant subjects. So, for example, there was a battle between the Nyakyusa living near Lake Nyasa and the German colonial governments, because the Nyakyusa were angry at their ill treatment. The Germans won, and afterward, in 1898, the Moravian missionary Theodor Myer remarked, as if the Nyakyusa were being somehow unreasonable, that "they will brook no authority. If anything crosses them, they throw submission to the winds. They obey only so long as they can gain anything by it. They want to be free; alas! too free."[32] Likewise, Monica Wilson noted that the value the Nyakyusa placed on the "truculence" of young men was problematic to the colonial authorities.[33]

Today, this reputation remains. Development projects report difficulties inducing local people to "participate," especially when participation is a euphemism for cash contributions. Rumor has it that four district commissioners have been forced to leave their posts since Kyela became a district in the 1970s. The most recent example was a district commissioner who was accused of seducing young women at a time when HIV was a major health problem. It was suggested to me that the old *mafumu*, the headmen who once advised and disciplined the chiefs, might have communicated to the troublesome district commissioners that their presence was no longer welcome. Such advice contains the threat of witchcraft—coincidentally, the imbepo sya bandu that is targeted by the bylaws.

These examples illustrate that Nyakyusa have often been considered by those in authority to be unreasonable, unruly, and even dangerous. Mark Leopold has shown how myths characterizing particular ethnic groups as warlike and belligerent are developed as a consequence of external preconceptions. There are advantages and disadvantages to such myths, but they can be used to justify particular modes of (dis)engagement by governments.[34] So long as the Nyakyusa (in Kyela) are viewed as backward, as uncooperative, or as not wanting development, any failure on their part to take notice of authority is rarely viewed as the critical judgment of a public but instead is perceived as reactionary.

Populations

Populations are the concern of and the product of government. Foucault observed that the work of a modern government centers on "the welfare of the population, the improvement of its condition, the increase of its wealth, longevity, health and so on."[35] Populations are created through efforts to manage life and, as such, are construed primarily as bodies. According to Ernesto Laclau, publics—in contrast to populations—are seen as "a dissemination of physically separated individuals *whose cohesion is entirely mental.*"[36] Publics have reason and are bound together by their minds, whereas populations are ideally composed of masses of ordered bodies. In public health, the concept of populations is important for any health intervention—bodies must be hygienic, healthy, productive, and docile. If public health officials are at all interested in minds, it is mainly to induce compliancy or biddability in the interest of welfare. These bodies have no political life; they are units—they are homogenous.[37] A population, unlike a public, does not disagree or debate, whereas a public (or a crowd) *can be* subversive and political.

A requirement of governments and public health is that populations must be legible. However, the population of Kyela shares some characteristics of what James Scott describes as a "non-state region"—it is, to an outsider, illegible.[38] Village settlements are invisible from the road, where public health officials travel, and once you leave the road for the densely inhabited villages, you must be accompanied by a local to find your way around. Similarly, individuals are not easily legible: most people do not have birth certificates or fixed surnames, only going to apply for the former and receive the latter when they are needed for some kind of official purpose.

This illegibility often leads to an authoritarian response from public health services, exemplified by Operation Safi (Operation "Clean"), an annual event in which public health inspectors tour the villages. These officials move from house to house to check up on various requirements of environmental hygiene; plots near houses must be kept free of weeds (to reduce the number of mosquitoes, although banana trees, cocoa trees, and other crop trees that serve equally as mosquito resting places are not seen as a problem); latrines must be adequately built; and household water must be boiled. Most people boil water to fill a bottle in advance especially for this purpose and do not boil the rest of the household drinking water, a strategy that the inspectors are perfectly aware of but ignore. Those who do not meet the required standards are fined. Although the inspection is purportedly to ensure adequate standards of hygiene in the village, local people see it simply as a money-making exercise to line the inspectors' pockets. The exercise also serves to naturalize the authority of the state, which encompasses and surveys the locality of the village.[39]

This authoritarian approach is carried through in the bylaws, which aim to direct the flow of the population through the funeral space: people must not gather for more than three days, only relatives and other genuinely "concerned" individuals can sleep or eat there, and the space must be kept clean and orderly. A hygienic and economic rationality is instilled—mourners must take care of their bodies and must not neglect themselves in the work of grief, and expenses and consumption should be kept at a modest level, so that economic resources are not diverted excessively from an individual's economic "development" and bodily welfare. Embodied in the figure of the village chairperson, the bylaws are a reminder that even this intimately "local" space is governed by the rational figure of the developmentalist state.

In sum, from the point of view of public health authorities, funeral crowds in Kyela are irrational, unruly, illiterate, unhygienic, and unreasonable. Public health officials, with the backing of the state, must act to create an orderly population, that is, legible, rational, productive, and healthy. The bylaws—as a public health intervention—construct the people of Kyela as "traditional," which allows the force of law to compel them to change their ways. This perspective does not see a public, or at least not a public with whom authorities can engage in a critical conversation. Public health in Tanzania requires a rational, legible population that will pay attention to authority, even engage in conversation with it, but ultimately acquiesce to its recommendations. However, this objective is complicated by the existence of an indigenous form of public health, to which I now turn.

The Public Control of Public Health
Indigenous Forms of Public Health

Murray Last has observed that "public health is not the invention of biomedicine; it is the primary outlook of most local medical systems. The community's health, 'the body politic,' is the central concern, with the immediate illness of an individual being taken *as a symptom of trouble in the community's well-being.*"[40] In East Africa, an indigenous public health that can be dated back to the precolonial period includes activities such as "rainmaking, identification of sorcerers, and control of infectious diseases, as well as public sanitation works and health education."[41] An understanding of the political nature of these indigenous public health activities as they have played out in Nyakyusa history sheds light on the significance of the most recent public health intervention—the bylaws against "misleading traditions."

Indigenous public health is as political as "official" public health, but as Steven Feierman has argued, scholars have often failed to recognize this fact. Feierman's important work has drawn attention to the role of public healers in precolonial and colonial Tanzania in addressing epidemics, fertility, famine, and the dependency of political leaders on "public healers." The work of public healers and prophets was carried out on behalf of a "political collectivity" to protect against misfortune. Their efforts could be either harnessed by political leaders to legitimize their authority or used against them by underlining the failure of a leader to safeguard the public health.[42]

This relationship between indigenous public health and political authority existed for the Nyakyusa. *Abanyafyale* (sing. *umwalafyale*, designated "chiefs" during the colonial period) were figureheads who depended on their advisors, *amafumu* (sing. *ifumu*, designated "headmen" during the colonial period), to keep the allegiance of the *abakiisu* ("people" of the country), who would not be shy of either removing or shifting allegiances from any inadequate umwalafyale. Political authority was highly contingent and depended on medicines and public health for its success. The very body of the umwalafyale depended on the medicine *ifingila* "to make the chief fearful 'so that the men obey him'"[43] and was necessary to keep the land and people healthy and fertile. The nails and hair of the umwalafyale symbolized fertility and growth and were kept to make medicines, and when he approached death, the amafumu were said to suffocate him so that he died with his breath in his body and, by extension, in the land.[44]

Anthropologist James Ellison has documented the public health measures taken by the abanyafyale at times of disease and famine. In reaction to the influenza pandemic and the subsequent famine of 1917–18, they suspended funerals and feasting to reduce contagion. They worked with healers to spread medicines containing their hair and nails on the land, and they supplied rainmakers with cattle to sacrifice in the "sacred groves" to restore health and fertility to the land.[45] However, by the 1930s, the abanyafyale would no longer sacrifice cattle to avert the famine that had been brought by swarms of red locusts.[46]

What led to this change? First, the abanyafyale's allegiance had switched to the colonial rulers, who paid them a salary and guaranteed their authority. They no longer needed to keep their followers to maintain their position. Second, the colonial government had become very nervous about public healing following the *maji maji* rebellion against the Germans, and the government cracked down on sacrifice. This was so sensitive that Monica Wilson wrote of her book *Communal Rituals* that it dealt with rituals that "provide the sort of background from which Mau Mau and the Basutoland ritual murders have sprung," but she went on, "I *do not wish this last point publicized*. It would cause acute embarrassment to the Government of Tanganyika as well as to me personally if it were."[47] The abanyafyale had been respected partly because of the work they did for the public health of the country. Once they could and would no longer do so, they lost the support of many local people, who still recalled their indifference to famine with anger in the 1990s.[48]

This also had implications for healers and other ritual specialists. Concerning themselves with public health became politically risky: colonial authorities used the antiwitchcraft ordinances to punish healers who exercised "sovereign power by deciding on life or death issues, or on questions of public order."[49] Healers could work only with the health of private individuals and families. The message is clear: nonstate actors in the realm of public health are potentially subversive.

The Government Are the People!

The other major indigenous public health activity is the control of witchcraft. In the past, this was the responsibility of the amafumu, who would watch over their village for witches at night. Their ability to do this served to both protect and discipline people, including the abanyafyale, who were said to be especially vulnerable to witchcraft, because they had no powers in this arena. One kind of witchcraft, known as imbepo sya bandu—the words of the people—is important to us here.

Imbepo sya bandu are the angry words of the community that target a miscreant and can make that person, or his or her relative, seriously sick or even die. Imbepo can be seen as an expression of public disapproval, and the magical power of their words (or "murmuring," as Monica Wilson puts it) gains momentum from the collective.[50] Imbepo and their invocation by ordinary people and amafumu to control and discipline play a complex role in indigenous public health. They can be used, and publicly sanctioned, to prevent and control antisocial forms of behavior. They underline the contingency of the umwalafyale's power and authority—if he overstepped the line, then he could be killed and replaced.[51] They manage matters of public concern and are in the hands of ordinary people. However, they could also be abused or get out of hand, and the amafumu were responsible for watching out for imbepo at night and taking steps against their misuse.

At independence, the new government abolished the system of chiefs and their assistants, because they considered these authorities to have been too close to the colonial system. This has left a vacuum, in which there is no authority to take responsibility for the control of imbepo sya bandu. One man from a family of amafumu told me that he would be afraid to take on the work of defending the community from witchcraft, because the government does not recognize his position. This was a matter of great concern for him, because the number of people dying indicated that there was some kind of crisis. One possible explanation for this was that imbepo sya bandu had sprung out of control. With no authority to oversee them, imbepo were being used to serve the greed of witches who wished to fill their stomachs at funerals and other feasts.

We can recall that one of the concerns of indigenous health is "symptoms of trouble in the community's well being."[52] Central to this in Kyela are many of the "misleading traditions" legislated against by the new bylaws. Public attendance at funerals, gift exchanges, and feasts related to birth, marriage, conflict, bereavement, and inheritance generally acts to maintain good relations between relatives, in-laws, friends, and neighbors. If this public "work" is neglected, then social ties can be broken off.[53] Failure to contribute to these events is sanctioned by imbepo sya bandu and the consequent sickness or even death. It was a widely held opinion that these sanctions had gone too far. On the one hand, imbepo were being used to enforce community well-being and could be seen as falling within the realm of indigenous public health, ensuring that standards of sociality and reciprocity would not slip. On the other hand, many felt very strongly that imbepo were sometimes being implemented so that the "murmurers" could earn the customary feast provided to placate and reverse ill feeling. These people felt that measures should be put in place to prevent imbepo but that the amafumu were powerless to do anything about it. The community was divided on the matter.

These misleading traditions are the "matters of concern" that are debated in Kyela. This is no new debate; the Wilsons' field notes from the 1930s reveal great uncertainty about the morality of funeral and other customs. At the time of the Wilsons' research, people were discussing and arguing over what kind of music and dancing there should be at funerals, how much wailing and crying was acceptable, how long the funeral should last, what (if anything) should be buried with the deceased, who should be fed at the gathering and with what, and how many cattle should be slaughtered. These debates had been stimulated by education and new Christian morals introduced by missionary teaching. Today, there are people who wish to shed traditions that they see as destructive.[54] Some have tried to take refuge in the Moravian and Lutheran churches as a way of removing themselves from traditional obligations,[55] but this has proven insufficient to protect them from imbepo sya bandu. Pentecostal churches now attract new members who wish to shelter from tradition.

The bylaws concerning these widely debated traditions have been widely seen as contributing to the reduction of imbepo sya bandu.

Quite simply, most of the "misleading traditions" listed in the bylaws are those that are sanctioned by imbepo sya bandu if they are not observed. Legislating against them removes the obligation to observe them (in theory), which by extension removes the sanction of imbepo exercised against those who do not observe custom, and thus (theoretically) will reduce the incidence of sickness and death associated with imbepo sya bandu. However, the bylaws attempt to make this a "matter of fact," through the prism of public health and hygiene, that the traditions are "misleading." Any debate for or against is closed.

This stance is not shared by everyone. There are those, such as Mzee Johnson, for whom this kind of indigenous public health was so important that he felt it would override any authority of the government to legislate against it. Crucially for him, it had the weight of "the people" behind it. He told me, "The government cannot stop the traditions; only the Nyakyusa people can decide to stop them. Nobody can forbid another person from following the customs, because they must carry them out themselves. The leaders cannot forbid people and say, 'Now stop bringing gifts of food to funerals,' because the people will tell him, 'If you forbid us, you will die.' So the leader must be afraid. We are afraid of the people more than the government, because, as they say, 'The government is the people' ['Serikali ni watu']." When Mzee Johnson says that someone will die if they do not "follow the customs," he is referring to imbepo sya bandu, and it is through this magical form of sanction that the "people's" authority is exercised. His phrase "the government is the people" appropriates the language of the developmentalist state, which uses the same language to imply that the will of the government and of the "people" are one and the same.[56] Nonstate actors have once again entered the realm of public health, and the bylaws are intended to displace them.

What Kind of Public Is There in Kyela?

With few exceptions, all of the "misleading traditions" referred to in the bylaws can be sanctioned by imbepo sya bandu if they are not fulfilled. This suggests two things. The first is that imbepo sya bandu pose a serious threat to public health in the form of illness caused by witchcraft. The bylaws are thus an ingenious intervention against witchcraft in a context in which officially witchcraft does not exist. The second is that there is a tension between two realms of public health—official (biomedical) public health and an indigenous, popularized form of public health, and the bylaws are an attempt to appropriate the authority of the latter. In a double move, however, the bylaws have been appropriated by the "public" of both indigenous and state forms of public health.

Funerals have provided a space in which a public assembly has been provoked. This assembly is "concerned" with the morality of sociability and its "double edge," a debate that has been going on at least since the Wilsons worked in the region. In this ongoing debate, matters remain open and unresolved. There is therefore a public in Kyela, who engage in rational-critical debate about themselves, but they cannot bring this to bear directly on the field in which public (or state) authority operates, because neither public health services nor state officials are able to participate fully in a debate about imbepo sya bandu. For the government and its representatives, imbepo sya bandu cannot exist. Instead it must focus on the space of funerals as unhygienic and unruly and as a suitable arena in which to intervene and "make" an orderly population of productive and healthy bodies.

The function of the bylaws appears to take the ambiguity out of these "matters of concern" and transform them into "matters of fact." Whether this certainty about what "traditions" are or should be will lead to a reduction in the transmission of infectious disease seems to me, at least, to be unlikely. I suggest that it will not succeed in closing down debate about how life should be lived in Kyela, either.

Notes

1. Melissa Parker and Ian Harper, "The Anthropology of Public Health," *Journal of Biosocial Science* 38, no. 1 (2006): 1–5.

2. Jürgen Habermas, *The Structural Transformation of the Public Sphere: An Inquiry into a Category of Bourgeois Society*, trans. Thomas Burger (Cambridge, MA: MIT Press, 1989).

3. This is a familiar form of statecraft in Tanzania; see, e.g., Kelly Askew, *Performing the Nation: Swahili Music and Cultural Politics* (Chicago: University of Chicago Press, 2002); Leander Schneider, "Colonial Legacies and Postcolonial Authoritarianism: Connects and Disconnects," *African Studies Review* 49, no. 1 (2006): 93–118.

4. Deborah Durham, "Love and Jealousy in the Space of Death," *Ethnos* 67, no. 2 (2002): 155–80; Deborah Durham and Frederick Klaits, "Funerals and the Public Space of Sentiment in Botswana," *Journal of Southern African Studies* 28, no. 4 (2002): 777–96.

5. Eric Gable, "The Funeral and Modernity in Manjaco," *Cultural Anthropology* 21, no. 3 (2006): 385–415; Peter Geschiere, *The Perils of Belonging: Autochthony, Citizenship and Exclusion in Africa and Europe* (Chicago: University of Chicago Press, 2009), 190–211.

6. Stefano Boni, "'Brothers 30,000, Sisters 20,000; Nephews 15,000, Nieces 10,000': Akan Funeral Ledgers, Kinship and Value Negotiations, and Their Limits," *Ethnography* 11, no. 3 (2010): 381–408, esp. 385; Marleen de Witte, "Money and Death: Funeral Business in Asante, Ghana," *Africa* 73, no. 4 (2003): 531–59, esp. 552.

7. Durham, "Love and Jealousy," 156.

8. Boni, "Brothers 30,000"; de Witte, "Money and Death."

9. Monica Wilson, *Rituals of Kinship among the Nyakyusa* (Oxford: Oxford University Press, 1957); Wilson, *Communal Rituals of the Nyakyusa* (Oxford: Oxford University Press, 1959).

10. Monica and Godfrey Wilson Papers (BC880), University of Cape Town, South Africa (hereafter cited as Wilson Papers).

11. National Malaria Control Programme, *Plan of Action for Accelerated Implementation of Malaria Control in Tanzania* (Dar es Salaam: Ministry of Health, United Republic of Tanzania / World Health Organization, 1999), 13.

12. Rebecca Marsland, "The Modern Traditional Healer: Locating 'Hybridity' in Modern Traditional Medicine, Southern Tanzania," *Journal of Southern African Studies* 33, no. 4 (2007): 751–65.

13. Wilson Papers, folder marked "Nyakyusa Research: Death Ritual."

14. Peter Geschiere, *The Modernity of Witchcraft, Politics and the Occult in Postcolonial Africa* (Charlottesville: University of Virginia Press, 1997); Jean Comaroff and John L. Comaroff, "Occult Economies and the Violence of Abstraction: Notes from the South African Postcolony," *American Ethnologist* 26, no. 2 (1999): 279–303.

15. Harry G. West, *Ethnographic Sorcery* (Chicago: University of Chicago Press, 2007), 37.

16. These debates about the morality of "tradition" are discussed at length in my forthcoming book, *The Words of the People*. For a discussion of witchcraft as a critical discourse about "tradition," see Todd Sanders, "Reconsidering Witchcraft: Postcolonial Africa and Analytic (Un)certainties," *American Anthropologist* 105, no. 2 (2003): 338–52.

17. Stacey A. Langwick gives an excellent history of the antiwitchcraft ordinances in Tanzania, which necessarily denied the existence of witchcraft and thus were inadequate to control it; see Langwick, *Bodies, Politics and African Healing: The Matter of Maladies in Tanzania* (Bloomington: Indiana University Press, 2011), chap. 2.

18. Charles L. Briggs and Clara Mantini-Briggs, *Stories in the Time of Cholera: Racial Profiling during a Medical Nightmare* (Berkeley: University of California Press, 2003).

19. Andrew Burton and Michael Jennings, "The Emperor's New Clothes? Continuities in Governance in Late Colonial and Early Postcolonial East Africa," *International Journal of African Historical Studies* 40, no. 1 (2007): 1–25; Michael Jennings, "'A Very Real War': Popular Participation in Development in Tanzania during the 1950s and 1960s," *International Journal of African Historical Studies* 40, no. 1 (2007): 71–95; Rebecca Marsland, "Community Participation the Tanzanian Way: Conceptual Contiguity or Power Struggle?" *Oxford Development Studies* 34, no. 1 (2006): 65–79; Schneider, "Colonial Legacies."

20. Habermas, *Structural Transformation*, 27, 43, 83–85.

21. Michelle Zimbalist Rosaldo, "Woman, Culture and Society: A Theoretical Overview," in *Woman, Culture and Society*, ed. Michelle Zimbalist Rosaldo, Louise Lamphere, and Joan Bamberger, 17–42 (Stanford: Stanford University Press, 1974).

22. Hannah Arendt, *The Human Condition* (Chicago: University of Chicago Press, 1998), 45.

23. Michel Foucault, *The History of Sexuality*, trans. Robert Hurley, vol. 1, *An Introduction* (1978; repr., London: Penguin, 1990), and vol. 3, *The Care of the Self* (1986; repr., London: Penguin, 1990).

24. Steven Feierman, "Struggles for Control: The Social Roots of Health and Healing in Modern Africa," *African Studies Review* 28, no. 2/3 (1985): 73–147; John Janzen, *The Quest for Therapy: Medical Pluralism in Lower Zaire* (Berkeley: University of California

Press, 1978); Julie Livingston, *Debility and the Moral Imagination in Botswana* (Bloomington: Indiana University Press, 2005).

25. Bruno Latour, "From Realpolitik to Dingpolitik or How to Make Things Public," in *Making Things Public: Atmospheres of Democracy*, ed. Bruno Latour and Peter Weibel, 14–41 (Cambridge, MA: MIT Press, 2005).

26. Noortje Marres, "Issues Spark a Public into Being," in *Making Things Public: Atmospheres of Democracy*, ed. Bruno Latour and Peter Weibel (Cambridge, MA: MIT Press, 2005), 216.

27. Michael Warner, *Publics and Counterpublics* (New York: Zone Books, 2002), 9–10.

28. Karin Barber, *The Anthropology of Texts: Persons and Publics, Oral and Written Culture* (Cambridge: Cambridge University Press, 2007), 143.

29. Durham and Klaits, "Funerals and the Public," 778.

30. Ernesto Laclau, *On Populist Reason* (London: Verso, 2005), 47.

31. George Rudé, *The Crowd in History* (London: Serif, 2005).

32. Myer quoted in Marcia Wright, *German Missions in Tanganyika, 1891–1941: Lutherans and Moravians in the Southern Highlands* (Oxford: Clarendon Press, 1971), 62.

33. Monica Wilson, *Good Company: A Study of Nyakyusa Age Villages* (London: Oxford University Press, 1951), 80.

34. Mark Leopold, *Inside West Nile: Violence, History and Representation on an African Frontier* (Oxford: James Currey, 2005).

35. Michel Foucault, "Governmentality," in *The Essential Works of Foucault, 1954–1984*, vol. 3, *Power*, ed. James D. Faubion (New York: New Press, 2000), 216–17.

36. Laclau, *On Populist Reason*, 44. Italics added for emphasis.

37. Peter Redfield, "Doctors, Borders and Life in Crisis," *Cultural Anthropology* 20, no. 3 (2005): 328–61.

38. James Scott, *Seeing Like a State: How Certain Schemes to Improve the Human Condition Have Failed* (New Haven, CT: Yale University Press, 1998).

39. James Ferguson and Akhil Gupta, "Spatializing States: Toward an Ethnography of Neoliberal Governmentality," *American Ethnologist* 29, no. 4 (2002): 981–1002.

40. Murray Last, "Understanding Health," in *Culture and Global Change*, ed. Tim Allen and Tracey Skelton (London: Routledge, 1999), 75. Italics added for emphasis.

41. Gloria Waite, "Public Health in Precolonial East-Central Africa," in *The Social Basis of Health and Healing in Africa*, ed. Steven Feierman and John M. Janzen (Berkeley: University of California Press, 1992), 213.

42. Feierman, "Struggles for Control," 116; Steven Feierman, "Colonizers, Scholars, and the Creation of Invisible Histories," in *Beyond the Cultural Turn: New Directions in the Study of Society and Culture*, ed. Victoria E. Bonnell and Lyn Hunt, 182–216 (Berkeley: University of California Press, 1999); Steven Feierman, "Healing as Social Criticism in the Time of Colonial Conquest," *African Studies* 54, no. 1 (2010): 73–88; Langwick, *Bodies, Politics and African Healing*, 41–42.

43. Wilson, *Communal Rituals*, 57.

44. For similar practices among the Bemba, see Meghan Vaughan, "'Divine Kings': Sex, Death and Anthropology in Inter-war East/Central Africa," *Journal of African History* 49 (2008): 383–401, esp. 386.

45. James G. Ellison, "Transforming Obligations, Performing Identity: Making the Nyakyusa in a Colonial Context," unpublished PhD thesis, University of Florida, 1999, 105–31.

46. Ibid., 198–209.

47. Wilson Papers, Uncatalogued box no. 1, letter from Monica Wilson to Chairman of Editorial Board, University of Cape Town, 19 September 1957. See also Vaughan, "Divine Kings."

48. Ellison, "Transforming Obligations," chaps. 2–3.

49. Feierman, "Struggles for Control," 118; see also Langwick, *Bodies, Politics and African Healing*, chap. 2.

50. Wilson, *Good Company*, 91–108.

51. Godfrey Wilson's field notes contain numerous examples of chiefs who had been displaced by amafumu because they did not provide food for their people. Likewise, the missionaries Merensky and Schumann wrote that the chiefs were very much at the mercy of their headmen: Simon Charsley, *The Princes of Nyakyusa* (Nairobi: East African Publishing House, 1969), 69.

52. Last, "Understanding Health," 75.

53. Similar processes have been reported in Botswana: see Durham and Klaits, "Funerals and the Public."

54. Local critiques of tradition are also reported in Gable, "Funeral and Modernity," 406, and James H. Smith, *Bewitching Development: Witchcraft and the Reinvention of Development in Neoliberal Kenya* (Chicago: University of Chicago Press, 2008).

55. In Kenya, Luo widows avoid inheritance customs by finding alternatives within the church: Ruth J. Prince, "Public Debates about Luo Widow Inheritance," in *Christianity and Public Culture in Africa*, ed. Harri Englund, 109–30 (Athens: Ohio University Press, 2011).

56. Schneider, "Colonial Legacies," 112.

THREE

The Qualities of Citizenship

Private Pharmacists and the State in Senegal after
Independence and Alternance

NOÉMI TOUSIGNANT

IN MAY 2008, ORGANIZATIONS OF SENEGALESE PRIVATE PHARMACISTS called a general strike. Rising pharmacy thefts put their lives and livelihoods at risk. In press releases, media interviews, and requests for audiences surrounding the strike, pharmacy leaders addressed their claims directly to public authorities.[1] Pharmacists connected pharmacy thefts to an undisciplined illicit market fuelled by stolen, contraband, and diverted medicines. Emphasizing the linked menace to profitable business, ethical professionalism, and the public's health, they reminded the government of its responsibilities while equating legitimate trade with quality control. In their demands for public protection and collaboration, private pharmacists have reasserted their work to be a concern of the state and guided by a commitment to the public good. As Aboubakrine Sarr, president of the Syndicate of Private Pharmacists, explained in a press release announcing the strike, pharmacists "are the guarantors of the quality of medicines; it is a heavy responsibility and a citizen's duty to be the legal custodians of pharmaceuticals."[2]

As I followed newspaper coverage of pharmacists' recent activism, I was reading documents from the late 1960s and 1970s that outlined the Senegalese government's plans for the pharmaceutical sector. I was struck by similarities between the use of citizenship by private pharmacists in the late 2000s—as an assertion of the public value of their expertise and a call for the state's reinvestment in its protection—and earlier justifications for spending public resources on pharmaceutical production and distribution in the 1970s. In that earlier decade, a development-oriented government had enlisted pharmacists, both public and private, in a shared project for making medicines generative of economic growth. Given the subsequent disinvestment of the Senegalese state from public health and security, it seemed surprising, in the late 2000s, that pharmacists would evoke a sense of citizenship so closely connected with government responsibility.[3] The privatization and globalization of previously national, public services in the past decades have been associated with the emergence of new forms of citizenship; responsibilities, entitlements, and allegiances are increasingly articulated as personal, communal, or transnational rather than national.[4] Why, then, are Senegalese pharmacists still, or once again, turning to the state to secure their futures as responsible citizens and "guarantors of quality"?

This chapter first explores this question through historical analysis: How have pharmacists' livelihoods, professionalism, and entrepreneurial qualities been intertwined with state futures and projects in the past? I suggest that pharmacists' recently expressed ethos of citizenship be located as part of a longer history of dense, if changing, traffic of people, values, and resources between public and private pharmaceutical sectors in Senegal. I focus on two moments of particular intensity in this traffic. The first, which I call "citizenship of the plan," refers to the enlistment of private pharmacists to fulfill the objectives of centrally planned economic development in the mid-1970s. Then, following a period of crisis in public pharmaceutical supply that also fuelled the expansion (for some, the overcrowding) of private markets, private pharmacists were once again connected to government goals and capacities in the name of the public good in the mid-1990s. This articulation of the value of pharmacists' managerial and entrepreneurial qualities as part of neoliberal solutions to the public health-care crisis in addition to their professional crisis is what I call "citizenship of crisis."

Following A. Sarr's location of pharmacists' sense of civic duty in "quality work" (the work pharmacists do to guarantee that medicines conform to standards of quality), I link this recent activism to the notion of "citizenship of quality." Pharmacists' recent demands intertwine with discourses on drug quality and have implications for relations between pharmacists, the state, and the "public" of public health. As an emergent global health issue, poor-quality medicines are often presented as the outcome of histories of weak public health-care and regulatory systems. What accusations against the state do Senegalese pharmacists articulate around the problem of drug quality? What kinds of solutions and futures does quality work entail? How might quality work lead to new arrangements between government regulation, business values, professionalism, and the public good?

My primary sources were produced by those most vocal in making claims for pharmacists' civic roles and qualities. These sources are not simply informative; they are also sites in which envisioned relations between pharmacists, publics, and the state are imagined and performed. Most recently, leaders of professional organizations (the Order of Pharmacists and the Syndicate of Private Pharmacists of Senegal) have actively sought media coverage of their activities and opinions. Especially since 2005–6, they have frequently released press statements to advertise protests, strikes, and conferences; have written open letters to public authorities; have spoken with journalists; and have resolved to systematically alert the press in the case of seizures of illegal medicines "to avoid that these affairs be buried under pressure and other agreements."[5] In this newspaper-mediated activism, pharmacists publicly imagine their collective futures with the state, simultaneously addressing demands to the state and presenting themselves as a collective whose concerns are relevant to the public. In addition to several interviews with pharmacists, I also followed discussions about quality and Senegalese pharmacists' public responsibility within an online forum on essential medicines, E-med.[6]

Other voices dominate older sources, revealing past perspectives on why and how private pharmaceutical activities should be of public concern. In the 1970s, the government of Senegal produced or sponsored reports that justified public investment in private pharmaceutical distribution and production.[7] In the 1990s, studies were sponsored by the World Health Organization (WHO) and the U.S. Agency for International Development (USAID) to evaluate the actual and potential role of private pharmacists in meeting public health goals; such reports describe but also informed the neoliberal reform of health care during this period.[8]

These sources provide new information on how structural adjustment and privatization have affected the experiences of African health professionals. Previous studies show that public-sector professionals have suffered from loss of status and motivation as government health facilities have deteriorated; they also document the "privatization" of these professionals' activities.[9] Changes have also been observed in experiences of work, ethics, social relations, and temporality.[10] These analyses point to the usefulness of situating the past three decades in contrast—but also in connection—to a more finely analyzed "developmentalist" era of state health planning in the postwar and postindependence decades. Transformations in the state thus seem to be experienced not only as shrinking budgets and deteriorating conditions but also as diminished expectations of the state as a frame for action, ethical engagement, and directionality through the imagination (and planning) of collective futures. By emphasizing quality work, might Senegalese private pharmacists be trying to revive this sense of shared future and projects with the state? If so, what kind of future do they envision?

Citizens of the Plan: Pharmacists and Development in the 1970s

Now retired, Doudou Ba remembers the early 1970s as a time when there was space in the state for Senegalese pharmacists. He describes himself as one of four pioneers who, upon returning from advanced studies in France, were hired by the Faculty of Pharmacy of the state university Cheikh Anta Diop and have since occupied high-level positions in the Ministry of Health.[11] Two had tried and failed to open private pharmacies but were reintegrated in the public system "because," Ba explains, "we couldn't lose people that Senegal had paid to educate."[12] By the end of the decade, Mounirou Ciss could still escape the impossible dilemma he associated with private practice—the need to choose between demanding family members (and suffer bankruptcy) and wealth (only to be rich alone)—by using his academic skills to obtain a university post and public service positions.[13] Ndeye Diénaba Fall, first president of the Order of Pharmacists in 1976, had worked in the public supply pharmacy before opening her own shop, "unlike," as she says, "the new wave of pharmacists."[14]

The first generation of Senegalese pharmacists could choose and move between the public and private sectors because there were few of them. The report of a 1969 survey of the Senegalese pharmaceutical sector identifies the scarcity of experts as the most pressing policy issue, and the majority of pharmacists in the country were not of Senegalese nationality.[15] The state was also expanding, creating civil service jobs as well as subsidizing and partially nationalizing private business.[16] By the end of the first postindependence decade, the government's initial strategy of investing in peanut cultivation and rural political support from religious leaders was being threatened by drought, falling peanut prices, and student protests. Thus, in the 1970s, new economic policies focused on the diversification, industrialization, and Senegalization of the economy, while seeking political support and technical expertise of the growing local university-educated elites.[17] Pharmaceuticals were made part of this new policy of economic planning that reached deeper into the private sector. Senegalese pharmacists and populations were redefined—by virtue of their capacity to produce, distribute, and consume pharmaceuticals—as citizens participating in national development.

Sub-Saharan markets for pharmaceuticals were also expanding rapidly. Yet rising drug importations continued to benefit the European pharmaceutical industry after colonial independence. French companies in particular sold a growing proportion of their products to ex-French African colonies.[18] Within Senegal, pharmacies and drug depots were mainly French and Lebanese owned. The network of urban French-owned private pharmacies and rural depots run by French trading companies and a few Lebanese merchants in peanut-trading centers grew rapidly beginning in the 1930s and accelerated in the 1940s and 1950s, creating a private drug market that was more extensive than in other colonies. It had functioned fairly autonomously from the colonial government.[19] Before the 1950s, only certain categories of pharmaceuticals, those distributed as part of mass campaigns against endemic diseases (malaria, sleeping sickness, leprosy, and syphilis/yaws), had been defined as relevant to public health and government planning.[20]

The convergence of an expanding market for medicines with the political goals of the 1970s tied together (in theory) the therapeutic and economic properties of pharmaceuticals, making them particularly valuable for national development. Harnessing this market meant overcoming the weak investment and purchasing power of Senegalese citizens. Two projects in the 1970s sought to address these obstacles. The first aimed to stimulate local pharmaceutical production. After commissioning several feasibility studies, the government of Senegal signed an agreement with a European pharmaceutical firm to create the SIPOA, a mixed public-private production facility, in 1973.[21] This was one of seventy parastatal enterprises created between 1970 and 1975 as part of the strategy of industrialization and Senegalization.[22] Pharmacy ownership was also Senegalized through a program of low-interest loans

provided by the treasury to Senegalese pharmacists to set up private re-
tail and bulk distribution pharmacies; three years after this program was
launched, 80 percent of private pharmacies were Senegalese-owned.[23]
The state thus sought to draw the profitable actions of producing and
selling pharmaceuticals into national development and promised to
make it easier to make a living as a Senegalese pharmacist.[24]

What kind of citizens did pharmacists become and serve in this
process? Irving Markovitz describes a shift in conceptions of national
development and citizenship in his study of the political philosophy
of Senegal's first president. Leopold S. Senghor had initially defined
development not simply as economic growth but as a broad social and
cultural process. Such development was nourished by and generative of
a new type of Senegalese "man [sic]": an individual who would acquire
the sense of ethics and will to form a group of "conscientious citizens"
able "to transform their collective situation." But by the mid-1960s, the
perceived need for political and economic stabilization had begun to
draw in the goals of development around economic growth. According to Markovitz, the Senegalese citizen-in-the-making was no longer
theorized by Senghor "in the abstract; instead, he posits as a principal
goal of the [economic and social development] plan the training of men
[sic] capable of promoting economic growth. Now, men count primarily
insofar as they can help fulfill the plan's objectives."[25] Citizenship and
development remained closely tied, but both were redefined in terms of
economic growth. The purpose of the state shifted from providing the
conditions for realizing citizens' full potential as human beings to those
for participating in a planned economy.

This more narrowly defined citizen was described in 1977 by Babacar
Ba, minister of finance and economic affairs, as the target of government
intervention in the pharmaceutical sector. Ba opened and concluded his
speech to the national assembly by stating the goal of pharmaceutical
policies: to render "Senegalese man [sic]" capable of fully and actively
participating in national development.[26] Producing a healthy citizenry
meant state-facilitated access to essential, or "social," pharmaceuticals,
notably, through the regulation of drug prices. But the affordability of
medicines was also presented in government documents as the outcome
of joint efforts by pharmacists and the state.[27] This collaboration was
negotiated. After the government lowered allowable profit margins on
a list of two hundred "social medicines" in 1963, using the French system of price controls that had been extended to West Africa in 1958,

pharmacists lobbied to raise them again.[28] Although profit margins were again reduced in the early 1970s, the state was soon seeking a strategy to minimize the effects of inflation on private profits. Government was willing to make this "sacrifice" on revenues, especially at a time when, Babacar Ba explained in 1977, "the Senegalisation of the sector [was] being undertaken."[29] Legislation was passed to eliminate import duties on pharmaceuticals in 1978.[30] The allocation of public benefits—in the form of investment, tax cuts, and a protected market—to local pharmaceutical firms was also justified in terms of the link between access to medicines and a population fit for the work of development.

Yet the power of pharmaceuticals to make citizens through better health was only one—and not the central—objective of private-sector stimulation. Even then, whether local production and price controls could really improve the accessibility of medicines in the private or public sector was unclear.[31] Also, even in the 1960s and 1970s, public budgets and policies did not prioritize health care, especially not the distribution of pharmaceuticals.[32] The development value of pharmaceuticals was in generating jobs, industrialization, and successful Senegalese professionals, that is, in economic rather than health-care planning. Was the pharmacist's citizenship enjoined in state-protected futures at the expense of the citizenship of the potential consumer of pharmaceuticals? Which public was constituted by pharmaceutical policies justified in the name of public health? Private pharmacists may have benefited the most from pharmaceutical policies, making them its primary public (on health authorities as, by virtue of their benefiting from public health monies, their "own public," see Murray Last's chapter in this volume). But these policies also opened a space for private pharmacists to actively negotiate with the state regarding issues such as drug prices, positioning them as the public that "reflects critically on the work of public health authorities" while relegating potential consumers of pharmaceuticals to the role of a passive target population (for a discussion of the distinction between *public* and *population,* see Rebecca Marsland's chapter in this volume).

By 1979, economic crisis had pushed Senghor to become the first African president to request a loan from the International Monetary Fund (IMF). Soon, the types of spending and regulation that had connected pharmacists to national development were cut by the austerity and adjustment measures implemented by Senghor's successor, Abdou Diouf.[33] Freezes on public-sector hiring created unemployment among pharmacists and weakened the state's ability to regulate pharmaceutical imports and sales; by 1997, there was still only one pharmacist working for the inspection services.[34] The government also disengaged from local pharmaceutical production (the parastatal firm SIPOA was taken over by Rhône Poulenc/Rohrer in 1987).[35] Pharmacists could no longer count on the state for jobs, loans, or even the legal protection of their professional rights. How would this change pharmacists' conception of citizenship?

Citizens of Crisis: Privatization and Devaluation in the 1990s

Aboubakrine Sarr, president of the Syndicate of Private Pharmacists, remembers 1994, when the Communauté financière africaine [African Financial Community] franc was devalued by 50 percent, as a time of renewed collaboration with the state and commitment to the public good. In 2008, Sarr reminded "the Authorities" of how private pharmacists had, in 1994, "voluntarily accepted a reduction of their profit margin by almost 5%," thus performing "a highly memorable gesture of great citizenship . . . the only goal of which was to support the distraught public authorities and relieve the population whose purchasing power had been brutally assaulted."[36]

Sarr's memory of devaluation is one of a shared experience of crisis, out of which could emerge new links between pharmacists and the state. For pharmacists were also, according to some, experiencing a crisis after the steady growth of licit and illicit private pharmaceutical markets. Indeed, A. Sarr's colleague Emmanuel Sarr remembers 1994, when "devaluated" profits and a shrinking market were shared among a rapidly multiplying number of actors, as the intensification of this crisis, ushering a decade of "upheavals" in the profession.[37]

In response to cuts in government spending during the 1980s, more and more Senegalese opened private pharmacies. Although pharmacy education was controlled by the state, student numbers were not restricted on the basis of estimated need as they were in the similar French system.[38] Drug shortages in the public sector and the practice of sending patients from public facilities to fill prescriptions in private pharmacies expanded the private medicines market.[39] Opportunities were seized not only by qualified pharmacists, who could no longer seek public employment, but also by those seeking opportunities in urban informal commerce.

Analyzed by Didier Fassin in the 1980s, this informal sector was dominated by Murid religious leaders and their disciples.[40] The Muriddya, a Sufi order indigenous to Senegal, has a long-standing history of mediation between the population and public authorities. During the colonial period, they helped expand peanut cultivation for export and, with independence, to legitimate the new state for rural populations. During the postindependence decades, Murid leaders continued to recruit votes, especially in rural areas, for the governing Socialist Party.[41] With the decline of the peanut economy, Murid economic networks shifted to urban, often informal commerce, including that of pharmaceuticals.[42] The government's tolerance of this illicit market was, Fassin argues, part of a larger set of interactions with the Muriddya aimed at securing its loyalty to the party, a political strategy that remained important despite the new technocratic rhetoric of Diouf's government (see Murray Last's chapter in this volume).[43] Thus, reduced health-care budgets were combined with the political consequences of adjustment to reshape the social relations of pharmaceutical distribution and create new opportunities for private pharmaceutical activities in the 1980s.

In the early 1990s, the state attempted to address the deterioration of public health care by implementing the Bamako Initiative.[44] The sale of cheaper and generic drugs in public facilities was seen by some pharmacists as an additional source of competition in an already crowded market, according to a USAID-funded survey in 1994.[45] The report of a WHO-sponsored study described private pharmacists as left out of, and unwilling to engage in, debates about pharmaceutical policies including the Bamako Initiative. Both studies, however, describe devaluation in 1994 as the catalyst for renewed interaction between private pharmacists and the state. The threat of a 100 percent increase in the price of pharmaceuticals created a crisis for the public and private sectors, affecting both sales and the ability to restock. The large, well-organized private sector demonstrated its public value by bridging supply gaps and accepting a reduced profit margin, while the state intervened by cutting taxes, negotiating lower prices with suppliers, and accelerating the introduction of generic drugs. Thus, according to the WHO study, "pharmaceutical policies began to concern all actors, including [those] in the private sector,"[46] while the USAID study recommended both loosening private-sector regulations and allowing private pharmacists to distribute public health commodities.[47] Senegalese pharmacists requested the right to buy and sell generic drugs as cheaply as in the public sector, which would require a partial privatization of the national supply pharmacy.[48] Thus, privatization as a response to crisis allowed pharmacists to show how, as responsible citizens, they could engage with pharmaceuticals as public health objects.

The privatization of the pharmaceutical sector in Senegal does not trace a simple trajectory from "all public" to "mostly private," even if the private share of pharmaceutical distribution has grown.[49] In the postindependence decades, Senegal's government had opted to invest in the expansion and "Senegalization" of an already well-established private sector, rather than in the extensive development of public pharmaceutical distribution (in contrast with other African countries). During the 1980s, a new dynamic of privatization took place in the margins and in substitution of deteriorating public health care. Neoliberal solutions to crises in public pharmaceutical supplies and price increases proposed new forms of collaboration between an increasingly privatized government health-care sector and increasingly numerous private pharmacists beginning in the mid-1990s.

Citizenship of Quality:
Poisons, Partnership, and Public Health after Alternance

Since about 2000, the quality of medicines has become a growing focus of critiques of global pharmaceutical distribution in international medical journals.[50] The World Health Organization, U.S. Pharmacopeia, Fondation Chirac, and nongovernmental organizations (NGOs) such as ReMed have launched campaigns against substandard, illicit, counterfeit, and inappropriately donated medicines, especially in developing countries.[51] These medicines are unsafe because of the lack of quality control. "*Les médicaments de la rue, ça tue*" ("Street medicines kill") is the slogan of a campaign against illicit drug trading launched in 2002 by ReMed, while a joint WHO/Interpol operation against fake drugs advertises, "Counterfeit drugs kill."[52] The opposite of quality drugs is poisons.

This turn toward quality has drawn attention to the weakness of national regulatory systems in countries such as Senegal. According to the World Health Organization, "over two thirds of countries, including most low- and middle-income countries[,] lack fully functioning medicine regulatory systems," while authors of surveys on drug quality call for these countries to "improve their ability to detect substandard medicines."[53] A few observers, especially social scientists and especially in Africa, have been bolder in blaming the effects of neoliberal reforms on the state for the aggravation of drug quality problems. Enforced cuts in public spending—on health care, as well as public salaries and equipment for inspectors, scientists, and customs officers—have limited governments' ability both to ensure accessible health care and to regulate pharmaceuticals, while high unemployment and reduced purchasing power have affected populations' ability to demand and purchase medicines in legal, quality-controlled networks.[54] Medicines made deadly by poor quality control might thus be mobilized to critique the excessive privatization and deregulation of health and to argue for a reassertion of state control over pharmaceutical matters.

Senegalese pharmacists repeated ReMed's slogan "Street medicines kill" in local press releases; they carried it in protests, written on posters (produced by ReMed) of a luminous skeleton foregrounded by a young man holding up a plastic bag full of medicine boxes. In Senegal, deadly medicines have carried specific accusations of governmental failure and political neglect. When the nephew of a pharmacist was killed during a robbery in 2009, for example, newspapers once again filled with pharmacists' expressions of outrage at the state's failure to eliminate illicit pharmaceutical trading. Cheikh Oumar Dia, president of the Senegalese Order of Pharmacists, told a journalist from the newspaper *Sud quotidien*, "[I]ndifference, laxity, corruption and lack of will have killed again."[55]

"Again" may refer to the ongoing consequences of a poorly controlled illicit market. The dead nephew was linked to those, unidentified and uncounted, who might have been killed by poor-quality drugs sold by unqualified merchants in open-air markets. A. Sarr has called these "merchants of death, murderers of the national economy." But like Dia, A. Sarr sees this capacity to kill as authorized by the state, which provides unqualified drug sellers with "a free ticket to defy [its] authority."[56]

Indeed, Dia's "again" echoes a common idiom of political criticism that accuses the current regime of murder by corruption and neglect. In a controversial book published in 2004, Almamy Mamadou Wane situates Senegal between the literal shipwreck of the Senegalese ferry the *Joola*, in which at least 1,863 passengers died in 2002, and the figurative shipwreck of Abdoulaye Wade's "Alternance" government, elected in 2000.[57] Another book, this one by Mame Marie Faye, exposes a young woman's suicide as an act of murder by Wade's "criminal" government.[58] Readers of the Senegalese press would likely associate Dia's bold accusation of murder by corruption with this more general sense of disenchantment with the government of Alternance.

If pharmacists' struggle against street medicines and pharmacy thefts utilizes the transnational slogans involving poisonous medicines, its expressions are full of reminders of the specific promises of Alternance. *Alternance,* which can be translated as "changeover," is a reference to the election of Abdoulaye Wade, an opposition leader since the 1970s, to power in 2000 after four decades of Socialist Party rule. Wade's campaign slogan was *Sopi,* or change; it promised a clean break from the Socialist Party's political culture of opacity, clientelism, corruption, and mismanagement. The promise of Alternance was also in the dynamics that led to Wade's election: an increasingly diverse and critical press, the political mobilization of youths and women, and the refusal of voting instructions given by religious leaders, including Murid *marabouts,* by their followers.[59]

The liberalization of the press and the promise—if not the realization—of a new configuration of political and religious power have enabled open discussion of both Murid involvement in the illegal pharmaceutical market and the government's passive complicity. In 2001, the newspaper *Info 7* described how the illicit market was supplied by donations to religious schools and run by Murid leaders; the customs authorities knew about this but were powerless to act.[60] By 2006, even the minister of health could say, "[W]e need to have the courage to engage in the fight against the illicit market, because we have no right to play *la politique politicienne* [literally, "politician politics," meaning factionalism or clientelism] with health; that is[,] with people's lives."[61] Since about 2006, pharmacists' intensified campaign against illegal pharmaceutical trading—and journalists' generally supportive rendering of their claims—has continued to make explicit this link between potentially deadly medicines, clientelist relations between the state and religious leaders, and the impunity of illegal drug traders.

Yet overall, pharmacists' protests have emphasized the state's potential strength rather than its weakness. By evoking the threat of poisonous medicines, they continue to imagine a future they share with the state: a future of professionalism, democracy, legality, and mutual responsibility for pharmaceutical quality. Accusations of inaction are doubled by urgent invitations to restore the functionality of the state in pharmaceutical matters and thereby reconnect pharmacists' future as "guarantors of quality" to the future of the Senegalese state as legal and democratic. Poisonous medicines threaten both these futures, as expressed by Aline Kane, vice president of the Syndicate of Pharmacists, in an impassioned text he posted on the *E-med* forum: "We dream of a pharmacy profession that stands up as one to say 'no' to the illicit pharmaceutical market, 'no' to those who, in the circles of political or [religious] power, think that pharmaceuticals are harmless products." If nothing is done to stop this "trivialisation" of medicines, the Senegalese will "watch the pharmacist become a museum piece" but also, by extension, lose hope in the possibility of democratic and lawful government.[62] But this hope is still alive, asserts Dia: "[T]he State *can* close down Keur Serigne-Bi if it wants."[63] Keur Serigne-Bi was a large, well-known (and identifiably Murid) site of illegal drug trade in the commercial center of Dakar, which the state needed to act upon because "the medicines of the street are poisons[;] . . . it is the responsibility of the state to do everything possible so that populations have access to good quality medicines."[64] The closure of the market a few months later was treated by government and the media as a highly political operation, announced and negotiated in the top circles of power, involving the president, prime minister, and khalife general of the Muriddya.[65]

Pharmacists' claims as "guarantors of quality" are not limited to police raids on illicit medicine markets; they have also requested a more active role in public programs of pharmaceutical distribution.[66] This second set of demands clarifies that pharmacists are not simply seeking to restore past legislative agreements with the state or recalling a time when the state was more successful in protecting public health and security; they are also actively negotiating a new type of arrangement. Sarr describes the "pharmacist of the third millennium" as "a new type who works in the private sector, but who is also involved in a partnership with the public in order to get closer to the population, and to whom a secure profession is guaranteed."[67]

In complaining about being shut out from public health initiatives, pharmacists are projecting their future relationships with the state in terms of public-private partnerships. Here, the quality of medicines is not just a responsibility of the state toward its population but also a potentially profitable business value. Recently, an argument broke out in the *E-med* forum between pharmacists and the head of the Senegalese national malaria program following the announcement of an initiative to distribute antimalarial drugs at heavily subsidized prices through community organizations and agents. One Senegalese pharmacist complained, "Public health in Senegal . . . suffers from a confusion with health in the public sector. . . . Medicines are protected by a monopoly that is defeated by the very same agent that is supposed to protect it, that is, the state. In our country, health policies are equated with programs that dispossess the pharmacist of her role in the healthcare system. . . . Pharmacovigilance is . . . a chain . . . in which the pharmacist is the essential link."[68]

Aline Kane asked the head of the malaria program directly, "Is the health-care system limited to the public sector?"[69] Finally, a third colleague proposed, "In Senegal, the private pharmaceutical sector could be in charge of the distribution of almost all the 'medicines' controlled by the public sector at comparable costs and with better availability and a better quality assurance."[70]

In this debate, Senegalese pharmacists are using the notion of quality to blur boundaries between public and private pharmaceutical distribution—its spaces, practices, resources, and responsibilities. These boundaries became more ambiguous with the reforms of the 1990s: first the sale of medicines in public structures, and then the lobbying of pharmacists to purchase and sell generic drugs, medicines previously associated with public health. In the later 2000s, pharmacists sustain this blurring of boundaries to engage with the state in areas of recently improved material capacities such as malaria treatment.

In 2005 and 2008, the Ministry of Health signed agreements with the Global Fund to Fight AIDS, Tuberculosis and Malaria for grants of nearly US$30 million for malaria programs with strong treatment components. In the first two-year program phase, nearly US$15 million was to be spent on purchasing antimalarial drugs (half this amount accounts for roughly 10 percent of Senegal's total health-care budget for the year 2006).[71] The scaling up of malaria treatment and prevention has been showcased as a signature program of the government's health-care policy, alongside the near tripling of the health budget, the expansion of health-care facilities, an increase in public employment (from 70 to 107 pharmacists), and three salary increases since 2000.[72] Increased donor funding merges with demonstrations of national political commitment to health, enabling the state to restore its image (at least in some areas, such as reduced malaria mortality and free antimalarial treatment) as a health-care provider.[73] Health-care professionals are generally aware that high-level ministry staff must continually vie for external funding to uphold this image. Yet for pharmacists, such programs have made the state newly relevant as an interlocutor in addressing their claims for opportunities and security.

Donor funding to the malaria program has also helped tie Senegalese drug distribution to global concerns and mechanisms in matters of drug quality. Agreements signed with the Global Fund include clauses about quality in the procurement and distribution of pharmaceuticals; recipients must either obtain their medicines through UN agencies, which have the obligation to purchase medicines prequalified by the World Health Organization, or reinforce local quality control systems.[74] USAID, through the President's Malaria Initiative (PMI), has funded the U.S. Pharmacopeia to run studies of antimalarial drug quality and to provide technical assistance in the form of minilabs for on-site quality testing (which were only recently extended to the testing of other drugs), as well as supporting training for drug-monitoring and communications campaigns on the dangers of informally traded medicines.[75]

Such flows of money, norms, and terminology have certainly influenced how Senegalese pharmacists can and do work as "guarantors of quality." They now use international standards and guidelines for drug procurement and control procedures, manipulate expensive laboratory equipment, participate in seminars and courses run by foreign experts, discuss in online forums, and pronounce imported slogans and statistics in their fight to improve the quality of medicines distributed in Senegal. Yet both private and public pharmacists' concerns about quality seem to exceed the largely technical and regulatory practices that are targeted by these forms of assistance and exchange. In petitioning the state for better regulation and greater collaboration, pharmacists are also using quality to describe a professional ethic: a way of working with medicines that is not purely commercial yet not incompatible with business values and private profit.

Upholding this ethic is a political process; it depends not only on a functional state, one capable of testing and regulating, but also on the political prioritization of pharmacists' professional privileges over clientelist relations and potentially risky forms of access to medicines in the informal market or even community public health programs. This means recognizing pharmacists as special kinds of citizens by virtue of their commitment to quality, while pharmacists describe quality as a public responsibility they are willing to share with the state but also a form of service and satisfaction that justifies the involvement of private actors in public health. As Sarr puts it, "The client or patient is also a consumer; a consumer of health so the pharmacist must take the lead by guaranteeing not only quality products, but also quality services."[76]

What kind of citizenship do they promise this consumer? On one hand, pharmacists are claiming the entitlement of all national citizens to quality-controlled medicines. Quality should not be a luxury or a choice: it is a standard of public safety to be upheld by the state. On the other hand, the consumption of quality becomes a matter of customer satisfaction, justifying the participation of an increasing number of private actors in state-run public health. As a citizen's right but also a customer's exigency, as a service provided by the state, but one increasingly run like a private business, quality control has ambiguous connections with accessibility. It is not clear whether quality, as a joint responsibility of state and private pharmacists, will broaden or restrict the notion of pharmaceuticals as public health objects, that is, objects to which a public can claim access as well as critically debate the meaning of.

So what do private pharmacy leaders mean by citizenship and by quality? Pointing to their duties "as citizens" evokes past moments and possibilities for relationships between private pharmacists and the state. In the 1970s, state support for private-sector stimulation was justified by all citizens' need to participate in national development, but it was mainly pharmacists' citizenship that was enrolled by these policies, orienting them toward a future they would share with the state as agents of development. In the 2000s, private pharmacists' use of the term revives this notion of joint futures that will be better protected by government financial and regulatory capacity. Yet they also recall a more recent moment of citizenship: when, after devaluation, private pharmacists stepped in to help the state and the population through a pharmaceutical crisis. In this citizenship of crisis, entrepreneurial qualities emerged as crucial in securing public health provision, while state health care opened up to expanded commercial opportunities.

The notion of quality builds on these pasts to help pharmacists define a finer intertwining of public regulation, private actors, entrepreneurial values, and government-channeled resources in Senegal's pharmaceutical sector. In justifying their claims for stronger measures against illicit pharmaceutical trading and for their integration in public health programs, private pharmacists define the quality of medicines both as a government responsibility (toward public safety and health) and as a business commitment (to consumer service and satisfaction). Private pharmacists address the state as concerned citizens, on behalf of a vulnerable public, and as responsible citizens who are entitled to state protection. Yet the values of quality also position them as efficient citizens who are capable of providing better (higher-quality) services than public-sector actors are. They need a state that is stronger in its ability to regulate and to subsidize but one that opens itself, in its dedication to quality, to their interests and abilities as "private agents of public health."

In articulating their claims, Senegalese private pharmacists describe drug quality as much more than the application of standards to medicines; quality work must be performed by qualified actors under appropriate political conditions. Senegalese and other African pharmacists have placed themselves at the forefront of local quality battles. Yet they are largely absent from internationally published accounts of quality control. Their specific vision of quality work is not the only possible avenue toward safe and accessible medicines for resource-poor populations. It nevertheless invites a more careful examination of how potential state capacities, civic, professional, and entrepreneurial values, and public protection and private interests are mobilized and reconfigured in the fight for quality medicines.

Notes

All translations in the text are mine.

1. E.g., El Hadji Massiga Faye, "Marché illicite du médicament, cambriolages: Les pharmaciens baissent rideau," *Le soleil,* 30 April 2008, www.lesoleil.sn; "Vendredi, jour de grève des pharmacies: Une ordonnance contre l'insécurité et la démission de l'état," *Le quotidien,* 22 July 2009, www.lequotidien.sn.

2. Quoted in Issa Niang, "Vol dans les pharmacies: Des pertes estimées à plus de 21 millions en 2007," *Walf Fadjiri,* 30 April 2008, www.walf-groupe.com/.

3. Meredeth Turshen, *Privatizing Health Services in Africa* (New Brunswick, NJ: Rutgers University Press, 1999); Jean-François Bayart, Stephen Ellis, and Béatrice Hibou, *The Criminalisation of the State in Africa* (Indianapolis: Indiana University Press, 1999).

4. Aihwa Ong and Stephen Collier, eds., *Global Assemblages: Technology, Politics, and Ethics as Anthropological Problems* (Malden, MA: Blackwell Publishing, 2005).

5. Abdoulaye Dieng, "(3) Sénégal: Saisie de médicaments d'une valeur de plus de deux millions de francs," *E-med: Le forum francophone sur les médicaments essentiels,* ed. ReMed, 19 May 2008, www.essentialdrugs.org/emed/archive/200805/. I searched the online searchable archives of major newspapers for articles on pharmacists, medicines, and quality. The comprehensiveness or representativeness of this set of sources is difficult to determine, yet it indicates a strong mobilization of private pharmacists and a consistent range of statements.

6. I performed Senegal-related keyword searches of the online archives of *E-med* going back to December 1997. Most of the current discussants are francophone African pharmacists and members of the ReMed staff, who moderate the group.

7. These reports were collected from the Bibliothèque nationale du Sénégal and its Centre de documentation and are cited hereafter under the file name *Dossier pharmacie.*

8. Pascale Brudon et al., *Le secteur pharmaceutique privé au Sénégal: Dynamiques de développement et effets sur l'accès aux médicaments essentiels*, Série de recherche no. 23 (Geneva: World Health Organization, 1997); James Knowles et al., "The Private Sector Delivery of Health Care: Senegal," Major Applied Research Paper no. 16, ed. United States Agency for International Development (Washington, DC: USAID, 1994).

9. Turshen, *Privatizing Health Services*; Pieter Streefland, "Public Health Care under Pressure in Sub-Saharan Africa," *Health Policy* 71, no. 3 (2005): 375–82; Susan Reynolds Whyte, "Pharmaceuticals as Folk Medicine: Transformations in the Social Relations of Health Care in Uganda," *Culture, Medicine and Psychiatry* 16 (1992): 163–86; reprinted in *The Art of Medical Anthropology: Readings*, ed. Sjaak van der Geest and A. Rienks (Amsterdam: Het Spinhuis Publishers, 1998). See also John Iliffe, *East African Doctors: A History of the Modern Profession* (Cambridge: Cambridge University Press, 1998).

10. Whyte, "Pharmaceuticals as Folk Medicine"; P. Wenzel Geissler, "Parasite Lost: Remembering Modern Times with Kenyan Government Medical Scientists," in *Ethos, Evidence and Experiment: The Anthropology and History of Medical Research in Africa*, ed. P. Wenzel Geissler and Catherine Molyneux (New York: Berghahn Books, 2011); Kenneth Ombongi, "The Historical Interface between the State and Medical Science in Africa: Kenya's Case," in Geissler and Molyneux, *Ethos, Evidence and Experiment*.

11. Cheikh Anta Diop University in Dakar is a state university; its teachers are therefore government employees. Professors in the Faculty of Pharmacy generally have a second appointment at the Direction of Pharmacy or as managers of public pharmaceutical structures.

12. Interview with Doudou Ba, Académie des sciences et techniques du Sénégal, 27 January 2009.

13. Interview with Mounirou Ciss, Laboratoire national de contrôle des médicaments, 22 March 2010.

14. "5e réunion de l'Ordre des pharmaciens: 100 millions pour la 'Maison du pharmacien,'" *Le soleil*, 4 July 2005, www.lesoleil.sn.

15. Michel Attisso, "Contrôle de la qualité des médicaments au Sénégal: Rapport de mission, 1–22 juillet 1969," ed. Organisation mondiale de la santé (World Health Organization) (Geneva: OMS / WHO, 1970). The report states that at the time, 15 out of 62 pharmacists were Senegalese and 6 out of 11 were employed by government (while 20, preferably more, were needed).

16. *Nationalization* here means both the promotion of Senegalese nationals to positions of influence and ownership by the state.

17. Mamadou Diouf, "Le clientélisme, la 'technocratie' et après?" in *Sénégal: Trajectoires d'un état*, ed. Momar-Coumba Diop (Dakar: CODESRIA, 1992).

18. "Produits pharmaceutiques: Un marché en rapide expansion," *Le moniteur africain du commerce et de l'industrie* 519, no. 9 (September 1971): 8; Noel Ngouo Ngabission, "Tout savoir sur . . . l'industrie pharmaceutique," *Jeune Afrique* 612, no. 30 (September 1972): 51–65. Colonial legislative legacies and continued cooperation between the countries maintained colonial patterns of importation.

19. While government authorization for the sale of pharmaceuticals was required, applications were granted with very few exceptions; see files HS 119–28 in the Archives nationales du Sénégal (ANS), Dakar.

20. For an analysis of French colonial logics of pharmaceutical distribution in Vietnam, see Laurence Monnais, *Médicaments coloniaux: Distribution, circulation et consommation de produits pharmaceutiques au Viêt Nam, 1905–1940* (Paris: Indes Savantes, 2013).

21. République du Sénégal and SOFFIN, "Convention d'établissement entre le gouvernement du Sénégal . . . et la société 'Soffin,'" [c. 1972], in *Dossier pharmacie*.

22. Diouf, "Le clientélisme, la 'technocratie.'"

23. Babacar Ba, "Communication à l'Assemblée nationale sur les produits pharmaceutiques," *Le point économique* 11 (1977): 34–39. Using a repertory of health regulation and legislation compiled by Charles Becker, I found sixteen "ministerial decisions" between July 1975 and December 1976 for loans from the treasury to pharmacists.

24. Ibid.

25. Irving Leonard Markovitz, *Leopold Sedar Senghor and the Politics of Negritude* (London: Heinemann, 1969), 164.

26. Ba, "Communication à l'Assemblée nationale," 34 and 39.

27. Attisso, "Contrôle de la qualité."

28. Ba, "Communication à l'Assemblée nationale," arrêté no. 1181/SE of 17 April 1958 and arrêté no. 16813– MFAE/SEFAE/C Eco of 3 December 1963.

29. Ibid., 38.

30. Loi no. 78-50 du 14-8-1978 exonérant de tous droits et taxes à l'importation des produits pharmaceutiques (position tarifaire 30-30), *Journal officiel de la République du Sénégal*, 1978, 4653: 1042.

31. SEDE, *Possibilités d'implantation d'une usine de fabrication de produits pharmaceutiques au Sénégal* (Paris: Ministère du plan et de l'industrie, 1969); SONEPI, *Perspectives de l'industrie pharmaceutique au Sénégal: Problèmes et solutions* (Dakar: Ministère du développement industriel, 1970); Ba, "Communication à l'Assemblée nationale."

32. République du Sénégal, Ministère du plan, du développement et de la coopération technique, "Propositions de planification dans les domaines de l'hygiène et de la santé publique," Dakar, 1961, document Br 5097 C, Archives nationales, Section Outre Mer, Aix en Provence, France; Momar-Coumba Diop, "Introduction: Du 'socialisme' au 'libéralisme'; Les légitimités de l'état," in *Sénégal: Trajectoires d'un état*, ed. Momar-Coumba Diop, 13–38 (Dakar: CODESRIA, 1992). Diop points out that Senegalese public investments in health were already in decline before the impact of structural adjustment programs.

33. Makhtar Diouf, "La crise et l'ajustement," *Politique africaine* 45 (1992): 62–85.

34. Brudon et al., *Le secteur pharmaceutique privé*, 11.

35. Knowles et al., "Private Sector Delivery."

36. Aboubakrine Sarr, "Indignation," *Sud Online*, 23 July 2008, www.sudonline.sn.

37. Fara Diaw, "Dr Emmanuel Sarr, pharmacien: '20% des officines dans la tourmente . . . ,'" *Le soleil*, 19 May 2004, www.lesoleil.sn.

38. Interview with Doudou Ba, Académie des sciences et techniques du Sénégal, 27 January 2009.

39. Knowles et al., "Private Sector Delivery"; Brudon et al., *Le secteur pharmaceutique privé*; M. Diouf, "La crise et l'ajustement"; Didier Fassin, "Du clandestin à l'officieux: Les réseaux de vente illicite des médicaments au Sénégal," *Cahiers d'études africaines* 25, no. 2 (1985): 161–77.

40. Fassin, "Du clandestin à l'officieux."

41. Donal Cruise O'Brien, "Le sens de l'état au Sénégal," in *Le Sénégal contemporain*, ed. Momar-Coumba Diop, 501–6 (Paris: Karthala, 2002).

42. Diouf, "Le clientélisme, la 'technocratie.'"

43. Didier Fassin, "La vente illicite des médicaments au Sénégal: Économies 'parallèles,' état et société," *Politique africaine* 23 (1986): 123–30; Diouf, "Le clientélisme, la 'technocratie.'"

44. The Bamako Initiative was adopted at a regional health meeting by African health ministers in 1987. It was implemented in Senegal beginning in the early 1990s. See Ellen E. Foley, *Your Pocket Is What Cures You: The Politics of Health in Senegal* (New Brunswick, NJ: Rutgers University Press, 2010).

45. Knowles et al., "Private Sector Delivery."

46. Brudon et al., *Le secteur pharmaceutique privé*, 34.

47. Ibid., 35; Knowles et al., "Private Sector Delivery."

48. 27-8-1999—Arrêté ministériel no. 99-851 portant érection de la Pharmacie nationale d'approvisionnement en établissement public de santé, *JORS*, 1999, 5882: 1259. The status of "établissement public de santé" (public health establishment) allows establishments offering a public service to manage their budgets autonomously from the central government, which gives them a greater incentive to "sell" these public services.

49. In 1967, the public and private sectors spent roughly the same amount for imported medicines. By the 1990s, the private sector covered 80 percent of the official market for medicines. SEDE, *Possibilités d'implantation*; Brudon et al., *Le secteur pharmaceutique privé*."

50. According to the results of searches in the database *Pubmed*.

51. WHO, *Continuity and Change: Implementing the Third WHO Medicines Strategy, 2008–2013* (Geneva: World Health Organization, 2009); U.S. Pharmacopoeia, "USP in Developing Countries," www.usp.org/worldwide/; Fondation Chirac, "Accès à une santé et à des médicaments de qualité," www.fondationchirac.eu/programmes/acces-aux-medicaments/; ReMed (*Réseau médicaments et développement* [Network for Medicines and Development]), www.remed.org.

52. ReMed, "ReMed s'engage contre le marché illicite des médicaments," www.remed.org/html/marche_illicite_de_medicaments.html; Peter Aldhous, "Counterfeit Pharmaceuticals: Murder by Medicine," *Nature* 434, no. 7030 (2005): 132–36; WHO, *Impact Brochure* (Geneva: World Health Organization / Interpol, 2008), www.who.int/impact/FinalBrochureWHA2008a.pdf.

53. WHO, *Continuity and Change*, 18; J. M. Caudron et al., "Substandard Medicines in Resource-Poor Settings: A Problem That Can No Longer Be Ignored," *Tropical Medicine and International Health* 13, no. 8 (2008): 1062. See also Abdinasir A. Amin and Gilbert O. Kokwaro, "Antimalarial Drug Quality in Africa," *Journal of Clinical Pharmacy and Therapeutics* 32, no. 5 (2007): 429–40.

54. Fassin, "Du clandestin à l'officieux"; Majid Yar, "The *Other* Global Drugs Crisis: Assessing the Scope, Impacts and Drivers of the Trade in Dangerous Counterfeit Pharmaceuticals," *International Journal of Social Inquiry* 1, no. 1 (2008): 151–66; Abdou Salam Fall et al., "Gouvernance et corruption dans le système de santé au Sénégal: Rapport provisoire," ed. Forum Civil CRDI, 2004; E-med, "Forum pharmaceutique de Dakar," *E-med*, ed. ReMed, 2001.

55. Assane Mbaye, "Vente illicite des médicaments: L'Ordre des pharmaciens riposte et contre attaque," *Sud quotidien*, 24 July 2009, www.sudonline.sn.

56. Sarr, "Indignation."

57. Almamy Mamadou Wane, *Le Sénégal entre deux naufrages? Le Joola et l'alternance* (Paris: L'Harmattan, 2004).

58. Mame Marie Faye, *L'immolation par le feu de la petite fille du Président Wade: Crimes, trahisons et fin du régime libéral* (Paris: L'Harmattan, 2008).

59. Tarik Dahou and Vincent Foucher, eds., *Sénégal, 2002–2004: L'alternance et ses contradictions*, Politique africaine 96 (Paris: Karthala, 2004).

60. Pape Diop, "Société: Pharmacies clandestines; Touba, plaque tournante du traffic de médicaments," *Info 7*, 11 January 2001, in *Dossier pharmacie*.

61. Eugene Kaly, "Accès aux médicaments: Abdou Fall pour une stratégie nationale de promotion de génériques de qualité," *Le soleil*, 14 December 2006, www.lesoleil.sn.

62. Aline Kane, "Re: Wade dit niet à Serign Bara," *E-med*, ed. ReMed, 3 August 2009.

63. Zahra, "Le président de l'Ordre des pharmaciens sur la vente illicite de produits pharmaceutiques à Keur Serigne Bi: 'L'état peut fermer 'Keur Serigne-Bi' s'il le veut,'" Nettali.net, 25 June 2009. Italics added for emphasis.

64. Ibid. Dia also defines access to quality drugs as a public entitlement that falls under the state's responsibility in the following interview: "Entretien avec . . . Cheikh Oumar Dia, président de l'Ordre des pharmaciens au Sénégal," *Le quotidien*, 22 July 2009, www.lequotidien.sn.

65. Idrissa Sane, "Sénégal: Vente illicite de médicaments à Keur Serigne-Bi—Les vendeurs acceptent de se conformer à l'interdiction," *Le soleil*, 29 July 2009, www.lesoleil .sn; "Poursuite des activités de Keur Serigne Bi: Wade dit Niet à Serigne Bara," *Walf Fadjiri*, 1 August 2009.

66. Maimouna Gueye, "Partenariat public-privé: Les pharmaciens demandent leur implication dans les programmes de santé," *Le soleil*, 27 April 2007, www.lesoleil.sn.

67. Maimouna Gueye, "Entretien avec . . . Dr Mamadou Ndiadé (président de l'Ordre des pharmaciens) et Dr Aboubakrine Sarr (président du Syndicat des pharmaciens): 'Dire que des pharmaciens ne sont pas impliqués dans le marché illicite du médicament est une contrevérité,'" *Le soleil*, 8 May 2007, www.lesoleil.sn.

68. Talla Diop, "(4) Programme de distribution des antipaludiques au Sénégal à 150 fcfa pour les enfants et 300 fcfa pour les adultes," *E-med*, ed. ReMed, 18 December 2008, www.essentialdrugs.org/emed/archive/200812/.

69. Aline Kane, "(7) Programme de distribution des antipaludiques au Sénégal," *E-med*, ed. ReMed, 19 December 2008, www.essentialdrugs.org/emed/archive/200812/.

70. Ndiouga Diallo, "(13) Programme de distribution des antipaludiques au Sénégal," *E-med*, ed. ReMed, 5 January 2009, www.essentialdrugs.org/emed/archive/200901/.

71. Global Fund, "Program Grant Agreement between the Global Fund . . . and the Ministry of Health of the Government of the Republic of Senegal," www.theglobalfund. org/grantdocuments/4SNGM_813_0_ga.pdf; Global Fund, "Senegal," grant portfolio, http://portfolio.theglobalfund.org/en/Grant/List/SNG. For Senegal's health-care budget for 2006, see République du Sénégal, "Note à la très haute attention de M. le PM sur l'évolution du secteur de la santé de 2000 à 2010," formerly available at www.sante .gouv.sn (accessed 10 October 2010).

72. République du Sénégal, "Note à la très haute attention."

73. Mamadou Cisse, "Luttre contre le paludisme: Le traitement graduit à partir du 1er mai," *Le soleil*, 27 April 2010, www.lesoleil.com.Various programs of free health care have been announced in recent years, including free perinatal care (2005), "le plan SESAME" providing free medicines for the elderly (2006), and free Caesarian sections (2010); see www.sante.gouv.sn.

74. Global Fund, "Program Grant Agreement between the Global Fund . . . and the Ministry of Health."

75. President's Malaria Initiative, "Malaria Operational Plan: Year Four—Fiscal Year 2010 Senegal," 2010, http://pmi.gov/countries/mops/fy10/senegal_mop-fy10.pdf.

76. Quoted in Faye, "Marché illicite du médicament."

PART TWO

Regimes and Relations of Care

FOUR

Regimes of Homework in AIDS Care

Questions of Responsibility and the Imagination of Lives in Uganda

LOTTE MEINERT

IS A NEW "HOMEWORK" REGIME EMERGING IN PUBLIC HEALTH? IF SO, what implications does this have for lives and homes, as well as for public health? This chapter explores these questions based on long-term fieldwork and a case about a woman I call Anna, who has been a client in a U.S.-funded Home-Based AIDS Care research project in Uganda since 2003.[1]

"Homework" is not a term used by the project, but rather an analytical lens I suggest we employ to examine what is happening to health care in a new light. The "homework" concept has been developed by a group of anthropology colleagues working in Denmark, the United States, and Uganda focusing on various chronic conditions.[2] We propose the notion of homework to highlight the kind of care work that patients and families are given by health authorities and are expected to carry out in their home contexts. We opted for the educational metaphor of homework (rather than health-systems concepts of home care and self-care) as a heuristic tool to enable us to focus on specific aspects of the relationship between patients, families, and health authorities. The intention behind the homework notion is to invite critical reflection on recent tendencies in the treatment of chronic illnesses, including how health systems relate to their patients and wider publics and vice versa. Concretely, homework may involve patients and family members carrying out such tasks as taking (and giving) medications, monitoring bodily signs, and changing everyday habits of eating and drinking, as well as altering social and sexual relations. Patients and families receive training by clinical experts in the various tasks they are supposed to perform at home and sometimes report to experts.

The homework perspective draws attention to the point that there is an element of teaching and giving homework assignments implicit in contemporary chronic health care. The practice of care thus becomes the responsibility of the pupils (patients) at home. There is an obligation on the patient side to do the homework—for their own sake—and to comply with the regime. Thinking about "homework" as a way of organizing and motivating health care raises a range of questions regarding responsibility for health as a public, social, and private good. It raises questions about the relationship between patients as citizens and the state as authority when international organizations with specific ideas about individuals, homes, and lives enter the health-care scene. The homework regime has implications for how patients and homes are imagined by health authorities and organizations; conversely, the homework relation impinges on how patients and their families imagine and relate to health authorities. Through Anna's case I explore some of the conflicts, dilemmas, and hopes that this type of homework creates over time. I approach these changes with a focus on the possibilities, vulnerabilities, personal struggles, and existential questions that the concept of homework allows us to explore. In this chapter, my attention is primarily on the patient/pupil side of doing homework.[3]

A range of theoretical concepts is potentially applicable to the analysis of what is happening in this historical era of public health in Africa. A Foucauldian approach to biopower emphasizes the disciplining of individuals and the formation of subjectivity.[4] Paul Rabinow introduced the idea of biosociality, the formation and practice of social identity on the basis of genetic characteristics, biomedical diagnoses, or treatments.[5] The notions of biological and therapeutic citizenship draw our attention toward how illness identities and claims concerning medical treatment may mediate relations between the individual and the state or other political entities.[6] But "homework" orients us toward homes, and in Uganda that means domains of interaction that are fundamental to aspects of life beyond the biomedical. The methodological approach of this study, which is based on long periods of fieldwork over a decade (1997–2010) in family homes, and in Anna's life world specifically, has led me to see "homework assignments" within the realm of everyday family life. By taking this ethnographic, experience-near life-world perspective, I foreground ambiguities characteristic of the realities of neoliberal health care that are less visible from a biopower, governmentality, and biological citizenship perspective.

Homework in public health is not a new phenomenon in Africa; Christian missions, schools, and colonial and postcolonial governments have all attempted to change people's practices concerning health, healing, and hygiene by teaching and preaching. Nonetheless, homework in curative practices seems to have a shorter history. Moreover, the role of the state and foreign entities or global assemblages in relation to the schooling of patients and citizens has also changed in significant ways.[7]

AIDS and ART in Uganda[8]

The AIDS epidemic that hit Uganda in the 1980s completely overwhelmed a health system that was already stretched to the limit by structural adjustment programs, decades of civil war, and the burden of various other infectious diseases. With an HIV infection rate of around 20 percent,[9] the human and material resources in the health care system to deal with the disaster proved insufficient. The Ugandan state had to find new ways of helping large numbers of sick and dying people and preventing new infections. The openness of the government and the leadership it took in confronting the AIDS epidemic are legendary.[10] By the late 1980s and early 1990s, self-help groups, NGOs, faith-based organizations, and donors were already active in providing education, support, and some health care. A mosaic of government, nongovernmental, and international actors was established early on and has grown more complex over the years.

The advent of antiretroviral therapy (ART) must be seen against this background; unlike countries such as Brazil and Botswana, whose programs are governmental, Ugandans access ART from a variety of sources. The first antiretrovirals (ARVs) in Uganda were offered through the Joint Clinical Research Centre (JCRC) in 1996, but the price was so high that only the wealthy could afford treatment. A 1999 UNAIDS (Joint United Nations Programme on HIV/AIDS) initiative called Medical Access Uganda ensured a supply of AIDS drugs to JCRC and other treatment centers. But treatment was still costly: at US$700 a month for triple therapy,[11] even the rich could not always remain adherent.

Things began to change in 2001 when generics came onto the market. An Indian pharmaceutical company began offering triple therapy for US$350 a month,[12] and prices continued to fall from that point on, including for patented drugs. A few programs were offering free ART by 2003, and some people were lucky to be enrolled in research projects that supplied ARVs. There were heated discussions in international forums about the provision of free ART in Africa. But this did not become a reality on the ground in Uganda until 2004 when funding from President's Emergency Plan for AIDS Relief (PEPFAR) and the Global Fund to Fight AIDS, Tuberculosis and Malaria allowed organizations that were already providing AIDS care to add ART to their services. The AIDS Support Organization (TASO), born in 1987, was able to start giving ART to some of its long-standing clients by the end of 2004. But even more groundbreaking was the establishment of HIV/AIDS clinics in government hospitals and upper-level health centers. Biomedical experts emphasized the overwhelming importance of adherence to a lifelong regimen of medication and regular examination. The nightmare they feared was treatment chaos and the development of drug resistance. Patients and their families took their strongest argument for strict control to heart: those who did not follow the regimen would die quickly. Control and survival were to be ensured by enrolling patients in ARV treatment programs. For all of these reasons, the landscape of health care blossomed with an array of programs, not just one package of care provided through the existing government health-care system. The programs also differed in their regimes of care. Most programs were clinic based; patients were required to come in for testing, monitoring, and treatment at the clinic. A few programs were home based in the sense that health staff monitored patients in their homes and delivered medicine to them. However, all programs included some kind of "schooling" of patients about HIV/AIDS, ART, and "living positively."

Imaginations of the Home

The idea that the home is an important site of health is not new in Uganda. As occurred elsewhere in colonial Africa, hygiene and domestic habits have played a prominent role in the colonial and postcolonial history of public health in Uganda.[13] Specific notions of "the good life" with reference to supposedly modern frameworks of wealth, aesthetics, and moralities have been promoted through school and church and were supposed to be realized in homes.[14]

However, in relation to curative practices, the home has been approached more critically. In colonial times, much effort was put into making people believe that hospitals and clinics were the right places for treating illness and that treatment should be done with biomedicine rather than herbal medicines and divination from home.[15] Despite these developments, the public health system remained underdeveloped until independence, and in Uganda at least, the result was a mushrooming of small, private medicine shops,[16] where people bought biomedicine and treated themselves and their family members from home.[17] From the 1980s to the 2000s, the Ministry of Health, on the background of information from the World Health Organization (WHO) and the Essential Drugs Management Program (1994), warned heavily against the treatment of diseases in homes with medicines bought from informal drug shops.[18] *Home treatment* and *self-treatment* were derogatory terms, and lay treatment at home was considered dangerous.

The situation and rhetoric changed considerably in the 2000s in relation to certain diseases and medicines. With the realization that the treatment burden of malaria and AIDS could not be borne by the health system alone, new health policies in relation to home treatment were introduced. This shift was conveniently paired with changing ideologies about the role of the state, from being the primary entity responsible for health care toward playing a minimal role.[19] Thus, there has been a lively development of home-based care programs, especially in relation to diseases such as malaria and AIDS.[20] With the introduction of the home-based programs, the rhetoric surrounding the home in relation to treatment shifted toward being a place of potential competence, partly because it was a cheap way—from the perspective of the health system—of filling in gaps in health care.

Teaching Home-Based AIDS Care (HBAC)

Anna was recruited by one of the home-based programs, which had started as a U.S. Centers for Disease Control and Prevention (CDC) research project funded by the U.S. Agency for International Development (USAID) and based at Tororo Hospital in eastern Uganda. The project was strict about home residence and enforced adherence by visiting people at home. Because it was also a research project, careful monitoring and testing were required by the various study protocols. In total, the project recruited just over two thousand subjects, mainly from the lists of TASO Tororo.[21] To be included, the client had to be a long-term member of TASO, had to have a CD4 count below 250,[22] and had to live and sleep seven days a week in the surveyed household. The project delivered medicine in the clients' home every week and provided options for counselling in the home on a monthly basis.

The hypothesis of the research was that more health care could be delivered at home for the same resources than through traditional clinic-based care. The study set out to demonstrate that frequent home visits by a trained layperson with a standard questionnaire are equivalent in terms of health outcomes to regular laboratory blood tests.[23]

When the HBAC project started, AIDS patients, families, health-care staff, and researchers were all excited. At that time, ARVs were available only at the neighboring district at JCRC, and at a very high cost. Patients and their families were eager and hopeful that they would be able to access the medicine and care through the project, because this was one of the first initiatives to make the ARV medicine available to poor rural people. In the beginning, the project was planned for only a three-year period, but surprisingly this was not a major worry for patients when they started treatment. Just getting access to treatment and having the prospect of surviving for some years seemed to overshadow concerns about the limited time frame of the project. However, this became a source of serious concern for many later on. The project was extended for another three years, and the implementation of the project has since been handed over to TASO with funding from CDC. (The funding of the project in the future became even more uncertain after the global financial crisis and consequent reduction of donor funding.)

The recruited "clients" were instructed to attend meetings at the newly built project office in the district hospital, where they were given information about the research protocol, AIDS, ART, and living positively by locally employed counsellors and health professionals. All the clients were told that the research would go on for three years, that they had to comply with the medicine regime, and that they were to stay in their homes seven days a week; otherwise, they would be removed from the study and consequently deprived of the medicine. The physical setup at these meetings resembled a school class, with pupils/patients seated behind desks (some of them taking notes) and a doctor or counsellor acting as teacher, giving lectures and sometimes using a blackboard or posters for illustrations.

Anna and Her Homework

Anna was in her early thirties when she enrolled in the program, after she had been living with and almost died from her infection several times over at least the previous decade. She had a daughter (age thirteen) who was staying with another family, but she lost her husband

and two other children to AIDS in the 1990s. Anna discovered her HIV status in the late 1990s after the death of her youngest child, when she finally went to have an HIV test done.

Before Anna joined the home-based program, she had to travel thirty kilometers to buy the medicine herself from one of the few government centers supplying ARVs. The transportation and medicine were a heavy economic burden as well as a constant source of worry. Anna managed to stay on the medication for six months and gradually improved significantly, but after a while she had to give up, mainly for economic reasons. She did not have a job, was hardly able to work, and had to rely on her brothers' donations for buying medicine, an arrangement that was not sustainable in the long run. After stopping the ARVs, she fell seriously ill with diarrhea and resistant tuberculosis. Fortunately, she had become a member of TASO by that time, from which the new home-based AIDS care (HBAC) project was recruiting patients. She was recruited and immediately hospitalized because of the seriousness of her condition, even though hospitalization was not the core idea of the HBAC project. This was when I first met Anna at the district hospital. She was lying in her hospital bed, unable to walk and eat, skinnier than I thought a live human being could possibly be. But she had an insistent look in her eyes. I spoke to her at length in the hospital, visited her several times, and recorded parts of her life story. After two months with hundreds of injections and withdrawals of water from her lungs, she was deemed well enough for "homework" and was sent home. However, Anna's home was not a straightforward matter, as I discuss later. Anna was educated with a group of patients at the HBAC project at the compound of the district hospital. The contrast was stark between the clean, air-conditioned, computerized HBAC facilities, including a teaching room with new furniture, and the completely worn-down, overcrowded, and smelly women's ward in the district hospital where Anna had been treated. A counsellor from HBAC also came to Anna's home to teach her and her stepmother about how Anna had to care for herself and be "compliant" and what her obligations toward the project were. When I asked Anna what the project had taught her, she was quick to list the tasks in what we later termed her "homework":

1. Take the medicine strictly every day on time, in the morning and evening.

2. Drink only chlorinated water.

3. Eat a healthy and varied diet.

4. Seek to have "peace of mind."

5. Socialize with people in your surroundings.

6. If you have sex, practice only safe sex.

7. Do not get pregnant.

8. Be available at home for the research team when they come to carry out their studies.

Anna told me about these instructions, and they resembled what I had overheard during the lessons I had attended.

After a couple of months at home, Anna had improved immensely. She commented on the project: "Right now I am under the care of HBAC. . . . They care for me right from home! They deliver drugs for me. In hospital I am given money for food and for transport back home." She was indicating with a wide smile that she considered this to be "excellent quality of care." Free medicine, money for food and transportation, and health workers "who come right up to your home—they really care!" This was Anna's perception and experience at the beginning of the project.

Some of the social aspects involved in homework were formalized in the HBAC project in the sense that each patient was asked to choose a "medicine companion" at home to observe his or her daily intake of the medication and sign for this on a paper form provided by the project. But in the first place, going home was a complicated issue for Anna. Anna had to move back to her childhood home, because her husband had died and she did not have a place of her own in Uganda. She had a small place in Rwanda, where she had been living with her husband, who had been a truck driver shuttling between Mombasa and Kigali. Yet to be part of the HBAC project she had to reside in the district. In Anna's childhood home, only her stepmother was still alive, and she was preoccupied with taking care of a handicapped grandchild and a few other grandchildren. Anna's father had passed away recently, and the stepmother had not yet found her feet. But Anna had no other home to turn to, and she felt she had to choose her stepmother as her medicine companion, "out of respect, since after all she was now head of the home." Yet Anna soon found it awkward and unnecessary to have her stepmother check on her, so they developed a secret system in which the stepmother would sign for all days once a week. They had a relatively straightforward relationship, by local standards, but to add a medical control aspect into this relationship complicated issues.

The initial miracle of the medicine that Anna, her family, the HBAC project, and her friends had hoped for was realized. During the first year at home, Anna's body transformed completely: she gained twenty kilograms, and her immune system improved tremendously. Every week a fieldworker delivered a package of medicine and asked her how she was feeling. Once a month a counsellor visited her at home and interviewed her about compliance and issues that concerned her. The counsellor also reminded her about the importance of living positively in all aspects—in other words, of "doing her homework."

Anna found parts of the homework easy (at least in the beginning): taking the medicine regularly, drinking her chlorinated water, not having sex, not getting pregnant. None of those tasks presented a problem to Anna. She was used to swallowing the medicine; the chlorinated water was provided by the project; she was not interested in sex and doubted that she ever would be; consequently, having children was a nonissue. Other aspects proved difficult right from the beginning, such as eating healthy and varied food in a home where supplies often ran short and where relatives moved in and out in a rather unpredictable manner. Anna tried to plan her shopping and buy the right food, but when visitors came, as they often did, they had to be served with the best food in the home, according to local customs, often leaving Anna with no or little food for the following days.

The task of seeking peace of mind also proved difficult. "To be bored in the village is not the same as having peace of mind," Anna said with a twisted smile. She was not merely bored and lonely in the village home with her stepmother and the handicapped niece; she also got worried when her CD4 count started going up and down. In addition, she was unsure about the future of the HBAC project, which was initially framed as a three-year program, and uncertain about the provision of medicine after that.

The HBAC clients were also advised to socialize with people in their local contexts. "But you know, Lotta, when you have this disease and you walk past the drinking places in the village, you feel people's eyes on you, you see them talking quietly to each other while they look at you and laugh. And you imagine what they say: 'This is the one who got AIDS, when she was "working" in Malaba, and her husband died and two baby girls, but look at her now. It is like a dead body walking . . . ' Some people are very good and happy that you are alive, but others still fear you and look at you as someone who should have been dead. So it is not easy." Even socializing with family members who had earlier taken care of and paid for Anna's medicine was complicated. Anna felt indebted, yet at the same time she felt that these were the same people who had given up on her at some point and had stopped paying her medicine. The social wounds were not healed by the miracle medicine.

Living positively in the village and being open about her status turned out to be a major challenge. After the first couple of years at home in the village, Anna had become bored and lonely and wanted to start working. Her hoped-for trajectory changed over time as she got better physically and realized that the kind of future she wished for was not compatible with the village. She was neither interested in nor very skilled in farming, which was the only real option in the rural home with her stepmother. She wanted to go back to an office job or travel to sell clothes. Yet to qualify for the HBAC project, she had to stay home seven days a week, so she had to give up her business plans. She tried to start a small business selling sandals imported from Rwanda, but there was no real market for these products in the village. She tried baking and selling bread to schoolchildren, but when rumors started that she was spreading HIV in this way, she gave up, disillusioned.

Anna talked to her counsellor and applied to the project for a cleaning job at their offices or "any kind of work," even though she was overqualified. The counsellor and other project staff were sympathetic but hesitated to employ her, perhaps because she was also a client in the project and becoming an employee would dissolve the borders between patients/pupils and doctors/teachers in challenging ways. The project told Anna that her application had simply been received too late. Whatever the reason, Anna took the rejection of her application to heart. She interpreted the gestures of the project "caring right from home" as a real interest in the clients' lives and well-being but was disappointed to find out that the project's interests had specific limits. The project's interest in securing the survival of the clients was not merely for the sake of the medical research, but this research interest obviously played an important role in the project's rationale. Anna's desire to be recognized not only as a medical success story but also as a full person—a citizen who participated in the job market, contributed to others' lives, and had some freedom of consumption—was thwarted. Anna's experience resonates with the analysis of Rosalind C. Morris from South Africa, where a young boy involved in an HIV project articulated a similar sentiment:[24] "You are saving us for dying. We want to make a living."[25] To make a living is more than having a life, mere physical life, or simply surviving. In Anna's quest for a job and for the young people Morris describes, there is an implicit demand for recognition of full personhood through work—for recognition as a person and not simply a patient. Anna decided to ask the project for permission to move to the district town while still remaining a client in the project, even though she would not be staying at home. She was granted permission and moved to town and started going to college to "upgrade my education—now that I have a future," as she said. The HBAC project wanted to deliver the medicine at her new home, the college dormitory, as a service and also to prove that the home-based care concept worked. However, Anna felt that the new social context raised some of the stigma issues that she had hoped to leave behind in the village. The attitudes of other students changed when they saw the HBAC project deliver medicine to her and they realized what this meant. Some of the students no longer wanted to cook and eat food with her. She decided to move away from the dormitory and into another student house. After this experience, Anna managed to negotiate a new arrangement with the HBAC project so that she would pick up her medicine from the clinic, because she did not want her new fellow students to know that she was HIV positive and receiving medicine.

Questions of Responsibility

Anna's experience of being given a life chance by a project that offered treatment of a life-threatening disease was significant for the development of the relation between Anna as dependent and responsible and the project as a kind of patron in caring control. The development of the strong link to the project had consequences for how Anna perceived the government health-care system and also for how she thought about the importance of her kin relations. Until Anna was given this chance by the HBAC project, she had been trying to buy the medicine herself with the help of her kin from a parastatal health organization that, although successful in some respects, exhibited the weaknesses of the public health-care system: the authorities often ran out of medicines, and patients had to buy the medicine at a high price that excluded the majority of citizens. The idea of a health-care system that provided health for the whole public had been promoted in Uganda as part of President Museveni's campaigns, but in reality the public health-care system had been decaying for years and did not live up to expectations, partly because of the AIDS epidemic. When the ART projects such as the one Anna was part of entered the public health scene in Uganda, they were perceived as "saviors entering a graveyard," as Anna phrased it. The fact that the ART medicine works (for most patients) in a dramatic, fast, and completely transformative way confirmed this perception of the projects as miraculous. Anna thus talked about the project with a special kind of dedication; she was grateful in an existential sense. Anna had a dream one night with a divine revelation. God told her to help others who were HIV positive and assure them that they could become part of the miracle as well. Anna was not usually a very religious person, but her experience of having been saved from dying started a spiritual calling. So whenever Anna heard about someone who was HIV positive and about to give up, she made an effort to spend time with this person and persuade him or her that there would be a "project with medicine for them, too, in the near future." The HBAC project took advantage of her great counselling skills when they had difficult clients who were not taking their medicine or not complying with their homework tasks in other ways and seemed to be beyond the reach of the professional counsellors in the project. Anna was never employed by the project, nor was she remunerated as a so-called volunteer, but all the same she seemed happy to be used by the project in informal ways. The existential experiences of what could be seen as resurrection from the grave, that is, becoming human and valuable to others again, no doubt established a special tie between Anna and the project. "I am one of their people" and "I belong to the project," Anna would say proudly, and just as she was dedicated to the project, so too did she feel that it was dedicated to her and provided "excellent care." This moral tie between patient and health provider is important for the homework because it imparts a feeling of obligation and responsibility to conform with project rules and ideas. The relationship of mutual obligation is well known in Uganda from various patron-client associations.[26] Anna is familiar with this type of relationship and knows how to play the role of the devoted and dependent client who evokes the patron's feelings of obligation.

The clients and staff in the HBAC project did not perceive the project to be part of government health care at all, even though the project office was located in the district hospital compound and much of the staff had previously been employed in clinics and hospitals under the Ministry of Health. They perceived the HBAC as an American project that set a different standard for health care. When we asked one of the foreign employees at the project why they did not collaborate more with the government health system, he answered provocatively, "Which health system?" indicating that in his view, the government health system was close to nonexistent.

The kind of projectification of health that takes place in a project such as HBAC raises questions about who is responsible for the health and treatment of the patient. Is it the individual patient? The family? The state? The project? The donor agency? These questions are constantly being opened up for all parties involved, because projects by definition do not last forever. While the intention of many projects is ultimately to be integrated in the public health-care system, for good reasons, this seldom actually happens.

Imagined and Real Homes

A striking feature in Anna's case is the home-based care concept's implicit assumptions about homes. I argue that there has been a historical shift in how the home is perceived and used in Ugandan and international health policies and projects. Only ten years ago, the Ugandan health authorities, as well as other health authorities in the region, were in strong opposition to people treating illness at home. Home treatment and self-treatment were considered highly problematic phenomena leading to "drug-abuse and drug resistance."[27] The National Drug Authorities in Uganda carried out campaigns against home treatment and small, illegal drugstores selling medicine that people used for self-medication. In reality, people were forced to do home treatment because access to the health system was limited in most rural areas, and very often the health clinics had run out of their relatively small supply of medicines. Despite—or possibly because of—this reality, the rhetoric of the government health authorities was strongly influenced by a modernization discourse about getting people out of their "primitive homes," that is, away from traditional herbal treatments, diviners, and biomedical home treatments and into the modern institutions and power relations of biomedicine. In this modernist discourse, "the home" and "the village" are imagined as backward and primitive places from which biomedicine should maintain a distance. As mentioned earlier, the change of ideas about the home also happened at a time when donors and international organizations were introducing ideas about the state and the individual that are now associated with neo-liberalism.[28] While the change in the view of the home had positive sides (such as acknowledging that the work families do in relation to health and treatment is valuable), there is still a great distance between the imagined home and real homes in which patients are to carry out homework. Home as a safe and resourceful haven of "therapy management groups" belongs to the fantasies of policy makers, clinical staff, and patients.[29] In Tanzania, Steven Feierman argues, support networks changed significantly in this period and had been gravely affected by the HIV/AIDS epidemic and their projects, as well as by increasing poverty and unemployment. Feierman points to the problematic focus in health policy on individual decision making because it misses the fact that most health-care decisions are made by the family and friends. This fact was not supported by health policy and initiatives, and this made the crucial social networks weaker.[30] Thus, political assumptions about homes and "the African family" as stable, well-functioning units may be both stereotypical and outdated. The actual homes people try to establish are often temporary, conflicted, and sometimes lonely, and this affects the homework that people are supposed to do in relation to their illness.

For Anna, the first problem was that she did not have a home and had to move back to her natal home, where her stepmom resided. It is not unusual in this part of Uganda for a woman who is HIV positive to move back into her paternal home after her husband has died.[31] Having her stepmother as medicine companion and staying in her home village paradoxically turned out to be an *unheimlich* (uncanny) experience because Anna sensed that the people she was supposed to socialize with gossiped about her behind her back and called her "a dead body walking" and "the whore from Malaba who killed a husband and two baby girls." When Anna moved to town to start afresh, the social aspects of homework visits from the HBAC project again turned into an experience of stigmatization. Anna was caught up in new dilemmas; ideally, she wanted to be open about her HIV status, which was encouraged by the "living positively" project jargon, and she wanted to be a good example of home care. At the same time, she wanted to be recognized as a normal, respectable person, a student with a promising future, and perhaps a potential girlfriend.

From Biological Survival to Living a Life

As people gain strength on ART, their concerns shift from barely surviving to wanting to live a fuller life: to becoming a whole person again, with sexual and reproductive desires as well as other aspirations. Thus, the temporality inherent in specific regimes of care may conflict with the temporality of patients' lives as their focus shifts from a concern with biological survival to their social lives. This tension is inherent in Anna's story.

The future Anna hoped for changed over time, and her new hopes became ultimately incompatible with the home-care concept: For Anna, the home-care concept was excellent care for a long time (two to three years) and she appreciated the "home" part of the care concept. She carried out her "homework" with pride, while feeling comfortably obligated to the project. But as Anna gained weight, strength, and agency, she began to hope for more than simply surviving. This brought her into conflict with the home-based care concept. She hoped to be able to get a job and have a home of her own, even a partner. With time, Anna might also wish to have children, as have other HIV-positive women who have regained their strength. Yet having children would be considered explicitly problematic within the framework of the project, because of the risk of infecting the baby. Anna wanted to be able to move around, and she wanted to be able to decide who got to know about her HIV status. Yet she could not control this when the project cared for her "right from home." So the initial success of the concept of home-based care allowed for new hopes that have produced new aspirations—which have since then produced new dilemmas and double binds.

The health workers and researchers in the HBAC project were aware of and worried about the issue of how their patients' perspectives, appetite for life, sexuality, and desire for children changed with time. Yet the project seemed to stick to the biological survival dogma, stressing the rather puritanical homework rules of eating and drinking appropriately, practicing only safe sex, and avoiding pregnancies. Paradoxically, the patients' successful healing processes, which are due to the treatment and homework, made them feel vulnerable and uncertain because their new desires disqualified them as responsible patients in the project.

The Intimate Relation between Care and Control

Homework had been part of public health in Uganda for a long time, especially in terms of preventive and health promotion initiatives in colonial and postcolonial times. I argue that the focus on homes for curative practices was a relatively new development that was perhaps symptomatic of these neoliberal times. With the development of homework as a regime of treatment, homes and families became central entities in health policies and interventions. This was not a return to an "original state" of home care and cure (as Kleinman's notion of the popular sector suggested in 1980).[32] The aim of home-care policies and interventions was to govern, manage, and guide *how* home care was conducted by patients, families, friends, and neighbors, so that it followed the ideals laid out by the professional health-care sector. The professional sector was still the realm of expertise—schooling the patients, providing knowledge and treatment. However, the patient and the home had become responsible for the outcome of treatment, which made a difference partly because the professional assumptions about the homes and lives in which the treatment should took place were unrealistic. Patients might therefore not be able to live up to the responsibility of treating themselves correctly at home, but they had no one to turn to with this concern, because it was *their* homes and *their* lives that were regarded as the problem and they were held responsible.

As health care and treatment in homes had become expert driven, what was formerly backstage health work hidden from the authorities had become a front-stage, official sphere: health workers and counsellors could enter patients' homes and comment on intimate practices. In the HBAC project, the counsellors routinely checked the medicine dispensers of the patients, the kitchen, the sleeping place of the client, and the family latrine. The relation between care and control was experienced as intimate and ambiguous; it was surveillance, but for one's own sake, reminding us of Foucauldian governmentality. When ART projects such as HBAC entered the Ugandan health-care landscape, this landscape was perceived to be an eroded desert by many patients. The strict rules, surveillance, and control that many of the ART projects applied were experienced as "excellent care," providing hope and life in a very literal sense. Yet even though projects such as HBAC considered their regime of care to be rational and economically sound and believed that they would be able to scale it up to a national level, in reality this was unlikely. Few consider the official health-care system worth collaborating with, and most have an idea that externally funded projects would have to patchwork to cover the needs of the population. Yet with the financial crisis it became painfully clear how vulnerable this health projectification strategy was. The large majority of Uganda's ART provision had been generously funded by the United States,[33] but with the financial pressure these budgets were cut back tremendously, which meant that new patients were able to start treatment only if another patient stopped or died. Out of the 500,000 patients who needed treatment by 2010, only 200,000 were getting it.[34] The hope that the new ART programs had evoked about being able to live a life with HIV was proving somewhat chimerical.

Much recent anthropological research on AIDS argues that new regimes of care promote novel forms of citizenship, in the sense of rights/obligation relationships between individuals and political entities. The notion of "therapeutic citizenship," which argues that citizenship has been reduced to the ability of some individuals to make claims and access treatment by invoking their HIV status, has gained ground in academic circles and has made us aware of new forms of rights consciousness and activism (in some parts of Africa) that have been created by access and lack of access to ART.[35] Rabinow's concept of biosociality has been instrumental in helping us to identify and formulate transformations in social relationships and identities based especially on new genetic knowledge in relation to a variety of diseases, as well as Nikolas Rose's idea of biological citizenship and Adriana Petryna's work with this perspective in Ukraine after Chernobyl.[36] In Brazil, João Biehl makes us aware of the "pharmaceuticalization of citizenship" as a consequence of how the state provision of ARVs intersects with NGOs and other institutions in a way that exacerbates health inequities.[37]

The citizen concepts, biosociality, and biopolitics approaches foreground a discourse on rights in societies: equal, individual rights and social activism organized around disease and treatment. The studies that have applied a citizenship perspective have mainly focused on clinics and moments of transformation. There are no doubt aspects of these processes of transformation and development of new ideas about being a citizen in Uganda as well. However, as described elsewhere, in various respects Uganda is a different context (from Brazil and South Africa) with relatively little history of social activism and where ideas about patron-clientship and related moralities are more prominent than ideas about rights and citizens.[38] My colleagues and I have suggested a "therapeutic clientship" perspective to complement the citizen perspective,[39] to encourage the examination of patients' family and social relations on their own terms. The citizen perspectives emphasize individual rights in a polity and their implications for shaping subjectivity. A citizen perspective may be more useful for understanding the positions of the donors, activists, advocates, policy makers, and to some extent providers. They are the ones offering inclusion; they feel they have an obligation to help; and they make claims on (or at least appeals to) the state or the international community on behalf of the hundreds of thousands in need of ARVs.[40] But most people on ART in Uganda do not talk about their rights and claims in the abstract sense. When following a person like Anna over a long time, it becomes apparent that becoming a citizen in a biological, therapeutic, and pharmaceutical sense is only one aspect of living with ART. The social aspects of living with ART—including desires to be a full person participating in the local economy, family, sexuality, and reproduction—are more sustained concerns. Following Anna closely over many years has made the truth of this banality clear: perspectives change over time. Funding of ART programs fluctuates; relationships with family members are challenged, confirmed, and sometimes broken; wishes to have children may appear impractical at one point in time but the only right thing at another time. Gratitude for surviving may turn into bitterness about not being recognized as a real person. These changes over time challenge short-term snapshot analyses that overlook how many issues—stigma is one of them—belong to specific historical and personal times and contexts. The changes over time in Anna's case show that questions about responsibility for health are never settled once and for all.

Notes

1. This chapter draws on my long-term relationship with an extended family in a village in eastern Uganda where I have done intervals of fieldwork since 1997. I also build on work done by the Living with ART research group under the TORCH Project including Phoebe Kajubi, David Kyaddondo, Hanne Mogensen, Godfrey Siu, Jenipher Twebaze, Michael A. Whyte, and Susan Reynolds Whyte. Even though the specific case in the chapter is not drawn from our common study, many of the insights were developed with this group of researchers. I have continued to follow Anna over the years, and last saw her in April 2013. One of my students, Marlene Møller, has done fieldwork while staying with Anna and her family. The chapter is also partly based on analytical work done with Grøn and Mattingly about chronic homework; see Lone Grøn, Cheryl Mattingly, and Lotte Meinert, "Kronisk Hjemmearbejde: Sociale håb, dilemmaer og konflikter i Uganda, Danmark og USA," *Tidsskrift for forskning i sygdom og samfund* 5, no. 9 (October 2008): 71–95, and Cheryl Mattingly, Lone Grøn, and Lotte Meinert, "Chronic Homework in Emerging Borderlands of Healthcare," *Culture, Medicine, and Psychiatry* 35, no. 3 (2011): 347–75.

2. Grøn, Mattingly, and Meinert, "Kronisk Hjemmearbejde."

3. For a more pronounced focus on the health worker and health authority side, see Susan Reynolds Whyte, Michael A. Whyte, and Betty Kyaddondo, "Health Workers Entangled: Confidentiality and Certification," in *Morality, Hope and Grief: Anthropologies of AIDS in Africa*, ed. Hansjörg J. Dilger and Ute Luig (New York: Berghahn Books, 2010). See also Lotte Meinert, "The Work of the Virus: The Cutting and Creation of Kin Relations in an ART Project," in *Para-states of Science: Ethnographic and Historical Perspectives on Life-Science, Government, and the Public in Twenty-First-Century Africa*, ed. P. Wenzel Geissler (Durham, NC: Duke University Press, forthcoming).

4. Michel Foucault, "Governmentality," in *The Foucault Effect: Studies in Governmentality*, ed. Graham Burchell, Colin Gordon, and Peter Miller, 87–104 (Hemel Hempsted, UK: Harvester Wheatshcad, 1991).

5. Paul Rabinow, *Artificiality and Enlightenment: From Sociobiology to Biosociality; Essays on the Anthropology of Reason* (Princeton: Princeton University Press, 1996).

6. Adriana Petryna, *Life Exposed: Biological Citizens after Chernobyl* (Princeton: Princeton University Press, 2002); Nikolas Rose and Carlos Novas, "Biological Citizenship," in *Global Assemblages: Technology, Politics and Ethics as Anthropological Problems*, ed. Aihwa Ong and Stephen J. Collier, 439–63 (Malden, MA: Blackwell Publishing, 2005); Vinh-Kim Nguyen, "Antiretroviral Globalism, Biopolitics, and Therapeutic Citizenship," in Ong and Collier, *Global Assemblages*, 124–44.

7. Aihwa Ong and Stephen Collier, eds., *Global Assemblages: Technology, Politics, and Ethics as Anthropological Problems* (Malden, MA: Blackwell Publishing, 2005); James Ferguson, "The Uses of Neoliberalism," *Antipode* 41, no. 1 (2009): 166–84.

8. This section builds largely on the introduction by Susan Reynolds Whyte in Susan Reynolds Whyte, ed., *Second Chances: Surviving AIDS in Uganda* (Durham, NC: Duke University Press, forthcoming).

9. Helen Epstein, *The Invisible Cure: Africa, the West and the Fight against AIDS* (London: Penguin Books, 2007), xxi.

10. Ibid.; Carolyn Green, *Handbook on Access to HIV/AIDS-Related Treatment: A Collection of Information, Tools and Other Resources for NGOs, CBOs and PLWHA Groups* (Geneva: UNAIDS / World Health Organization / International HIV/AIDS Alliance, 2003); Justin O. Parkhurst, "The Ugandan Success Story? Evidence and Claims of HIV1 Prevention," Lancet 360, no. 9326 (2002): 78–80; Justin O. Parkhurst and Louisiana Lush, "The Political Environment of HIV: Lessons from a Comparison of Uganda and South Africa," *Social Science and Medicine* 59, no. 9 (2004): 1913–24.

11. John Iliffe, *The African AIDS Epidemic: A History* (Oxford: James Currey, 2006), 148–49.

12. Ibid., 149.

13. John L. Comaroff and Jean Comaroff, *Ethnography and the Historical Imagination* (Boulder, CO: Westview Press, 1992).

14. See Lotte Meinert, *Hopes in Friction: Schooling, Health and Everyday Life in Uganda* (Charlotte, NC: Information Age Publishing, 2009).

15. Megan Vaughan, *Curing Their Ills: Colonial Power and African Illness* (Oxford: Polity Press, 1991); John Iliffe, *East African Doctors: A History of the Modern Profession* (Cambridge: Cambridge University Press, 1998).

16. Richard O. Adome, Susan Reynolds Whyte, and Anita Hardon, *Popular Pills: Community Drug Use in Uganda* (Amsterdam: Het Spinhuis, 1996).

17. S. R. Whyte, "Medicines and Self-Help: The Privatisation of Health Care in Eastern Uganda," in *Changing Uganda: The Dilemmas of Structural Adjustment and Revolutionary Change*, ed. H. B. Hansen and M. Twaddle, 130–48 (London: James Currey, 1991).

18. Uganda National Drug Authority, National Drug Policy and Authority Statute (Entebbe: Government Printer, 1994).

19. Susan R. Whyte et al., "Therapeutic Clientship: Belonging in Uganda's Mosaic of AIDS Projects," in *When People Come First: Critical Studies in Global Health*, ed. João Biehl and Adriana Petryna (Princeton: Princeton University Press, 2013); Jean Comaroff, "Beyond Bare Life: AIDS, (Bio)politics, and the Neo-liberal Order," in *Morality, Hope and Grief: Anthropologies of AIDS in Africa*, ed. Hansjörg J. Dilger and Ute Luig (New York: Berghahn Books, 2010).

20. Lotte Meinert et al., "Faces of Globalisation," *Folk* 45 (2004): 105–25; N. Nshakira et al., "Appropriate Treatment of Malaria? Use of Anti-malarial Drugs for Children's Fevers in District Medical Units, Drug Shops and Homes in Eastern Uganda," *Tropical Medicine and International Health* 7, no. 4 (2002): 309–16; Susan R. Whyte et al., "Treating AIDS: Dilemmas of Unequal Access in Uganda," in *Global Pharmaceuticals: Ethics, Markets, Practices*, ed. Adriana Petryna, Andrew Lakoff, and Arthur Kleinman, 240–62 (Durham, NC: Duke University Press, 2006); Paul J. Weidle et al., "Adherence to Antiretroviral Therapy in a Home-Based AIDS Care Programme in Rural Uganda," *Lancet* 386, no. 4 (2006): 1587–94; Ministry of Health, Republic of Uganda, *Implementation Guidelines for the Home Based Management of Fever Strategy*, 1st ed. (Kampala, Uganda: Ministry of Health/UNICEF/BASICS/DISH, 2002).

21. TASO: The AIDS Support Organization was one of the earliest AIDS NGOs in Uganda, formed in 1987 with the slogan "Living positively with HIV and AIDS"; see Noerina Kaleeba, with Sundanda Ray, "We Miss You All: AIDS in the Family," in *HIV and AIDS in Africa: Beyond Epidemiology*, ed. Ezekeil Kalipeni et al., 259–78 (Oxford: Blackwell Publishing, 2004).

22. An indication of a seriously lowered immune system.

23. http://clinicaltrials.gov/ct/show/NCT00119093.

24. Rosalind C. Morris, "Rush/Panic/Rush: Speculations on the Value of Life and Death in South Africa's Age of AIDS," *Public Culture* 20 (2008): 199–231.

25. Ibid., 205.

26. Whyte et al., "Therapeutic Clientship."

27. Adome et al., *Popular Pills*; Lotte Meinert, "Usund Viden? Sundhedsundervisning og medicinsk praksis blandt itesobørn i Uganda," *Tidsskriftet Antropologi* 38 (1998): 65–78; Nshakira et al., "Appropriate Treatment of Malaria"; P. Wenzel Geissler et al., "Children and Medicine: Self-Treatment of Common Illnesses among Luo School Children in Western Kenya," *Social Science and Medicine* 50 (2000): 1771–83; P. Wenzel Geissler et al., "Self-Treatment by Kenyan and Ugandan Schoolchildren and the Need for School-Based Education," *Health Policy and Planning* 16, no. 4 (2001): 362–71.

28. Comaroff, "Beyond Bare Life"; Steven Feierman, "Chaoala, History, and Health Care Today" (paper presented at "The Publics of Public Health Conference" in Kilifi, Kenya, December 2009).

29. John M. Janzen, *The Quest for Therapy: Medical Pluralism in Lower Zaire* (Berkeley: University of California Press, 1978).

30. Feierman, "Chaoala."

31. Susan Reynolds Whyte, "Going Home? Burial and Belonging in the Era of AIDS," *Africa* 75, no. 2 (2005): 154–72.

32. Arthur Kleinman, *Patients and Healers in the Context of Culture: An Exploration of the Borderline between Anthropology, Medicine and Psychiatry* (Berkeley: University of California Press, 1980), 50.

33. Donald G. McNeil, "At Front Lines, AIDS War Is Falling Apart," *New York Times*, 9 May 2010.

34. Ibid.

35. Nguyen, "Antiretroviral Globalism"; Comaroff, "Beyond Bare Life."

36. Rabinow, *Artificiality and Enlightenment;* Rose and Novas, "Biological Citizenship"; Petryna, *Life Exposed.* See also Sahra Gibbon and Carlos Novas, *Biosocialities, Genetics and Social Sciences* (London: Routledge, 2008); Monica Konrad, *Narrating the New Predictive Genetics: Ethics, Ethnography and Science* (Cambridge: Cambridge University Press, 2005).

37. João Biehl, "Pharmaceuticalization: AIDS Treatment and Global Health Politics," *Anthropological Quarterly* 80, no. 4 (2007): 1083–1126.

38. Lotte Meinert, Hanne O. Mogensen, and Jennifer Twebaze, "Tests for Life Chances: CD4 Miracles and Obstacles in Uganda," *Anthropology and Medicine* 16, no. 2 (2009): 195–209; Meinert et al., "Faces of Globalisation."

39. Whyte et al., "Therapeutic Clientship."

40. Ibid.

FIVE

"Home-Based Care Is Not a New Thing"

Legacies of Domestic Governmentality in Western Kenya

HANNAH BROWN

Community-based public health projects in Kenya build upon a legacy of developmental practices, structures, and ideas that became hegemonic during the colonial period.[1] This legacy has shaped an endeavor founded on conceptualizations of difference that can be mediated through flows of expertise, knowledge, and resources. It has also shaped many of the specific, localized practices and activities undertaken by people involved in such projects. International development and public health initiatives for HIV care resemble previous attempts at social improvement, in terms of the practices that enact them, the forms through which people engage with them, and the philosophies underlying them.

This chapter draws upon ethnographic data collected during fieldwork with a community-based organization in western Kenya during 2006–7 and places this material alongside secondary sources from nongovernmental organizations (NGOs) and the Kenyan Ministry of Health, as well as historical accounts.[2] Viewed together, this material highlights how certain aspects of older interventions appeared to resurface in a contemporary public health project. The community group in question was involved in carrying out home-based care—an HIV/AIDS intervention that extends hospital care into the home—work that revolved in part around enduring governmental renderings of the domestic realm, alongside an allied conceptualization of women as both objects and agents of improvement.

In this chapter, I argue that the specific activities that came together as part of home-based care occurred partly because of the historical longevity of similar groupings of practices and ideas. Simultaneously, practices in circulation around home-based care were shaped by more recent international responses to the HIV epidemic. In the intersection between its relations to the past and its extensions around the world, home-based care gained political and practical traction in Kenya. Public health interventions in Africa and elsewhere must be examined in the light of these past and present associations if one is to make sense of the hopes, aspirations, and motivations of those who become involved in them.

Home-Based Care

Nyanza Province, Kenya, is one of the regions of Sub-Saharan Africa that has been most severely affected by the HIV/AIDS pandemic.[3] One important response has been a health intervention called home-based care. Policy literature describes home-based care, also referred to as community home-based care (CHBC), as "any form of care given to ill people in their homes."[4] However, in Kenya, as elsewhere in Africa, the term *home-based care* has come almost invariably to imply the care at home of people who are suffering from HIV/AIDS-related illnesses, through a recognized set of interventions.

By the year 2000, numerous community groups, particularly those that described themselves as "women's groups," were organizing such activities in Nyanza Province.[5] These initiatives mushroomed in 2001 when the Kenyan government began to fund small groups directly through the National AIDS and STI Control Programme (NASCOP).[6] More recently, with the introduction of free antiretroviral therapy,[7] home-based care has increasingly been formalized at a national and international level and has become part of a wider set of strategies known as "comprehensive HIV care" and "care across a continuum."[8] This has involved a concurrent shift in emphasis away from a so-called good death and appropriate terminal care to ambitions around "living positively," including drug adherence and nutritional support.

Home-based care programs in Kenya are typically led by a clinical officer or nurse based at a rural health facility or by a "community leader" who supervises a group of "community health workers." Unlike the Ugandan project described by Meinert in this volume, the Kenyan national home-based care strategy did not involve delivering medications and other clinical services to the home. Instead, community health workers were envisaged as supporting the government health sector in

the management of clinical HIV care by tracking patients and introducing and referring them to hospital-based support centers where
patients received medication, thus creating a link between the health
facility and the home. Community health workers also assisted with
what were referred to as the "social" needs of patients: providing counselling, nutritional advice, and support for familial caregivers of those
who are sick at home.[9] The work of community health workers was thus
simultaneously integral to "comprehensive HIV care" and peripheral to
or "supportive" of clinical care.

Home-based care has been widely praised as broadly beneficial to
people with AIDS illnesses and their families.[10] Some scholars emphasize
the organic, spontaneous, and communitarian nature of early forms of
home-based care in Africa.[11] However, critics of the growing endorse-
ment of home-based care have labeled the policy as making a virtue
out of community compassion in a way that hides the toll on individual
community members, particularly women.[12] These analysts argue that
home-based care developed largely "in an effort to fill the 'care-gap' left
by the retreating public sector" and claim that the policy allows the state
to absolve itself of responsibilities to citizens by relying on the unpaid
labor of mostly female family members in lieu of adequate funding and
support for the health sector.[13]

Such analyses sit within a wider literature on the experience of
neoliberalism and structural adjustment in Africa, which describes
NGOs—the "voluntary sector" writ large—as moving into the vacuum
created by the "rolling back" of the state, if such spaces are filled at all.[14]
It is certainly true that Kenya has experienced a process of "NGO-
ization" over the past thirty years, which has included the deliberate
transfer of responsibility for some aspects of curative health care from
the state to NGOs and has resulted in patchy and inequitable coverage of health resources.[15] However, an overwhelming emphasis upon
rupture and discontinuities caused by new forms of political economy in
Africa risks obscuring material, ideological, and discursive continuities
across time.[16] More importantly, it potentially distracts attention from
attempts to understand how innovations and imaginaries of the new
intersect fruitfully—and powerfully—with the past.

This chapter argues that the political and practical traction of home-
based care rests in the kinds of connections that it mobilizes with
other governmental forms. These connections extend spatially, through
new, globalized, NGO-centric economies that draw those who do

home-based care into international relations inflected by the prestige of "development." At the same time, these governmental connections also extend temporally through previous interventions focused upon the domestic and women's labor. My argument does not seek to undermine the claim that the cuts in public services resulting from structural adjustment agreements were detrimental to the health and economic development of people in Kenya. Nor is it at odds with the commendable effort to highlight the way in which the grim reality (and gendered burden) of caring for people who are dying from AIDS at home can become hidden in idealized descriptions of home-based care. My aim is rather to show that as a tactic of government, in a Foucauldian sense,[17] home-based care is in as many ways "old" as it is "new." Although home-based care involves new governmental configurations,[18] in many respects, home-based care is a new category that acts as a blanket for a range of activities, some of which are new but many of which are enduring and mirror previous organizational forms. For these reasons, rather than being symptomatic of the "withdrawal" of the state, doing home-based care allows people, primarily women, to position themselves as actors with a relationship to the state using a long-standing set of techniques.

A Meeting at Kagot Development Group

In a pair of small rooms behind a row of shops in Kagot town, a few kilometers from Lake Victoria in western Kenya, lie the offices of a small community-based organization.[19] Handwritten posters and faded health education materials cover the walls of the single-story building. A sewing machine sits in one corner. Large sacks of maize are piled high in another next to a stack of plastic chairs ready for use at meetings and by visitors. A couple of young women chatter and tell stories while one fills out a tedious record sheet; another woman enters and greets them, asking them to decipher a prescription she has for the sickly baby wrapped tightly on her back. In dribs and drabs, more women arrive to attend a meeting as the sheets of *mabati*—the corrugated iron that forms the roof—slowly cook the air inside the small rooms.

Kagot Development Group was formed by a small group of local residents in 2001, with two women the driving force behind the foundation and ongoing management of the organization. Elizabeth, who had fashioned the smaller of the two rooms into her office, was responsible for the day-to-day running of the group. The second woman,

Philomena, was a retired teacher and widow who owned a large bar-cum-hotel and several rental properties in the town, including one that the organization used free of charge as an office. She was mostly absent from the office but played an important role in the writing of reports and funding proposals and meeting guests and visitors.

Both women were openly "living positively" (that is, with HIV) and told me that they had started the organization because they "saw the way that the youths were dying." Elizabeth explained, "From that time we have been doing home-based care, although we didn't realize it at first, we were just doing it, but after a time we came to know that it was home-based care." For Elizabeth, home-based care was a broad concept under which, in addition to carrying out home visits, she provided counselling and nutritional advice, donated school uniforms and raised money for school fees for orphans, dispensed basic drugs from her office, and encouraged income-generating activities. All the work that went on in the organization was completely voluntary; Elizabeth, Philomena, and the two "office girls" who carried out menial work within the organization did not receive a salary for their work.

The women who had begun to arrive at the office were members of a group referred to interchangeably as the "support group" and the *nyamreche* (sing. *nyamrerwa*), or community health workers, coming to attend their weekly meeting. Most of them were widows, older women who did not have very young children to care for at home. Many were themselves HIV positive. They came dressed in long skirts or dresses and wore cheap "rubbers" on their feet (plimsolls—so called because of the rubber sole), which carried the muddy signs of early morning farmwork and the walk from the village; their heads were covered by large scarves tied neatly in knots at the back of the neck. In their bags they carried a *leso*, a piece of fabric upon which they could sit and rest or cover up the items of food that they had bought at the market, and holding a few coins tied up in the corner. Some had received a partial secondary education, while others had little schooling at all. They spoke to one another in Luo, the local language, and all identified ethnically as *Joluo*, Luo people. Just over half of the group members had been trained as community health workers to provide home-based care.[20] When asked to define home-based care, these women, like Elizabeth, emphasized the idealized concepts of domestic care behind the model. They often said, "Home-based care is not a new thing, it has always been there. It is just the care that people are giving at home."

When the women had squeezed into the room, placing chairs in every available space until they begin to sit on the floor upon their leso, Joyce began the meeting with a short prayer. The agenda for the meeting included voting for a "chair of welfare" and a treasurer. They discussed obligations to one another when a family member died; should they make funeral contributions only for deaths of close family members? Purity reminded the group that there were those (like herself) without a husband or children. The women agreed that 150 shillings each was an appropriate amount.[21] The meeting slowed down as the women become hot, tired, and hungry. Elizabeth had said that she wanted to talk to them but had not yet arrived in the office.

When Elizabeth finally arrived, shining with enthusiasm in her smart suit tailored from colorful Ugandan fabric, hair salon-straight and smooth, Joyce, who had acted as secretary, stood up and read the minutes to her. Elizabeth had three more items to discuss: a new income-generating scheme that involved making mats from banana leaves; the repayment of a loan that had been made to the community health workers;[22] and her plans for an outing to visit another community group.

Last, Elizabeth started talking about the monthly reports that the community health workers had to fill in. She emphasized that it was important to fill the forms in properly because the information in the reports would "go up to provincial level" and "provide information for NASCOP." The forms were arranged in pairs, with the top sheet for female clients and the bottom one for male clients. Each A4-sized sheet had a space for the name of the client, the number of visits that were made in a month, and then, in small columns that filled the page, such things as ARV treatment—"you tick or write a dash, no blank spaces"—adherence counselling, educational support, tuberculosis medication, opportunistic infection prophylaxis, nutritional support, and so on. The community health workers found the reports very difficult to use, and Elizabeth began a didactic session, "What is a CHW?" They were silent until at last Beatrice offered, "*Nyamrerwa.*"

> Elizabeth: What is an O.I.?
>
> Beatrice: O.I. is opportunistic infection.
>
> Elizabeth: One kind of opportunistic infection is what?
>
> Joyce: Headache, cough.
>
> Elizabeth: They are things like chronic diarrhea, chronic cough, spots, vaginal discharge. Septrin is taken for O.I.'s. The TB column

is asking if they are on TB drugs. If they have it, put a tick, if they don't, a dash. Now, what is nutrition?

Elizabeth turns her head to look at Beatrice, who addresses Pauline: "It is just eating. If they eat well you can tick it."

Elizabeth: What are psychological problems?

Agnetta [slightly mocking]: I'm ready to tell you.

Elizabeth [ignoring Agnetta]: It is issues in somebody's head [*weche wich ng'ato*]. If you think deeply about something it is psychological.[23]

As the meeting ended, Purity handed out one hundred shillings to each woman, to reimburse them for transportation (although they all arrived by foot or bicycle). The women began to leave. Some requested drugs from the office. Susan, one of the office girls, put on a glove and counted out pills for them: Panadol for Purity's co-wife and Brufen for Agnetta, who had a chest pain.[24]

Income generation, funeral contributions, record keeping, health education, loans, pharmaceuticals—my argument is that home-based care is a legitimate and worthwhile activity, here, in Kagot, precisely because it includes all of these activities. Most analyses of home-based care focus on interactions and activities that take place within the home, describing the kinds of labor undertaken and the experience of involvement in home-based care from the perspective of caregivers and those in receipt of care.[25] While certainly useful for enriching understandings of the reality of caring for very sick people at home, many of the activities that these women associated with home-based care took place outside of the narrow confines of the home visit. The women who were members of Kagot Development Group also visited sick people at home; persuaded people to go for HIV tests; fetched water and delivered gloves, medicines, and high-protein porridge flour; and discussed drug adherence—the more conventional imaginings of home-based care. However, practices in circulation around home-based care extended well beyond these activities.

It is striking that the broad conceptualization of home-based care understood and practiced by members of Kagot Development Group was also underlined in policy documents. For example, see the enormous range of activities considered by the World Health Organization to be "essential elements of Community Home-Based Care":

TABLE 5.1. ESSENTIAL ELEMENTS OF CHBC

Category	Subcategory
Provision of care	Basic physical care; palliative care; psychosocial support and counseling; care of affected and infected children
Continuum of care	Accessibility; continuity of care; knowledge of community resources; accessing other forms of community care; community coordination; record keeping for ill people; case finding; case management
Education	Curriculum development; educational management and curriculum delivery; outreach; education to reduce stigma; mass media involvement; evaluation of education
Supplies and equipment	Location of the CHBC team; health-center supplies; management, monitoring, and record keeping; home-based care kits
Staffing	Supervising and coordinating CHBC; recruitment; retaining staff
Financing and sustainability	Budget and finance management; technical support; community funding; encouraging volunteers; pooling resources; out-of-pocket payments; free services
Monitoring and evaluation	Quality assurance; quality-of-care indicators; monitoring and supervision; informal evaluation; formal evaluation; flexibility

Source: WHO, *Community Home-Based Care in Resource-Limited Settings*, 34.

Meanwhile, in a key document on HIV/AIDS policy, the Kenyan Ministry of Health described the work of community health workers as follows:

> The CHWs' role is ever expanding to assist vulnerable families with food production and food security by referring the most vulnerable to emergency food programmes. They also link clients, caregivers and mature orphans with programmes that train or assist in food production. Strong links with microfinance programmes and income generating activities have been established for HBC recipients and families to help clients, caregivers, and guardians of orphans and vulnerable children (OVCs) with economic support. Strong links with health facilities and community-based support programmes have evolved, thus strengthening the 2-way referral system between community home-based care programmes and local health facilities.[26]

Like many other kinds of community-based projects, home-based care consisted of a wide range of practices and meanings simultaneously: a multiplicity that was necessary to make home-based care viable for the diverse groups who came together around it.[27] This multiplicity is partly what has enabled home-based care to remain a central part of HIV policy despite dramatic shifts in the organization of HIV care since 2006, allowing a change in emphasis to slightly different enactments of home-based care (from a focus on palliative care to concerns around drug adherence) while retaining an overall sense of coherence. However, equally significant in relation to this particular ensemble of practices is that its ability to enroll actors emerges from a long history as a modality of engagement with the domestic in this part of Kenya.

Women's Groups and Health Care in Historical Context

Across Africa, women's groups and other forms of voluntary association have a long history as "technologies" of government.[28] Throughout the colonial era, the domestic arena was understood as an appropriate and important site of intervention for governments and missionaries. The colonial encounter changed the domestic realm immeasurably, influencing everything from the shape of homes—which became square rather than round—and those things considered appropriate goods to buy for the home, to the manner in which and to whom one should be married, to how many children a woman should have and where and how she should have them.[29] Women were understood as key to domestic development, and as part of endeavors to achieve this, women's education in the colonial period revolved almost entirely around domestic science and homecraft.[30]

In 1940s Kenya, the training of women and the need to influence behavior in people's homes became the responsibility of social welfare officers. Social welfare was understood as central to economic development and as something that would be achieved "[f]rom the bottom up. The official line was that through associations, clubs and committees people could do this for themselves in their own way, receiving 'maximum of inspiration' and 'minimum of oversight.'"[31] By the 1950s, such clubs and associations had proliferated, and the gendered role of these kinds of groups was cemented in a range of tasks linked to women and the home. Consider the following suggested list of meeting topics prepared by the Department of Community Development

for Maendeleo ya Wanawake (Women's Progress/Development) meetings in the 1950s:

    1. bathing a baby

    2. health and hygiene in the home

    3. agriculture—rotation of crops

    4. children's play, training in character building

    5. clothing—choice of suitable clothes for climate, etc.

    6. how to build a mud stove (if the women have their own house)

    7. child welfare

    8. hygiene and health in the home

    9. recipes or cooking demonstration

    10. agriculture-compost and compost pits

    11. handwork [sic] or needlework demonstration

    12. tea party and concert

    13. talk on current affairs

    14. literacy classes should be held in addition to the club meeting[32]

The Maendeleo ya Wanawake (hereafter MYWO) clubs remain the
most famous women's groups in Kenya. Started by the wives of settlers
and government administrators in the early 1950s, the clubs were initially hugely popular, particularly in Nyanza Province, which had almost
ten thousand members by 1954.[33] In a series of activities that would be
echoed by future home-based care initiatives, activities in MYWO clubs
included instruction in child care, cleanliness, health and hygiene, farming, and the making of handicrafts for sale.[34] Church-based women's
groups such as the Mother's Union (an Anglican women's group widespread in Africa) also have histories of large membership across western
Kenya, and the configurations of contemporary women's groups—of all
kinds—owe much to Christian dogma and the legacies of the missionary endeavor.

    The argument that postcolonial development thought and interven-
tion is the legacy of a set of practices, structures, and ideas that became
hegemonic through the colonial period is made eloquently in Joanna
Lewis's historical study of administrative thought and the implementation of colonial welfare policy in Kenya from 1925 to 1952.[35] Lewis
identifies a broad-reaching legacy of ideas, practices, and infrastructure,

which include notions of the socialistic nature of "African" community (where communities by nature function for the good of all) and the preference for self-help as an instrument of intervention, which continue to underpin current conceptualizations of home-based care. Lewis argues that the social welfare programs introduced by the Colonial Office for 1940s Kenya were "built on two platforms: the modernized form of state intervention designed to regulate people's lives, and the traditional ways in which the labouring classes had collectively organized themselves . . . to improve their economic and political status through co-operative societies, social clubs and savings groups."[36]

Perhaps the best-known example of activities in Kenya that have built these assumptions is *harambee*. "*Harambee*," a Swahili term meaning "Let's pull together," was Kenyatta's rallying cry at independence. The harambee movement has successfully drawn upon ideals of community and the value of self-help in the achievement of development. Building upon traditionalist notions of communal labor, harambee activities were central to the building of community facilities, especially rural health facilities and schools, in the period immediately following independence.[37] Harambee fundraisers continue to be arranged in Kenya for everything from the payment of hospital bills and school and college fees to the improvement of schools and hospitals.[38]

While the object of intervention (HIV/AIDS) is relatively new, many of the assumptions underpinning home-based care about the nature of community and the value of the domestic sphere as a site of developmental intervention are much older. Public health projects around HIV/AIDS are influenced by the forms that previous interventions took, forms that are embedded in people's memories and have traveled through social practices and institutions such as MYWO, which continues to operate a branch office in the center of Kagot town and to which many of the members of Kagot Development Group, including Elizabeth, belong.

Women's Groups, Patron-Client Politics, and the Distribution of Resources

Although often idealized, in the Luo context the social configurations of associational life do not represent an egalitarian communalism. Involvement in groups tends to underline hierarchies of power, wealth, and flows of material resources, marking out sites for the development of individual distinction. Women's groups and similar kinds of association have long provided opportunities for people to play upon the complex dynamic between benefits to the self and the sustenance of broader networks of support and solidarity, within the context of changing governmental interventions.[39] For example, *harambee* meetings and financial contributions at weddings and funerals can emphasize an egalitarian ethos but are simultaneously "competitive donations."[40] Money and other items offered at such events are documented meticulously and contributions are read aloud to those present. These proceedings underline gradients of power and responsibility as attention is drawn to generous individuals and groups through public offerings.

Hierarchies are also articulated through more informal arrangements for collectively pooling agricultural labor. Plowing teams that form to share their resources will always plow the fields of those who own the plow and cattle before they plow those of people who merely assist them in their enterprise, often after the optimum time for plowing and planting.[41] As one informant explained of her son's attempts to earn a living through fishing, "Fishing is good if you have nets, lamps and boats, but if you are just having your hands it is not so good."

Like many other people in Kagot, most of the women involved in Kagot Development Group belonged to several different groups. Their involvement in groups fluctuated over time, reflecting the benefits they accrued by being a member of the group; the amount of time and money they were expected to contribute (sometimes group leaders required people to invest financially before joining); and whether they trusted the leader of the group to deliver promises and not to "eat" (that is, embezzle) money that belonged to the group.

In Kagot, groups often evolved into a power base for the individuals who led them. Analysts of Kenya's political economy identify patron-client politics, marked by the exchange of resources for political support, as a key motif of the postcolonial Kenyan state.[42] This is a pattern that repeats in the micropolitics of associational life. Group leaders are expected to procure resources for the group and to share them out fairly. In return, group members offer their names for membership lists, which demonstrates the size and importance of the group; attend meetings; and praise group leaders in public. Persila once complained, "There is a saying in Kenya that the wise eat the foolish [*Jofuwo gin chiemb jorieko*]. I tell you, Hannah, in Kagot Development Group we are the foolish!" She went on to complain about Elizabeth and Philomena, "They don't share the resources of the organization properly. Elizabeth used to be thin, but since starting Kagot Development Group she has become fat—but when we go to the office there is nothing!"

Despite these drawbacks, groups provided possibilities to make strategic connections outside immediate kin groups and offered access to valuable resources. In Kagot Development Group, the availability of donated objects was greatly appreciated by members; gifts of maize, beans, blankets, water storage containers, and school uniforms were received with gratitude and also became markers of success at negotiating the micropolitics of associational life. Furthermore, groups were sites of potential education. One informant had an envelope stored securely in the dresser of her sitting room bursting with prized certificates for training in everything from community nutrition and home-based care to the distribution of contraceptives and public speaking. Meanwhile, Purity, Joyce, and Beatrice had all used their growing connections as community health workers to start up profitable businesses selling pharmaceuticals. Nurses whom I worked with earlier in my fieldwork exclaimed, "Ay! Elizabeth Oyoo has become famous!" when I told them I was now doing research with her, for they were impressed at Elizabeth's ability to make connections and obtain resources through her group.

Ann Swidler and Susan Cotts Watkins have recently described people's involvement as volunteers within development projects in rural Malawi as a search for distinction, arguing that many involved in such groups aspire to leave the village rather than to live in it.[43] They point to contradictions between the individual aspirations of participants in development projects and presumptions of egalitarian reciprocity within "local communities." Building upon their insights, I argue that the ambitions of people involved in community-based health and development initiatives should further be understood as part of broader processes of differentiation that take place *within* villages. Located primarily within the framework of the small-scale politics of women's and other kinds of community-based groups, home-based care was enacted through modes of practice with deeply entrenched histories, along well-trodden paths shaped by aspirations for individual improvement.

Engaging Home-Based Care

Beyond the possibilities opened up in terms of local politics, involvement in home-based care linked women into relationships with wider extensions, articulating both connectivity and difference as it did so. Like many other community-based projects, home-based care felt "local" yet drew upon highly charged moral categories that were in much wider circulation. Home-based care entailed a range of conceptual connections to different international discourses, including the primary health agenda that stems from the Alma Ata declaration, the hospice movement, the experiences of initiatives such as TASO (the AIDS Support Organization) in Uganda, and the specific history of responses to the HIV epidemic in Africa—and elsewhere—which has enabled the organization of a range of public health and development interventions around a specific illness. Home-based care also involved more tangible connections through flows of resources from international NGOs, documentary tools that traveled outside of Kagot, and concrete relationships. For these women, such relationships included not only involvement with a British anthropologist—whom Elizabeth sometimes described as being "on attachment" at Kagot Development Group—but also, in 2005, a visit from the then UK secretary of state for international development, Hillary Benn.

Interested in "how universals work in a practical sense," Anna Lowenhaupt Tsing employs the concept of the "engaged universal" as a way of analyzing how categories employed across a variety of contexts work at the level of the specific to make actions meaningful.[44] Among Kagot Development Group members, recourse to international discourses created the sense of an involvement in a broader enterprise, which—in part—shaped a framework for group members to delineate "proper" modalities of home-based care. Thus, alongside concerns about poor medical services and strictly demarcated norms of care provision within families, particularly around expertise in managing the hands-on care of the dying body, women in the group encouraged their home-based care clients to "learn how to manage stress" and to eat "nutritious" food that was "affordable, accessible and available." The engagement of "universal" notions of sustainability and self-sufficiency and the use of developmental buzzwords by women in Kagot Development Group marked contours of power within home-based care that were morally and politically charged through relationships to other (often "developed") places.[45] Appearing to be strategically placed in these relationships to the outside world, involvement in home-based care had the further effect of rendering the women who worked within the group as themselves "developed" people.

Working through the intersection of the micropolitical processes of associational life and the global connections engendered by localized engagements of home-based care, women involved in Kagot Development Group therefore did not see themselves as doing the work of the state (or NGOs) at huge personal cost. Rather, doing home-based care was a means of making themselves visible so that they might be able to access the resources of the state (and the international development community) in exchange for their time and effort, and also a means of being drawn into the state's processes of legibility.[46] As I argue in the previous section, women's groups and similar associations have developed in part through their ability to materialize (often literally) relationships to the state. Building upon this history, activities such as the use of monitoring forms that "went up to NASCOP" were viewed promisingly by group members as demonstrative of greater involvement with the Ministry of Health and the growing importance of their group. Meanwhile, links to powerful political actors were seen as potential avenues for channeling the resources of the state down to individual group members.

Domestic Distinction

Also central to the way in which home-based care was engaged locally was its profound domestication. Success for Kenyan women seems necessarily to combine achievements in the domestic sphere (that is, as mothers) and extradomestically. Therefore, while powerful women do not carry out domestic tasks themselves, as wives and mothers they are responsible for managing the execution of domestic tasks effectively. Elizabeth employed "office girls" at Kagot Development Group partly because this constituted the proper management of menial work, such as cleaning, by a group leader.

For women in Kagot Development Group, doing home-based care allowed them to demonstrate achievements in the management of the domestic arena alongside connections to a wider political sphere. These women had come of age during a period of relative prosperity in Kenya. They had watched some of their female contemporaries complete secondary school and gain prestigious jobs as teachers and nurses for the postcolonial state. Although they themselves had not managed such attainments, they used their involvement with groups, churches, and similar organizations to access the resources of the state and NGOs as part of (albeit precarious) attempts to develop distinction by aligning themselves with progress, development, and education.

In Kagot, involvement in women's groups was one aspect of broader attempts to promote individual development and success alongside strategies to build connections with people within and outside one's own community. These individual achievements were further embodied in projects such as building a house with a tin (rather than grass) roof and sending one's children to school and perhaps ultimately to university and even overseas. Women's search for distinction through groups was thus thoroughly entangled with the prosperity of the home and the achievements of children. Introducing me to an old woman who had been active in the Mother's Union for more than twenty years, my informant gestured at the woman's clean, tidy sitting room full of well-cared-for furniture; "Don't you see that this is the house of a Mother's Union member!" she remarked enthusiastically.

In the context of a particular history of domestic governmentality, involvement in the activities of women's groups in western Kenya has thus become deeply intertwined with successful domestic management and women's status. In Kagot Development Group, doing home-based care became a marker of achievement in a context in which individual agency, the strategic management of networks of supportive others, and connections to the outside world were seen to demonstrate "development."[47] In an uncanny echo of the activities of MYWO during the 1950s, home-based care activities at Kagot Development Group were linked to concerns around power, status, and resources that were wider than the domestic. Yet through an association with a gendered domestic realm that encompassed, was produced by, and was aligned with women's responsibilities to care for family members and manage domestic processes, this broad range of activities became classed as "women's work" and as valuable pursuits for those women who did them. Such engagements were not without paradox, however: they transformed home-based care simultaneously into a move toward being a modern "developed" person while remaining an "appropriate local technology," or "just the care that people are giving at home." Something old, and something new.

Many recent contributions to the anthropology of development, policy, and the state have been influenced by Foucault's essay "Governmentality."[48] A key insight of this literature is that governmental practices bring certain realms of intervention into existence.[49] Using the example of home-based care in western Kenya, I argue in this chapter that the "rendering technical" of the domestic is a governmental project with substantial longevity.[50] This longevity exists not only in the way that the domestic sphere is imagined and mobilized but also in the ways in which those people who become positioned as the targets and agents of such projects have responded to these interventions and incorporated them within wider concerns of everyday life. What has been successful both in earlier inventions and in contemporary public health projects such as home-based care in this part of Kenya is the way they have complemented women's efforts to demonstrate their individual development and attempts to build supportive networks by joining and leading groups that are active beyond their immediate kin relations.

One signifier of the success of the synergy between governmental and personal concerns is the repeated bringing together of a range of different activities that are loosely linked to the home but extend beyond it, for example, into political domains. The broad repertoire of practices engaged around home-based care range from income generation activities to nutritional interventions, farming, and support for orphaned children. These divergent activities, which in an absolute sense have little in common, come together within these regimes of domestic governmentality so easily partly because they all gain traction within the synergistic space afforded by the meeting of governmental intervention and women's interests.

Furthermore, this set of practices is also powerful because of a longevity of correlation; these activities were put together previously and now appear to belong together. They are flexible enough to incorporate new ideas and practices, new methods of documentation and engagement with the state. At the same time, they are easily recognizable as activities that are to be done for or by women and relate to the management of the domestic sphere and to sites of opportunity for women's individual progress. "New" policies around HIV in western Kenya thus speak to enduring practices of domestic governmentality that date back to the colonial encounter and the "community development" initiatives of British colonial administration in Kenya dating from the 1940s,[51] as well as to long-term conceptions of individual gendered progress, even as they speak of a relationship to the rest of the world. Recognizing the embedded and relational texture of contemporary public health projects in Africa is particularly relevant to our understanding of public health in Africa today, because it is precisely within this tension between the old and the new that home-based care gains its power and traction as a public health intervention.

Acknowledgments

The Economic and Social Research Council generously funded the fieldwork and PhD scholarship upon which this chapter is based. I am grateful to all the members of "Kagot Development Group" who welcomed me into their organization. I also thank my collaborators at the Population Studies Research Institute, University of Nairobi, Lawrence Ikamari and the late A.B.C. Ocholla-Ayayo. I would like to thank Maia Green, Sarah Atkinson, Thomas Grisaffi, Pablo Jaramillo, Ruth Prince, Rebecca Marsland, and Wenzel Geissler for critical comments.

Notes

1. Joanna Lewis, *Empire State-Building: War and Welfare in Kenya, 1925–52* (Oxford: James Currey, 2000).

2. The fieldwork with Kagot Development Group was part of a wider piece of PhD fieldwork carried out during 2005–7.

3. NASCOP, *Kenya AIDS Incidence Survey 2007 Preliminary Report* (Nairobi: National AIDS and STI Control Programme, 2007), 14–15.

4. WHO, *Community Home-Based Care in Resource-Limited Settings: A Framework for Action* (Geneva: World Health Organization, 2002), 6.

5. Women's groups in this part of Kenya sometimes involve men as well as women, particularly at the higher levels of the organization.

6. Bethwell A. Ogot, *Politics and the AIDS Epidemic in Kenya, 1983–2003* (Kisumu: Anyange Press, 2004), 83–88, 96–99.

7. In the area I describe in this chapter, following a short period during which antiretroviral therapy was available only to those who could afford to pay a subsidy at the district hospital, first-line antiretroviral treatment was made free to those who met eligibility criteria in March 2006.

8. For the formalization of home-based care, see WHO, *Community Home-Based Care: Action Research in Kenya, September–October 2000* (Geneva: World Health Organization, 2001); Ministry of Health, Kenya, *Home-Based Care for People Living with HIV/AIDS: National Home-Based Care Programme and Service Guideline* (Nairobi: National AIDS/ STD Control Programme, 2002), hereafter cited as Ministry of Health, *Home-Based Care Service Guideline;* Olagoke Akintola, *Policy Brief: The Gendered Burden of Home-Based Care-Giving* (Durban: Health Economics and HIV/AIDS Research Division [HEARD], University of KwaZulu Natal, 2004); WHO, "Community Home-Based Care in Resource-Limited Settings"; Ministry of Health, Kenya, *Reversing the Trends: The Second National Health Sector Strategic Plan of Kenya—NHSSP II—2005–2010* (Nairobi: Ministry of Health, 2005), 24–25; John Iliffe, *The African AIDS Epidemic* (Oxford: James Currey, 2006), 110–11. For comprehensive HIV care, see Ministry of Health, Kenya, *AIDS in Kenya: Trends, Interventions and Impact,* 7th ed. (Nairobi: Republic of Kenya, 2005), 46–57. For care across a continuum, see WHO, *Key Elements in HIV/ AIDS Care and Support* (Geneva: World Health Organization / UNAIDS, 2000); Jessica Ogden, Simel Esim, and Caren Grown, "Expanding the Care Continuum for HIV/ AIDS: Bringing Carers into Focus," *Health Policy and Planning* 21, no. 5 (2006): 333–42.

9. Ministry of Health, Kenya, *Home-Based Care for People Living with HIV/AIDS: Home Care Handbook; A Reference Manual for Home-Based Care for People Living with*

HIV/AIDS in Kenya, 2nd ed. (Nairobi: National AIDS/STD Control Programme 2006), hereafter cited as Ministry of Health, *Home-Based Care Handbook;* see also Ministry of Health, *Home-Based Care Service Guideline.*

10. E.g., Olagoke Akintola, "Gendered Home-Based Care in South Africa: More Trouble for the Troubled," *African Journal of AIDS Research* 5, no. 3 (2006): 237–47, esp. 237; Alison Wringe et al., "Delivering Comprehensive Home-Based Care Programmes for HIV: A Review of Lessons Learned and Challenges Ahead in the Era of Antiretroviral Therapy," *Health Policy and Planning* (2010): 352–62, esp. 354.

11. Iliffe, *African AIDS Epidemic,* 98–111.

12. Soori Nnko et al., "Tanzania: AIDS Care—Learning from Experience," *Review of African Political Economy* 86 (2000): 547–57; Ogden, Esim, and Grown, "Expanding the Care Continuum."

13. Ogden, Esim, and Grown, "Expanding the Care Continuum," 23. See also Anesu Makina, "Caring for People with HIV: State Policies and Their Dependence on Women's Unpaid Work," *Gender and Development* 17, no. 2 (2009): 309–19; Akintola, "Gendered Home-Based Care"; Elsbeth Robson, "Invisible Carers: Young People in Zimbabwe's Home-Based Healthcare," *Area* 32, no. 1 (2000).

14. James Ferguson, *Global Shadows: Africa in the Neoliberal World Order* (Durham, NC: Duke University Press, 2006). For a similar perspective, see Jean Comaroff and John L. Comaroff, "Millennial Capitalism: First Thoughts on a Second Coming," *Public Culture* 12, no. 2 (2000): 291–343. This phenomenon is also elaborated by those who seek to describe the broader tenets of the "neoliberal turn" as it has played out around the world; see, e.g., David Harvey, *A Brief History of Neoliberalism* (Oxford: Oxford University Press, 2005), 177–79.

15. Julie Hearn, "The NGO-isation of Kenyan Society: USAID and the Restructuring of Health Care," *Review of African Political Economy* 25 (1998): 89–100.

16. Maxine Molyneux, "The 'Neoliberal Turn' and the New Social Policy in Latin America: How Neoliberal, How New?" *Development and Change* 39, no. 5 (2008): 775–97; Andrew Kipnis, "Neoliberalism Reified: Suzhi Discourse and Tropes of Neoliberalism in the People's Republic of China," *Journal of the Royal Anthropological Institute* 13, no. 2 (2007): 383–400.

17. Michel Foucault, "Governmentality," in Michel Foucault: *Power,* 201–22, vol. 3 of *Essential Works of Foucault, 1954–1984,* ed. James D. Faubion (London: Penguin, 2002 [1978]). Here I am particularly thinking of scholars whose work engages with the way similar practices of government are articulated across different versions of the state rather than through an evolutionary unfolding of different types of government as in the original Foucauldian imaginary. See, e.g., Tania Murray Li, *The Will to Improve: Governmentality, Development and the Practice of Politics* (Durham, NC: Duke University Press, 2007); Donald S. Moore, "The Crucible of Cultural Politics: Reworking 'Development' in Zimbabwe's Eastern Highlands," *American Ethnologist* 26, no. 3 (1999): 654–89.

18. See Meinhert's chapter 4, this volume.

19. Kagot is a pseudonym. This meeting took place in September 2006 and was typical of the many such meetings I attended at this organization in 2006 and 2007. All personal names are also pseudonyms.

20. They were trained by Mildmay (an NGO) and the Ministry of Health.

21. The contribution, 150 shillings, at the time of the fieldwork was equivalent to approximately £1.20 or one of the following: 2 kilograms of sugar, 1.5 kilograms of beef, or two bags of maize flour. Thus, it was a considerable amount of money for these women.

22. The community health workers had all been given micro loans of 500 shillings, approximately £3.20 at the time of the fieldwork. The loans were funded by the African Medical and Research Foundation.

23. I have translated this exchange into English, but the women all switched between English and Luo. For example, in the sentence from Elizabeth in which she describes some kinds of opportunistic infections, she worded it like this: "*gin kaka diep* chronic, chronic cough, *kaka* spots, *kaka* vaginal discharge." Septrin is the local brand name for the antibiotic co-trimoxazole, used in HIV care as a prophylaxis for some common opportunistic infections. Thinking deeply in this community is not a sign of academic propensity but is thought to be a sign of depression.

24. The money for transportation came from an NGO, Mildmay. The drugs (highly valued items in a community where many people have very limited buying power in the cash economy) largely came from a smaller NGO. Access to these funds and items was highly valued and a significant factor in the women's regular attendance at meetings. Elizabeth and Philomena spent much of their time writing proposals for small grants to continue such work.

25. In addition to literature cited earlier in this chapter, see, e.g., Phyllis Orner, "Psychosocial Impacts on Caregivers of People Living with AIDS," *AIDS Care* 18, no. 3 (2006): 236–40; Walter Kipp et al., "How Much Should We Expect? Family Caregiving of AIDS Patients in Rural Uganda," *Journal of Transcultural Nursing* 18, no. 4 (2007): 358–65; Hannah Brown, "Living with HIV/AIDS: An Ethnography of Care in Western Kenya," unpublished doctoral thesis, University of Manchester, 2010, chap. 3.

26. Ministry of Health, *AIDS in Kenya*, 57.

27. Maia Green, "Making Development Agents: Participation as Boundary Object in International Development," *Journal of Development Studies* 46, no. 7 (2010): 1240–63; Rebecca Marsland, "Community Participation the Tanzanian Way: Conceptual Contiguity or Power Struggle?" *Oxford Development Studies* 34, no. 1 (2006): 65–79; Susan Leigh Star and James R. Griesemer, "Institutional Ecology, 'Translations' and Boundary Objects: Amateurs and Professionals in Berkeley's Museum of Vertebrate Zoology, 1907–39," *Social Studies of Science* 19, no. 3 (1989): 387–420.

28. Michel Foucault, "Space, Knowledge and Power," in *The Foucault Reader: An Introduction to Foucault's Thought*, ed. Paul Rabinow, 239–56 (London: Penguin, 1991).

29. Kenda Mutongi, *Worries of the Heart: Widows, Family and Community in Kenya* (Chicago: University of Chicago Press, 2007), 59–60, 77, 135–38; Jean Comaroff and John L. Comaroff, "Home-Made Hegemony: Modernity, Domesticity, and Colonialism in South Africa," in *African Encounters with Domesticity*, ed. Karen Tranberg Hansen, 37–74 (New Brunswick, NJ: Rutgers University Press, 1992); Lynn M. Thomas, *Politics of the Womb: Women, Reproduction and the State in Kenya* (Berkeley: University of California Press, 2003); Nancy Rose Hunt, *A Colonial Lexicon: Of Birth Ritual, Medicalization and Mobility in the Congo* (Durham, NC: Duke University Press, 1999); Janice Boddy, "Remembering Amal: On Birth and the British in Northern Sudan," in *Beyond the Body Proper: Reading the Anthropology of Material Life*, ed. Margaret Lock and Judith Farquhar, 315–29 (Durham, NC: Duke University Press, 2007), esp. 321.

30. Lewis, *Empire State-Building*, esp. 52–68; Mutongi, *Worries of the Heart*, 119–21.

31. Lewis, *Empire State-Building*, 313.

32. Cited in Audrey Wipper, "The Maendeleo Ya Wanawake Organization: The Co-optation of Leadership," *African Studies Review* 18, no. 3 (1975): 99–120, list from 100.

33. Audrey Wipper, "The Maendeleo Ya Wanawake Movement in the Colonial Period: The Canadian Connection, Mau Mau, Embroidery and Agriculture," *Rural Africana* 29 (1975); 197–201; Lewis, *Empire State-Building*.

34. Wipper, "Maendeleo Ya Wanawake Organization."

35. Lewis, *Empire State-Building*.

36. Ibid., 75–76.

37. Barbara P. Thomas, *Politics, Participation and Poverty: Development through Self-Help in Kenya* (Boulder, CO: Westview Press, 1985), 8; Robert Maxon, "The Kenyatta Era, 1963–78: Social and Cultural Changes," in *Decolonization and Independence in Kenya: 1940–93*, ed. Bethwell A. Ogot and William R. Ochieng', 137–38 (London: James Currey, 1995); Martin J. D. Hill, *The Harambee Movement in Kenya: Self-Help, Development and Education among the Kamba of Kitui District*, London School of Economics Monographs on Social Anthropology 64 (London: Athlone Press, 1991). Hill also traces *harambee* to a colonial history of forced labor.

38. However, contemporary *harambee* seem to be less about emphasizing the idea of working together toward making Kenya a better stronger country (as was partly true in the period after independence) and more about coming together to help an individual or shared community facility as well as allowing wealthy Kenyans and politicians to build up networks of support.

39. E.g., Henrietta L. Moore, *Feminism and Anthropology* (Cambridge, UK: Polity, 1988), 155–64.

40. David Parkin, *The Cultural Definition of Political Response: Lineal Destiny among the Luo* (London: Academic Press, 1978), 216.

41. See Parker Shipton, *The Nature of Entrustment: Intimacy, Exchange and the Sacred in Africa* (New Haven, CT: Yale University Press, 2007).

42. E.g., Bruce J. Berman, "Ethnicity, Patronage and the African State: The Politics of Uncivil Nationalism," *African Affairs* 97, no. 388 (1998): 305–41; Roger Southall, "Re-forming the State? Kleptocracy and the Political Transition in Kenya," *Review of African Political Economy*, no. 79 (1999): 93–108.

43. Ann Swidler and Susan Cotts Watkins, "'Teach a Man to Fish': The Sustainability Doctrine and Its Social Consequences," *World Development* 37, no. 7 (2009): 1182–96, esp. 1189–90.

44. Anna Lowenhaupt Tsing, *Friction: An Ethnography of Global Connection* (Princeton: Princeton University Press, 2005), 7.

45. The process of recognizing oneself as "developing," or as a "development category" with a relationship of a particular kind to the "developed" world, has been debated by anthropologists. See, e.g., Stacy Leigh Pigg, "Inventing Social Categories through Place: Social Representations and Development in Nepal," *Comparative Studies in Society and History* 34, no. 3 (1992): 491–513; Akhil Gupta, *Postcolonial Developments: Agriculture in the Making of Modern India* (Durham, NC: Duke University Press, 1998).

46. In an inverse or response to the kind of practices of "seeing" described by James C. Scott in *Seeing Like a State: How Certain Schemes to Improve the Human Condition Have Failed* (New Haven, CT: Yale University Press, 1998), I was prompted to think about the dynamics of such inversions of processes of governmental visibility by Alice Street, "Seen Like a State: Transparency and Visibility in a 'Failing' Papua New Guinea Hospital" (paper presented at the conference "Hospital Ethnography: Institutions, Collaborations and Power," University of Sussex, 2009).

47. See Maia Green, "Participatory Development and the Appropriation of Agency in Southern Tanzania," *Critique of Anthropology* 20, no. 1 (2000): 67–89.

48. E.g., Cris Shore and Susan Wright, "Policy: A New Field of Anthropology," in *Anthropology of Policy: Critical Perspectives on Governance and Power*, ed. Cris Shore and Susan Wright, 3–34 (London: Routledge, 1997); Li, *Will to Improve*; Michael Watts,

"Development and Governmentality," *Singapore Journal of Tropical Geography* 24, no. 1 (2003): 6–34.

49. E.g., Scott, *Seeing Like a State;* Timothy Mitchell, *Rule of Experts: Egypt, Techno-Politics, Modernity* (Berkeley: University of California Press, 2002); Nikolas Rose, *Powers of Freedom: Reframing Political Thought* (Cambridge: Cambridge University Press, 1999).

50. For "rendering technical," see Li, *Will to Improve,* 7–8.

51. Lewis, *Empire State-Building;* Hill, *Harambee Movement in Kenya,* 23–29.

SIX

Technologies of Hope

Managing Cancer in a Kenyan Hospital

BENSON A. MULEMI

CANCER IS A GROWING PUBLIC HEALTH PROBLEM IN KENYA. HOWEVER, it is invisible at many levels: there is little government funding, and timely diagnosis is rare. The preventive measures, acute treatment technology, and care advances that are available in developed countries have not yet materialized in Kenya. This is due to insufficient resources such as infrastructure and trained personnel, as well as the unaffordable cost of chemotherapy drugs and other treatment technologies. The current focus of global health is on the "big three" preventable infectious diseases—tuberculosis, HIV/AIDS, and malaria—together with the "neglected" tropical diseases and not the prevention and management of cancer. In Kenya, the cancer problem is not on the Ministry of Health's list of priorities, even though it is the third leading cause of death after infections (including HIV) and cardiovascular diseases.[1]

The severity of the cancer situation in Kenya is worsened by the fact that cancers are often not diagnosed or are diagnosed too late. Too often, a patient must follow a long therapeutic path, in which district or even provincial health-care providers, who do not have the requisite levels of expertise, may make many incorrect diagnoses before cancer is identified. As a consequence, referral for treatment in hospitals often occurs at a late stage. When this happens, the symbolic value of the relatively advanced medical technologies available at the referral hospital generates hope in patients that their health will be restored. Sadly, even at this stage, the lack of diagnostic tools and treatments and the late presentation contribute to tensions between patients, their families, and hospital staff about how to manage treatment and care and how much or little information to communicate to the patient about his or her condition. Despite these drawbacks, all the actors in the management of the disease—families, nurses, doctors, and other hospital personnel—strive to keep hope alive, by emphasizing the potential of medical technology to cure cancer. The dominant message is that patients must acquiesce to treatment and cultivate the strength to endure the arduous treatment and care regimes. Cancer ward staff work hard to help patients achieve this with a variety of techniques designed to keep hope going in the most difficult circumstances.

This chapter is based on ethnography in a cancer ward, in Kenyatta National Referral Hospital (KNH), conducted between July 2005 and August 2006 with follow-up visits in 2007 and 2010. KNH is the largest public referral hospital in Nairobi and offers one of the few cancer clinics in the Kenyan public health system. It is often full, with long queues of desperate patients seeking admission and routine outpatient treatment. In this chapter, I examine the struggles of patients and their families, as well as doctors and nurses, to treat cancer in the context of limited resources, high costs of treatment, and low awareness about the disease. I trace how divergent and even conflicting forms of knowledge about cancer treatment and care shape how people—medical staff, patients, and their families—attempt to transform cancer from a mystery into a condition that is knowable and can be acted upon, often despite much less optimistic realities.

Medical staff often know when treatment is hopeless but regularly persist with it to prolong a patient's (false) hope. The tension between the desire to instill hope and the realities of the ability of medical science to cure cancer is not unique to Kenya. Not all cancers can be cured even in resource-rich countries, where there has also been debate about the advantages and disadvantages of communicating bad or uncertain news to patients, and the consequent effects on health outcomes.[2] Good communication behavior has been documented to have positive impacts on patient health outcomes.[3] In their desire to seek treatment, using the best available technology, families often insist on drastic treatments up until the end of the patient's life, even when this increases suffering. Nurses look for alternative solutions to the suffering endured by patients pursuing treatment against all odds, sometimes by recommending alternative therapies such as African or Chinese traditional medicine or by redefining the goals of successful care, aiming to improve the quality rather than the length of life. In these most constrained of circumstances, patients, their relatives, and medical staff struggle to find a balance between promoting hope of recovery and reducing suffering. Hope is an important aspect in attempts to understand the success or failure of disease prevention and treatment programs.[4] Health-care interventions produce varying degrees of hope, which shape challenges that face disease management initiatives and patient care struggles.

The Cancer Crisis

Records at the Nairobi Cancer Registry and at KNH indicate that diagnoses of new cancer cases in Kenya have doubled in the past decade; 82,000 new cases are reported annually, yet hospital treatment facilities are limited.[5] The five most common types of cancer, in order of incidence, among men are esophagus, prostate, non-Hodgkin's lymphoma, liver, and stomach cancers.[6] Cervical and breast cancers are the most common among women. Ovarian, non-Hodgkin's lymphoma, and stomach cancers also have a high incidence rate relative to other cancers afflicting women in Kenya.[7] Patients suffer protracted morbidity that undermines their quality of life, and many die from cancers that are preventable and manageable elsewhere in the world.

This picture, in which cancer has been invisible in both statistics and health policy, can be traced to the colonial era, when the incidence and frequency of the disease was assumed to be relatively low in African countries.[8] Indeed, until recently, cancer was thought to affect only the developed and industrialized world, an assumption out of step with the present reality of developing countries such as Kenya.[9] Despite the fact that cancer first emerged as a public health problem in Kenya in the late 1940s, coinciding with a steady flow of reports about the disease in Africa after the Second World War,[10] it remains a low-profile disease with minimal budgetary allocation for treatment, research, and registration today.

Kenyatta National Hospital began treatment of cancer through chemotherapy in the 1960s, but the first full-scale cancer research was conducted about ten years later in 1979, by Dr. Edward Kasili, whose studies suggested that cancer caused 20 percent of all adult and 9 percent of child deaths in Kenya.[11] His work highlighted how the suffering of people with cancer in Kenya was shaped by the difficulties of nursing chronically ill patients at home and the inadequate diagnostic and treatment procedures in regional hospitals. His observation that pain relief was grossly inadequate because effective analgesics are not available and that most doctors simply do not know what to do still hold true today.[12] Kasili was also one of the first to point to the usually fatal delays leading to treatment, a problem that is often compounded by poverty.[13]

The low priority afforded to cancer in the colonial period continues in health policy today. A national cancer control program was established in 1994 by the Ministry of Health, but it received little funding and was soon neglected. Just twelve hospitals provide cancer care, and these are in only four out of eight of Kenya's provinces. There were five clinical oncologists in Kenya during the main period of the ethnography, and this number has now increased to about twenty, most of whom are based in Nairobi. The numbers of pathologists and specialized radiographers are also low. Outside of the private sector, key medical technologies, especially radiotherapy machines, are found only in KNH. Inadequate supplies of effective analgesics in regional health facilities and in district and national hospitals continue to blight the care of terminally ill patients.

Rural health facilities or even district hospitals do not have any form of cancer expertise or diagnostic technologies, and so only a very small proportion of cancer patients arrive at KNH for specialized treatment.[14] Ms. Kadi,[15] whose brother was a patient on the ward, talked about the situation of patients she believed to be suffering from cancer in Thika District, which is one of the nearest rural catchment areas to KNH. The district hospital at Thika was hardly equipped to provide proper cancer diagnosis and treatment: "They keep the patients waiting and then at the end they refer them here (KNH) . . . when the disease has already eaten someone. One patient's cheek had been covered with a piece of cloth. You could see so many terrible wounds. . . . So I thought, is it not better for them to tell him to go [to another hospital] instead of dying on the queue? He came back late with a piece of cloth to wipe the pus, just saying there was no money [for treatment]" (Ms. Kadi, 11 May 2005).

KNH deals with enormous numbers of referral cases of relatively poor patients from government and private hospitals all over the country and beyond. Once they arrive, they are faced with overcrowding, low quality of care, and shortages of medical equipment and supplies, which hampered the efforts of the committed, well-trained staff.[16] The diagnostic tests and treatment machines that are available to them are unreliable, and to complicate this, professionals frequently hold divergent views about appropriate cancer care. As a result, the most accessible therapies—chemotherapy and radiotherapy—valuable for the management of conditions such as breast cancer are grossly underutilized.[17]

During the ethnography, hospital staff estimated that the cancer treatment center at KNH receives between 3,000 and 4,000 patients annually, but it did not have enough human and technical resources to handle the workload. The cancer ward admitted patients with head and neck, breast, cervical, colon, colorectal, prostate, esophageal, and gastric cancers. The hematology, obstetrics, and gynecology departments manage the other types of cancer. The cancer ward caters to patients on chemotherapy, radiotherapy, the two therapies combined, and supportive care. Supportive care includes intravenous feeding, handling chronic wounds, and general palliative care. The ward has five rooms and only thirty-two beds. About 150 patients seeking admission were reviewed at the clinic over a period of about one month, but only 32 could be admitted each week. The average length of stay for patients was between seven and fifteen days, but some stayed for over a month. Repeated hospitalizations were typical of the cancer treatment and care process. However, some patients had more frequent hospital visits and admissions than others, because of chronic pain, metastasis of cancer, and opportunistic infections acquired both in the hospital and during respite periods at home.

Data from the ethnography indicated that patients' social backgrounds, divergent caregivers' views about cancer management, livelihood vulnerability, and abilities to sustain subsequent treatment influenced treatment follow-up practices. This scenario contributed to the phenomenon of "unpopular decisions" that characterized treatment uncertainty, as I explain below. In addition, the daily experiences of patients and their caregivers in the hospital confirmed the reality of inadequate treatment follow-up duration. Hope for the survival of cancer patients became dismal with each treatment and admission.[18] Different actors in the hospital deployed different strategies to maintain hope and encourage patients to stick to the treatment program.

Hospital Ethnography of Cancer Management

Observation and informal conversations with patients, their families, and staff members at the KNH cancer ward were the main methods of data collection. I also conducted focused in-depth conversations and (recorded) interviews. The first part of the ethnography involved conversations with inpatients, their relatives, and hospital staff as well as observation in the adult cancer ward and the Cancer Treatment Centre. All the patients in the cancer ward and treatment center were participants, but only forty-two gave in-depth narratives of their lived experiences. The second part of data collection entailed follow-up home visits of ten patients to explore how they coped with cancer after or between hospitalization sessions.

Initial Hope in the Cancer Ward

The situation at KNH and its cancer ward is bleak. KNH is the only public health facility that offers chemotherapy and radiotherapy to both inpatients and outpatients. Only one of two radiotherapy (cobalt) machines was operational during my ethnography, and it was stretched beyond its capacity. Because of the overwhelming number of cases that needed radiotherapy, the machine handled 150 patients a day, instead of the recommended 40. The hospital's radiotherapy waiting list was about 500 and was increasing. The earliest that patients referred for chemotherapy would get their first session would be after about three months. Thus, arrival at KNH for both inpatients and outpatients introduced yet further delays as patients waited for diagnosis to be confirmed and treatment to begin. Despite this, many patients initially felt optimistic about the cancer ward's promise of proper treatment and care: "Their main interest is recovery. They come here with a hope that everything that was not possible elsewhere would be possible here. They believe that Kenyatta National Hospital is the only institution that holds their hope in life, since it is the biggest [hospital] within East and Central Africa. . . . So they have the belief that being sent here means that they will be healed. They believe that cancer is cured after one is admitted to this ward" (Mr. Bob, enrolled nurse, 10 May 2006). Like other cancer ward staff members, Mr. Bob remained silent about his reservations regarding patients' optimism. He reaffirmed the nurses' perception that "cancer by itself is a unique disease . . . It is a disease which is not treatable." Cancer ward staff members were dealing with people for whom prognosis was poor and treatment probably useless. The purpose of instilling hope in the patients was to facilitate therapeutic cooperation for any possible improvement in well-being.

Near the staff-changing room in the cancer ward is an ominous space labeled "private room," where bodies of patients who die lie before a porter takes them to the mortuary. The high frequency of use of the private room was a reminder of the low survival rates of cancer patients. Many patients feared going past it to their shared toilet and the nurses' desk. These grim facts were not obvious to patients and their kin when they first arrived, and despite or even because of their long and difficult therapeutic history, they felt fresh hope: "I was expecting that I would be diagnosed accurately. . . . Now I have been told that it is possible to cure the disease, because of the facilities in Kenyatta [Hospital]. . . . My expectations were that after [the initial courses of] treatment I would go back home a fully healed person to continue with normal life. . . . My hope is that I will be healed and continue with normal work, to serve my family, my church, and my community . . . and continue working until retirement age in good health" (Mr. Jabari, age 49, 10 February 2006). The patients' typical estimation of uninterrupted chemotherapy time was four to six months to complete the six courses, which they initially believed would cure them. These expectations would typically dwindle as they experienced the suffering and tensions that are part and parcel of treatment and care decisions at KNH.

Maintaining Hope in the Face of Uncertainty

Cancer incidence underreporting, missed diagnoses, and undertreatment during previous health-seeking trajectories were evident in narratives and experiences of patients who arrived at KNH. One, for instance, said, "Doctors would tell me it is malaria. . . . Then they referred me to the district hospital, where they told me, 'Oh! It is typhoid!' . . . They referred me to a bone specialist, . . . then to another referral [hospital]. . . . The doctor could not help because the referring doctor was senior to him. . . . He referred me back to our [district] hospital. . . . After surgery, the 'doctor did not see the disease.' . . . He took a small piece of flesh back to a Russian doctor. . . . 'He is the one who was good at looking.' . . . He said, 'Ah! . . . Where were you?'" (Mr. Kassi, age 64, 10 August 2005).

The national referral status of KNH embodies expertise and technology, and so patients initially expect it to be a place that will provide accurate diagnoses and offer adequate treatment. Patients and their families often entered the cancer ward with renewed hope, buoyed by their observations of well-attended consultant ward rounds and elaborate laboratory examinations. The biomedical technology and teamwork that the patients encountered at KNH were not available in facilities they had visited earlier. Their hope could be identified in their expectations of a precise identification of the primary cause of different cancers, prognosis, and proper treatment, all of which reinforced their idea of the hospital as an epitome of the power and "magic" of biomedical science.[19] Yet this hope quickly led to disappointment. Treatment decisions tended to take longer, machines did not function properly, and cancer treatments turned out to be increasingly arduous for already fragile bodies. Consider a patient's comment: "Even these people, . . . the doctors themselves, do not believe in their machines. . . . They may tell you go to the university [for more] laboratory tests. . . . [But] when you bring the results they say, 'No, we must compare it again,' . . . so they say, 'Go to Nairobi hospital' [for similar tests]. . . . They don't trust their own machines here. . . . So we wonder if the machines here are faulty" (Mr. Kassi, 12 August 2005). Patients and their relatives depended on the hospital professional staff to provide more knowledge and information that would reduce the mystery of cancer, to make it more knowable and manageable. Before arriving at KNH, patients typically experienced uncertainty, as the following excerpt shows:

> [It] started with the left breast. It came from the neck, and I did not know it would come to the breasts. . . . When I went to hospital they told me it was typhoid, and I was given medicine for typhoid. I was told it is that disease in milk and meat [brucellosis], and I was treated for it. . . . I was told it was flu or cold . . . and was treated. . . . I was told it was cerebral malaria. . . . I went to hospital a lot, and I took a lot of medicines. . . . I went and told them, I was put[ting] Norplant on this side. . . . They removed it. So I went and told [them I] was feeling a big gland [lump] in the breast. . . . It has not yet been removed. (Mrs. Gatoro, age 40, 3 October 2005)

However, the slow pace, missing results, and repeated diagnostic procedures led to disappointment and feelings of uncertainty about treatment and the likelihood of recovery. Many patients felt that laboratory tests and examination results were underutilized, especially when hospital staff did not refer to the tests they had ordered in subsequent therapeutic activities. Furthermore, there were difficulties in patient care communication, supervision, and proper monitoring of care and treatment activities. Some pharmacy interns and nurses set the intravenous chemotherapy apparatus but did not return to monitor the progress. On occasion, patients would bleed at points where intravenous lines were fixed, or the chemotherapy drugs would not flow consistently as expected, while other patients complained of swelling arms and delays in removing the chemotherapy lines.

Faced with this disillusionment and increased suffering, staff and relatives deployed a range of methods to prolong hope. Despite the considerable tensions around treatment and care decisions, health professionals saw the hospital and cancer ward as both a medical and a moral space that could inspire patients' determination to get well. They wished to encourage patients to "fight on" and sustain their determination to get through often-arduous therapy. The strategies they employed to achieve this were diverse and often contradictory, sometimes unwittingly increasing the suffering and anxiety of patients. Clinical staff would resort to what they described as "unpopular decisions" that went against protocol in order to help patients cope; both relatives and cancer ward staff struggled with communicating bad news to patients for fear that it would lead to despair, and nurses redefined the goals of cancer therapy—by referring patients to alternative practitioners and aiming to improve quality of life rather than pursuing unrealistic hopes of cure.

Unpopular Decisions

Junior hospital staff were left to their own devices to make treatment decisions, many of which the senior staff often openly contested and even reversed when they turned up. This complicated cancer treatment uncertainty as patients frequently witnessed tensions between junior and senior staff regarding patient care practices. Senior staff, such as consultant oncologists, for instance, rescinded their juniors' decisions about treatment, hospital discharge, or extension of hospitalization time on many occasions. The senior staff were often alert about what they dubbed "unpopular decisions" in cancer treatment. A decision was unpopular with main participants in patient treatment—clinical and patient support staff, and patients, by extension—when they perceived the decision as contradicting conventional protocol, observed lived experiences of patients, and the moral obligation to mitigate suffering. Senior staff scolded their juniors when they made unpopular decisions but were unable to recognize or stop implementation of similar decisions of their own. "Unpopular decisions" included sending patients for radiotherapy before they completed the recommended courses of chemotherapy, as well as ordering unnecessary laboratory tests. Some disagreements among hospital staff about medical and nutritional care were obvious to patients, even when they could not follow care and treatment discussions couched in medical jargon and the English language.

However, on many occasions, treatment and patient care alternatives were limited. Therefore, there was a silent expectation that hospital staff in the lower levels of the medical hierarchy would condone unpopular decisions made by senior staff. Senior staff relied on these measures as a last resort to cope with professional helplessness in the face of chronic cancer illness and to sustain hope among patients and their families. The following excerpt from my field notes partly illustrates this: "It is Friday, the day for the weekly consultant ward round. An oncology consultant announces that he is about to make an 'unpopular decision.' The patient on bed 18 is just finishing the first round of chemotherapy, but the doctor recommends that he be taken for radiotherapy 'marking' on Monday due to the continued swelling of his cheek. For the consultant and other ward round participants, this is an unpopular decision because typically, they conventionally expect a decision about radiotherapy to be made after completion of the required six sessions of chemotherapy" (5 December 2005). The consultant decided to terminate chemotherapy prematurely when it became apparent that the patient's condition was worsening despite the treatment. Consultants and other senior staff occasionally announced "unpopular decisions" to their colleagues during treatment and review procedures to preempt open opposition. Announcing such decisions implied that the consultants were aware of inherent contradiction but would proceed to implement them as a last resort when they had run out of other acceptable options. Some of the treatment decisions that generated silent or covert tension included "helping patients to abscond treatment or hospitalization." This occurred when doctors facilitated patients' exit from the hospital because they perceived that any further treatment was futile. Some decisions to change cancer treatment drugs, discontinue radiotherapy in order to start chemotherapy (and vice versa), or undertake radical interventions such as surgery were unpopular. The outcome tended to increase the suffering of already desperate patients.

Unpopular decisions reflected either inaccuracy in diagnosis and choice of treatment regimens or medical staff members' helplessness in the face of chronic illness and scarce resources. Doctors and other staff on occasion confessed to each other that they did not know what to tell patients who were in distress. A doctor, for example, reported to his colleagues during a ward round how his colleagues and he helped patients abscond treatment in such circumstances in the past:

> We could assess the patient in the first week of admission and if we found that he/she could not pay, we would help them abscond. . . . If the patient cannot pay and we are not doing anything for him/her, we would discharge them, give them the fare and tell them to go home. . . . You can help the patients to abscond in such a case. We would give them fare and escort them to the bus stop! That would save the hospital a lot of money if you help them abscond. . . . There is no need keeping the patient, doing nothing for him, yet he is eating. . . . You end up discharging him anyway, but who pays the other bills? (Dr. Samani, 6 June 2006)

Patients abscond treatment when they withdraw and terminate it clandestinely or without official release. Patients who are "assisted to abscond" after waiting for a long time for results of numerous diagnostic tests were often asked to "go home and rest" because "nothing was being done" for them. In such cases, doctors would indicate that they discharged a patient temporarily, pending a future review date, which they did not communicate to the patients. In view of the above extract, clinical staff would superficially ask patients to return for review or treatment, in principle, yet it was apparent that some patients would not make it back, because of their socioeconomic and physical vulnerability. They were given an appointment for clinic review after one to three months. This granted beset clinical staff some break from dealing with challenging desperate cases. Patients who could not afford the drugs and admission fees for timely care follow-up returned to the hospital or cancer ward in more critical condition, which posed a further challenge to available biomedical technology.

Sustaining the Will to Live

Hospital staff consistently wished to inspire hope even for cases whose outlook was apparently desolate. This seemed to be a method of ensuring therapeutic cooperation and hope for any possible improvement in well-being of patients. Some nurses, clinical staff, and patients alike testified that some patients who had seemed hopeless had their health revived, "miraculously," after sustained arduous treatment, assisted by what appeared to be their "will to live." Therefore, instilling hope was a way of protecting this will and determination to endure treatment, even to the end of life. This attitude underpinned the belief that cancer treatment technologies would be most effective when God worked with them. Maintaining one's belief in technology was reinforced by a belief in God and demonstrated the strength of one's faith. A miraculous recovery came from God's intervention as a reward for this demonstration of faith. Patients, their relatives, and medical personnel held on to hospital treatment as a method of hope—and they often persisted on hope in treatment, as in other circumstances of hope in adversity, despite experiences to the contrary.[20]

Thus, the maintenance of hope was a technique used to keep patients' focus on improving their health to give them the strength to endure the unpleasant side effects of treatment. Patients devised a "discourse of hope" regarding drastic interventions such as mastectomies, amputations, colostomies, and artificial rehabilitation technologies, which both alleviate and increase physical, social, and existential suffering.[21] Doctors also encouraged patients to interpret unpleasant or painful sensations as signs that the body was healing. For instance, they assured patients that pain was an ephemeral effect of either the inherent biochemical processes of effecting cure or the resistant responses of cancer cells as they succumb to the treatment.

Nondisclosure of Diagnosis and Treatment Prospects

Follow-up visits to KNH in 2007 indicated that lack of adequate cancer diagnosis and treatment knowledge among hospital health-care professionals continued to be an issue after admittance to the cancer ward. Moreover, there were tensions around communication about cancer and its management. While hospital staff shared information among themselves, they tended not to disclose diagnosis and prognosis to patients, often at the insistence of family members, who sometimes fought battles with staff to keep information from patients. This was mainly to safeguard patients' hope and treatment endurance and to prevent suicidal thoughts. A young woman diagnosed with nasopharyngeal carcinoma, for example, complained about a ward physician's unwillingness to reveal his diagnosis:

> He did not give me the information about the diagnosis. . . . Maybe he revealed [it] to my brother. . . . This is perhaps because the first doctor who had done the biopsy did not disclose what the exact disease was. . . . I went through the results and suspected cancer. . . . I was surprised he had told them [family members] and not me. . . . But they told me, "No, he has told us it is not cancer." . . . I forced

him to disclose the information to me. But I had given up. I had even wanted to commit suicide and had even bought the *triatix* poison. (Ms. Marina, age 24, 17 October 2006)

An oncologist acknowledged dilemmas about disclosure of cancer diagnosis and treatment prospects: "Unfortunately, a majority of the doctors don't inform patients that they have cancer. They just tell them, 'You have a growth and you need radiotherapy.' . . . The family tries to hide the information from the patient. . . . They say, 'No, they will know they are going to die, or they will be depressed.' . . . Sometimes they come to the doctor and say, 'Please, we know that he/she has cancer but don't tell that patient,' . . . but we still believe that the patient has the right to know what is happening" (Dr. Matina, 10 May 2006). In KNH, medical personnel and patient support staff understand the fact that cancer patients' hope is that there is a cure and they will make a full recovery. I found that although cancer patient caregivers in the hospital must deal with great uncertainty in the face of inadequate technologies, resources, and capacity, they made great efforts not to communicate their uncertainty, helplessness, and hopelessness in dealing with incurable or advanced cancer. Mrs. Ndunduri, for instance, had been in the cancer ward for over two months after being admitted with a condition diagnosed as squamous cell carcinoma. However, medical records indicated that the primary cause of her cancer had not yet been diagnosed. She often felt bitter toward the hospital caregivers for failing to provide adequate pain relief and treatment: "Then they saw that disease and they gave me some medicine. They told me this disease of yours is 'defeating the doctor.' . . . And I told that doctor, 'You are [a] doctor with high qualifications, tell me the things you should tell me. . . . If you see it is the disease you cannot treat and that I will die, just tell me [and] I [will] go home to die.' I am waiting for nothing here" (Mrs. Ndunduri, age 56, 19 September 2005). Exactly a month later, on 19 October 2005, Mrs. Ndunduri's son also complained that the doctors did not tell him about the prognosis of his mother's illness. For him, "there [was] guarded information," which the medical staff did not wish to disclose. He was aware that the primary cause of his mother's cancer type had not been identified, despite her prolonged hospitalization. He had been given a letter that he would take to the hospice so that the hospice staff could come to counsel his mother on the next course of palliative care. Mrs. Ndunduri, according to her son, expected to get well quickly on admission to KNH. This hope had not materialized, and she gradually became angry with and bitter toward doctors, whom she felt were not telling the truth about her illness.

Most nurses said that they were not permitted to talk about cancer diagnosis and prognosis to patients and relatives, unless a physician or consultant oncologist had already disclosed the news. Nurses feared that if they did so, they would be blamed if disclosure resulted in adverse reactions, such as absconding treatment or suicidal thoughts among patients. Meanwhile even among other hospital staff members, case discussions showed divergent and occasionally conflicting views.

Some patients overheard and either understood or misunderstood information about their condition. The words or expressions used to describe cancer conditions turned out to have significant effects on the process of patient care and the ability to sustain hope. On occasion, patients could read expressions of despair on the faces and hear it in discussions of hospital staff members. They were also alert to the fact that medical staff would not always agree about treatment decisions and choices. Clinical personnel often treat patients as passive parties to treatment and care encounters. Patients' voices, desires, and appraisals of therapy and care are marginalized during medical procedures and ward rounds. Several patients in the cancer ward, for instance, frantically tried calling doctors or nurses back for unanswered questions. Insufficient information and communication with patients aggravated despair, anger, and resistance.

Inadequate clarifications about effects of cancer and treatment—such as inability to eat or concurrent illnesses such as "ulcers," constipation, and mouth sores—worsened despair. This also worsened compliance when patients developed fears that their treatment might not be efficacious or even safe. However, because of the complicated nature of cancers, medical staff would not always have ready answers and information to help patients cope with their concerns. Doctors and nurses were often reluctant to divulge precise information not only because they lacked time, or because they did not consider the patient's point of view, but also because they did not know. They also concealed information from the patients because the news was rarely good news; treatment prognoses were usually ominous. Patient caregivers feel obliged to protect patients from bad news. This partly defines the context of the uneasy collusion among carers to keep guarded realistic cancer treatment information.

Giving information always involved, for the medical staff, a painful adjustment of patients' expectations to the often-grim reality not only of prognosis but also of the form of treatment that was actually available to them. Thus, what patients sometimes saw as a callous refusal to explain was partly due to staff members' identification with their pain and suffering and desire to protect them from the effects of knowing the details of their poor prognosis. Clinical staff hesitated to explain cancer treatment facts. They reserved information about the lethal effects of chemotherapy, for example, the possibility that chemotherapy drugs can destroy both cancerous and healthy body cells. Similarly, some patients and family members who insisted on continuing drastic treatment were not adequately informed about potential damage that chemotherapy could cause on body organs, such as the liver, kidneys, heart, and lungs. Many patients discovered only from informal talks among themselves that radiotherapy could also "burn" tissues and cause wounds or sores. For many patients, perceived negative effects of cancer treatment technology circulated among them as menacing rumors. These included perceptions about the possible failure of hospital treatment to cure cancer and the futility of prolonged chemotherapy and radiotherapy to eliminate tumors totally. In such instances, limited communication about treatment outcome intended to protect patients' resilience has the opposite effect of heightening uncertainty, fear, and disillusionment.

Cancer proved a mystery to patients, not only because of the difficulty of detecting it in most Kenyan medical facilities but also because of the absence of straightforward treatment regimens. As patients continued treatment, experiencing related pain and suffering, they revised their view of the technology. Some patients even speculated that clinical trial medicines were being used and that this was the reason for the high death rate in the cancer ward. Others believed that being treated with appropriate medicine and receiving good care was conditional on their relationships with hospital staff. Therefore, they strove to maintain the role of a trusting, cooperative, uncomplaining, and undemanding patient, to increase the prospect of receiving favorable treatment and care.[22]

Despite the best efforts of medical staff and relatives to conceal biotechnological truths from patients in order to maintain hope and compliance, there were many cases in which patients interrupted treatment on their own volition, as they could no longer bear the debilitating side effects. Several patients, for instance, resisted "medicines that hurt," which they hid after pretending to take them. Others would stop taking prescribed medicine and decided not to return to the hospital for scheduled appointments because of their perception that medical expertise would be futile in attempts to restore their health. Ms. Stella, a breast cancer patient, had been hospitalized for over five months for recurrence and metastasis. She decided not to buy the prescribed medicine for the next course of chemotherapy and did not intend to go back to the hospital: "Perhaps this is for 'enhancement chemotherapy.' . . . But I fear the medicine would kill me. I am tired. I wonder why chemotherapy is endless. I will stop the chemotherapy and continue with Chinese [medicines]" (Ms. Stella, age 47, 8 October 2005). Some patients' families and caregivers acted on the illness through continued treatment, even beyond the stage when it was useful. Hospital staff often sought to conceal information from patients that would have discouraged them from continuing to undergo treatment. Medical staff found this frustrating, yet they too struggled with the question of how and whether to tell patients the full extent of their diagnosis and prognosis. In doing this, they sought to safeguard the hospital as a symbol of hope for cancer victims.

Protecting the Hospital as a Symbol of Hope

There is often a stigma attached to working with patients whose prognosis is poor. Some cancer management hospital staff believed that colleagues in other units did not recognize their role in overall health improvement. For them, maintaining hope helped them to justify to themselves and others why they continued to take care of patients whose prognosis was already predetermined, or people who were "half dead," as some patients described themselves.[23] Doctors and nurses in such circumstances felt that they had a moral obligation to protect the image of the hospital, available technology, and patient care spaces as symbols of hope. They wished to protect confidence in biomedical technology and the hope this typically inspires among ordinary people.

Doctors in Kenya prefer to say very little to patients about their cancer management. In this context, informal interactions among patients, their kin, and hospital staff in lower hierarchies, such as nurses and ward assistants, reshape the discourse on hospital management of cancer, its potential to restore health, and limitations of available technology. Nurses and other hospital staff participate in this discourse because they want to hold the hospital space of hope open. This may account for the concealed resort to alternative therapies in the course of cancer treatment in the Kenyan hospital. This is part of a process in which patients and other participants seek to redefine cancer therapy and draw on available resources that may contribute to the desired synergy for management of cancer through biomedical technology.

Redefining Therapy

Simultaneous or sequential patterns of resort to hospital management and alternative therapy with the facilitation of nurses further defined the quest to boost hope in hospital treatment of cancer.[24] In the Kenyan cancer ward, nurses' and patients' experience of inefficacy, debilitating side effects, and having to "continue fighting on" reduced their faith in the biomedical management of cancer. Nurses' experience with taking care of chronically ill patients and cancer patients' experience of the disease unfold the limitations of biomedical technology as the main approach to restoration of health. Therefore, nurses recommended alternative therapies to increase the hope for positive outcome of hospital treatment. Thus, the hospital remains the arena of hope, where all possible strategies for the improvement of cancer patients' quality of life can converge for a fruitful synergistic interaction.

Unlike the clinical and other technical hospital staff, many nurses tended to attribute accelerated morbidity and mortality of cancer patients to the therapies available in the hospital, especially the toxicity of chemotherapy drugs. They associated surgical interventions with worsening bodily weakness. Nurses had to deal with increased suffering as part of their daily work. And so they sought therapeutic synergy or complementary care resources by encouraging patients and their families to draw on alternative therapies.[25] Doctors were aware of patients' use of alternative medicines and on occasion blamed these therapies for aggravating deterioration or treatment failure.

Nevertheless, nurses facilitated patients' clandestine resort to alternative therapies to increase prospects of positive outcomes of hospital treatment of cancer: "A nurse told me, 'This is the secret . . . this is the solution.' She said that here we give you chemo, but sometimes it does not work. She gave me the contacts of a 'doctor.' . . . When I returned to the ward, she asked me whether I had gone to see him, but when I said that I had not gone, she was disappointed. She said the 'chemos' are just chemicals. . . . She said the hospital may accuse her of spoiling their business" (Ms. Souda, age 40, 3 October 2005). Ms. Souda was readmitted for treatment of stage II cervical cancer and contemplated seeing the "doctor" dealing in African traditional medicine (ATM) and dietary supplements that two nurses had recommended to her. Nurses' attempts to link patients up with alternative therapies inside and outside the hospital were part of their own strategy of coping with the treatment and patient care crisis. Through this strategy, they strengthened their own hope and motivation to take care of patients with dismal prospects for survival or restoration of health.

Patients and their kin also resorted to traditional Chinese medicine (TCM) to substitute for or complement hospital treatment of cancer. TCM has become popular in Kenya's major urban areas as an important alternative health-care resource. Many respondents perceived TCM as effective in managing multiple illnesses, relatively cheap and having negligible negative side effects compared to biomedicine. In Dar es Salaam, Tanzania, TCM gained popularity among local residents because they perceived the medicine as an easy-to-consume and rapidly effective "advanced" "traditional" medicine because of its ready-made patent formula.[26] The proliferation of alternative remedies for cancer management is a free-market phenomenon in which people choose remedies they perceive as efficacious or contributing to therapeutic synergy within the rapidly growing medical pluralism in Kenya (see Whyte's chapter in this volume).[27]

Given the challenges to hospital management of cancer in Kenya, nurses defined successful patient care as having patients leave the hospital while still "whole" (even if they ultimately did not pull through), that is, walking and eating without support, talking, and without bed sores, while controlling anxiety and pain. Nurses saw their role as "adding life in their [that is, the patients'] days," rather than adding "[low-quality] days in their life" by means of biomedical technology. Nurses resorted to this adage to justify their cancer patient care efforts, including promotion of both biomedicine and alternative therapies in the ward, as part of their initiative to formulate a more realistic goal of cancer management. For nurses, job satisfaction depended on meeting patients' basic needs and, in the case of terminal illness, enabling a "good death." For nurses, cancer patient support professionals, and informal carers, a good death was characteristic of patients who would die with their skin and most of their body parts "intact" and not severely degenerated by the disease and treatment side effects. Similarly, quality of life in terminal cancer illness required minimizing the pain and suffering among patients and their families.

Curing, Caring, and Safeguarding Hope

Cancer management struggles at Kenyatta National Hospital in Kenya reflect the continuing challenge of cancer to biomedical science and technology. Insufficient human resources and medical facilities in Kenya contribute to the mounting hopelessness in cancer treatment, even after patients arrive at either public or private hospitals for proper medical care. When they arrive at the referral hospital for appropriate treatment and care, they are often already at an advanced stage of cancer but are full of optimism that they have found the right expertise to bring them back to health. As treatment progresses, patients undergo heightened physical deterioration, pain, and severe side effects. It is not surprising that patients struggle to stay positive under these conditions, and they must do so in a context in which the public perception is that cancer is incurable unless you have wealth and resources, in parallel to perceptions about HIV/AIDS in many African settings.[28]

In spite of or because of this, all the participants involved in managing cancer drew on strategies that were designed to safeguard hope. Clinical staff and relatives coped at times of crisis by discussing the disease, treatment, and prognosis among themselves, but they did not always choose to share this information with the patients, for fear of causing distress. Counter to their intentions, this choice to remain silent sometimes led to greater fear and anxiety among patients who could sense that bad news was being withheld. Clinicians sometimes resorted to changing treatment decisions against normal protocol to create an impression that more could be done. They encouraged patients to believe that pain and discomfort was a sign that the treatment was working. When a stay in hospital was causing unnecessary suffering, they even helped patients to "abscond." Nurses took a different approach, referring patients to alternative forms of therapy and moving the goals from cure to care. These strategies illustrate the lengths to which practitioners will go to sustain relationships of care.[29] This is a gesture of goodwill intended to improve the well-being of the sick.

Patients and hospital caregivers drew on a variety of sources of determination and hope despite many uncertainties about cancer treatment technologies. Examples of successful cases of hospital management of cancer inspired their hope. However, cancer and its management engender adversities that threaten to obliterate the hope. Proper treatment often coincides with intense suffering, which contradicts the hope people often associate with hospitals as symbols of the power of biomedical technology and science. Therefore, cancer management policy in Kenya should encourage earlier resort to palliative care to protect patients and their families from catastrophic effects of prolonged hospital treatment. Chronic terminal illness transforms the hospital into a space for convergence of different sources of hope, including biomedical technology. Patients, their kin, and nurses shared this perspective as they attempted to harness other resources for maintenance of hope and the synergy to complement biomedical interventions. Therefore, African and Chinese traditional medicine and faith healing find a complementary niche inside and outside the hospital to augment biomedical struggles for the improvement of cancer patients' quality of life.

The quests for hope in hospital cancer management in Kenya illustrate the crisis in caregiving that is experienced by professionals with limited access to resources.[30] The nurses' receptive stance about the use of alternative therapy in the cancer ward indicates the imperative for hospitals to open up to and tolerate alternative approaches to patient care. The cancer ward staff's persistence to protect hope against the odds demonstrates that the hospital is an intensely moral space—one in which the balance between hopelessness, suffering, and efforts to sustain optimism must be addressed every day. The hospital thus emerges as a stage where dramatic social and cultural divisions and moral dilemmas are played out against the backdrop of modern medicine's battlefield between life and death.[31]

Notes

1. Geoffrey Z. Mutuma and Anne Ruggut-Korir, *Cancer Incidence Report: Nairobi, 2000–2002* (Nairobi: Nairobi Cancer Registry, Kenya Medical Research Institute, 2006).

2. Jenenne P. Nelson, "Struggling to Gain Meaning: Living with Uncertainty of Breast Cancer," *Advances in Nursing Science* 18, no. 3 (1996): 59–76.

3. Neeraj K. Arora, "Interacting with Cancer Patients: The Significance of Physicians' Communication Behaviour," *Social Science and Medicine* 57, no. 5 (2003): 791–806; Elizabeth J. Clark, "Chemotherapy and the Issue of Patients' Rights," in *Psychosocial Aspects of Chemotherapy in Cancer Care: The Patient, Family, and Staff,* ed. Robert De-Bellis et al., 43–52 (New York: Haworth Press, 1987); Shelley E. Taylor, "Hospital Patient Behavior, Reactance, Helplessness or Control?" in *Interpersonal Issues in Health Care,* ed. Howard S. Friedman and M. Robin DiMatteo, 209–32 (Paris: Academic Press, 1982).

4. Astrid Blystad and Karen Marie Moland, "Technologies of Hope? Motherhood, HIV and Infant Feeding in Eastern Africa," *Anthropology and Medicine* 16, no 2 (2009): 105–18.

5. Human Rights Watch, *Needless Pain: Government Failure to Provide Palliative Care for Children in Kenya* (New York: Human Rights Watch, 2010).

6. Clare Sansom and Geoffrey Mutuma, "Kenya Faces Cancer Challenge," *Lancet Oncology* 3, no. 8 (2002): 456–58.

7. Ibid.; Mutuma and Ruggut-Korir, *Cancer Incidence Report.*

8. Frederick L. Hoffman, *Mortality from Cancer throughout the World* (Newark, NJ: Prudential Press, 1916).

9. D. Maxwell Parkin et al., "Part I: Cancer in Indigenous Africans—Burden, Distribution, and Trends," *Lancet Oncology* 9, no. 7 (2008): 683–92; Paolo Boffetta and D. Maxwell Parkin, "Cancer in Developing Countries," *CA: A Cancer Journal for Clinicians* 44, no. 2 (1994): 81–90.

10. C. A. Linsell, "Cancer Incidence in Kenya, 1957–63," *British Journal of Cancer* 21, no. 3 (1967): 464–73.

11. John Iliffe, *East African Doctors: A History of the Modern Profession* (Cambridge: Cambridge University Press, 1998), 142–43, 177–78.

12. Ibid.; E. D. Kasili, "Leukemia in Kenya," MD thesis, University of Nairobi, 1979; J. F. Onyango and I. M. Macharia, "Delays in Diagnosis, Referral and Management of Head and Neck Cancer Presenting at Kenyatta National Hospital, Nairobi," *East African Medical Journal* 83, no. 4 (2006): 85–91.

13. Kasili, "Leukemia in Kenya."

14. E.g., Onyango and Macharia, "Delays in Diagnosis."

15. I use pseudonyms to refer to study participants throughout this chapter.

16. David Collins et al., "Hospital Autonomy: The Experience of Kenyatta National Hospital," *International Journal of Health Planning and Management* 14, no. 2 (1999): 129–53; David Collins, Grace Njeru, and Julius Meme, *Hospital Autonomy in Kenya: The Case of Kenyatta National Hospital; Data for Decision Making Project* (Boston: Harvard School of Public Health, 1996); Kenyatta National Hospital, *Strategic Development Plan, 2005–2010* (Nairobi: Kenyatta National Hospital, 2005).

17. N. A. Othieno-Abinya et al., "Post-surgical Management of Patients with Breast Cancer at the Kenyatta National Hospital," *East African Medical Journal* 79, no. 3 (2002): 156–62.

18. Similar findings hold for the follow-up of breast cancer patients at KNH; see ibid.

19. Alice Street and Simon Coleman, "Introduction: Real and Imagined Spaces," *Space and Culture* 15, no. 1 (2012): 4–17; Benson A. Mulemi, "Patients' Perspectives on Hospitalization: Experiences from a Cancer Ward in Kenya," *Anthropology and Medicine* 5, no. 2 (2008): 117–31.

20. Hirokazu Miyakazi, *The Method of Hope: Anthropology, Philosophy, and Fijian Knowledge* (Palo Alto, CA: Stanford University Press, 2004), 9.

21. Mary-Jo DelVecchio Good et al., "American Oncology and the Discourse on Hope," *Culture, Medicine and Psychiatry* 14, no. 1 (1990): 59–79.

22. Judith Lorber, "Good Patients and Problem Patients: Conformity and Deviance in a General Hospital," *Journal of Health and Social Behavior* 16, no. 2 (1975): 213–25.

23. Benson A. Mulemi, *Coping with Cancer and Adversity: Hospital Ethnography in Kenya* (Leiden: African Studies Center, 2010).

24. Allan Young, "The Relevance of Traditional Medical Cultures to Modern Primary Health Care," *Social Science and Medicine* 17, no. 16 (1983): 1205–11.

25. In Tanzania, nurses have likewise been found to help patients gain access to traditional medicines. See Stacey Langwick, "Articulate(d) Bodies: Traditional Medicine in a Tanzanian Hospital," *American Ethnologist* 35, no. 3 (2008): 428–39.

26. Elisabeth Hsu, "'The Medicine from China Has Rapid Effects': Chinese Medicine Patients in Tanzania," *Anthropology and Medicine* 9, no. 3 (2002): 291–313.

27. Patients and their families would be blamed for substituting cancer medications with patented nutritional supplements. Such supplements are marketed by Golden

Neolife Diamite (GNLD) and Tianshi companies. GNLD is an international company that has attained global popularity for supplying health supplements. Many people in Kenya today associate nutritional supplements with faster recovery and healing from chronic illness. Some nurses and patients were marketing agents for the supplements in the hospital. Tianshi is a competitor to GNLD and uses biotechnology to mix traditional Chinese health regimes and modern medical material.

28. The construction of AIDS not only as incurable but also as an untreatable condition without hope, in South Africa, for instance, accounts for people's inclination not to undertake HIV tests or even use antiretroviral therapies; see Isak P. Niehaus, "Death before Dying: Understanding AIDS Stigma in the South African Lowveld," *Journal of Southern African Studies* 33, no. 4 (2007): 845–60, esp. 860.

29. Fredrick Klaits, "Faith and Intersubjectivity of Care in Botswana," *Africa Today* 56, no. 1 (2009): 3–19.

30. Ibid., 17.

31. Street and Coleman, "Introduction," 9–10.

PART THREE

Emerging Landscapes of Public Health

SEVEN

The Publics of the New Public Health

Life Conditions and "Lifestyle Diseases" in Uganda

SUSAN REYNOLDS WHYTE

IT WAS ONLY RECENTLY, ON DIABETES DAY, THAT I LEARNED THAT diabetes is a lifestyle disease. It is for the rich. The rich can buy medicine and get better. But even we poor people get diabetes, and we can't afford medicine.

Mr. Ajaliboye, the man who spoke these words at a meeting of the Gulu Diabetes and Hypertension Association, touched on the issue of class in relation to chronic disease. This chapter follows his lead by exploring the relevance of social and economic differences to "lifestyle diseases" in Uganda. Social differences—between rich and poor, urban and rural, more and less educated—play out in relation not only to treatment but also to the causes and prevention of diseases such as hypertension and diabetes.

Epidemiologists have focused on these differences far more sharply than have anthropologists. They relate the rapid increase in chronic noncommunicable diseases in Africa in part to rising rates of overweight and obesity, which in turn are connected to socioeconomic factors. A review of surveys in seven African countries showed that prevalence of overweight/obesity in women was three times higher in urban than in rural areas. Focusing on trends over time, the authors show that within a twelve-year period, prevalence rose by 35.5 percent in urban populations. While prevalence was consistently highest in wealthier women, the increase was greater among poorer women. Even more striking, prevalence increased by about 50 percent in women with only primary or no education, while it fell by almost 10 percent among women with higher education.[1] But how do people conceive of such differences in relation to the rising tide of diabetes and cardiovascular disease?

On the basis of fieldwork in Kampala, in rural eastern Uganda, and in Gulu town in northern Uganda, I describe how positioned members of the public perceive the causes, prevention, and treatment of chronic noncommunicable diseases (NCDs).[2] The basic assumption is that the "publics" of public health are multiple. Health promotion messages appeal to the more cosmopolitan public, which is also better able to access treatment. Exploring this differentiation ethnographically is particularly urgent at the current juncture in Uganda's history. Given the lack of government programs and donor support, prevention and treatment of NCDs are left to an assortment of private initiatives and commercial interests that seldom reach rural and poorer people. Healthy practices, risk factors, and management of NCDs form a prism in which we as researchers, like members of these publics, can see differences and inequalities in contemporary Ugandan society.

At a global level, the growth of NCDs in low- and middle- income countries is recognized as one of the major health challenges of our time.[3] The World Health Organization (WHO) adopted a Global Strategy for the Prevention and Control of Noncommunicable Diseases at its fifty-third assembly in 2000 and endorsed an action plan for implementing it in 2008. The WHO is bringing together a wide variety of actors—including member states, businesses, NGOs, philanthropic foundations, and academics—to control cardiovascular disease, diabetes, cancer, and chronic lung disease.[4] The WHO and global health researchers point to the "double burden of disease," consisting of both infectious and noninfectious conditions, borne by countries where AIDS, tuberculosis, and malaria exist side by side with cardiovascular disease, cancer, and diabetes.[5] Yet in most African countries, government attention has thus far been directed almost exclusively at the infectious part of the burden.

Chronic conditions other than HIV/AIDS have as yet attracted little donor support, and in countries such as Uganda that are highly dependent on external funding for health-care programs, government seldom takes new health initiatives on its own. The situation with regard to diabetes and cardiovascular disease differs somewhat from the general pattern Prince describes in the introduction to this volume, in that NGOs do not play a major role either. Business, the media, and to some extent patient organizations are the principal advocates in matters of both prevention and treatment.[6] The kind of "lifestyle" they promote for prevention is mainly relevant for the Ugandan "working class," those fortunate ones who have salaries and are more educated and cosmopolitan. Likewise, the medication they market is too expensive for most people. The nominally free government health services provide insufficient care for people with chronic diseases other than HIV.

In countries of the Global North, particularly those with national health-care systems, there has been for decades an enormous emphasis on health promotion and minimizing the risks of chronic disease. The term *"new" public health* denotes a turn in policy that can be dated to the 1970s. The "new" arguably continued many elements of the "old" in that its chief characteristic was a heavy emphasis on health promotion and prevention, rather than cure. With a sharper focus on chronic noncommunicable diseases, what was new, as many scholars underline, was that responsibility for cultivating health and avoiding illness was cast as a matter for individuals. They are called upon to change their behavior, particularly in relation to diet, exercise, and consumption of alcohol and tobacco. Just as people in chronic treatment are assigned "homework" to be undertaken in the realm of everyday domestic life (see Meinert's chapter in this volume), so too are publics called upon to prevent disease by homely practices of monitoring bodies and changing lifestyles.

In the scholarly literature, the term *lifestyle* is challenged by critics who assert that life conditions, not lifestyles, are the fundamental problems. One review sees these along a spectrum: at one end are "collectivist" perspectives that relate inequalities in health to economic, political, and social structural factors; at the other are "individualist free market perspectives" that conceive of individuals as freely choosing lifestyle options.[7] Social and economic inequalities constrain the choices of many people, particularly in Africa. Their conditions of life are such that they do not freely decide what to eat, any more than they have the realistic option of buying the medicine that has been prescribed. This has implications for primary prevention but also for secondary and tertiary prevention aimed at avoiding further development of disease in those who have already been diagnosed.[8]

Health promotion campaigns almost invariably interpellate, or call to, some publics rather than others; that is, they appear relevant, possible, and appealing to certain segments of the population.[9] An apt example appeared in a Ugandan newspaper piece on healthy living that advised smaller, more frequent meals. Under a picture of two children and their smart, casual parents eating a lunch of sandwiches in a modern dining room was a box titled "A meal schedule for [the] working class."[10] Both the timing (that is, dinner at 6:00 pm) and the content (smoothies, nuts, fruit yoghurt, and oatmeal) of the suggested plan were clearly irrelevant to the vast majority of Ugandans. While some campaigns explicitly aim at a defined target group, many do so implicitly in that they call for measures that can most easily be realized by people of a certain means. The emphasis on lifestyle may itself become "a vehicle of social differentiation . . . [serving] to dislocate and disaggregate population sectors into targeted, bounded and discrete units."[11] Living a healthy lifestyle becomes a matter of distinction.

Biomedical Authority

Not until 2006 did the Ugandan Ministry of Health establish a unit for prevention and control of NCDs. This coincided with the launching of the second Health Sector Strategic Plan, in which, for the first time, goals and guidelines were set for the control of NCDs.[12] Because there were no reliable figures on the prevalence of NCDs in Uganda, documenting their extent was the first point in the new strategic plan. Yet by 2012 the survey had still not been carried out, and the head of the NCD unit had been interdicted for failing to move the program ahead.

Biomedical authorities link the spread of NCDs to aspects of modern life. In an article in the *Daily Monitor* (31 March 2008) entitled "That Junk Food Will Make You Diabetic," the NCD head officer is quoted as saying, "Urbanization has forced people to change their lifestyle and has exposed them to the risk factors of diabetes like eating junk food. . . . [M]ost families in urban areas feed on junk food, hardly do physical exercise or work like jogging and digging and have no balanced diet." Professor Marcel Otim, endocrinologist and chairman of the Uganda Diabetes and Hypertension Association, likewise named lifestyle and rising obesity in a recent speech: "People are changing their lifestyles. Many no longer exercise, they do not work and instead of walking, they are driven in cars" (*New Vision*, 27 November 2009).

These statements are in line with a recurrent theme in the new public health: that modern life is unhealthy. As Deborah Lupton writes: "There is thus a shift from viewing ill-health as caused by an infective agent such as a bacterium or virus, to ill-health as a product of society, in which illness is viewed as expressing the condition of a group as a social entity. Illness is conceptualized as a 'symptom of the pathology of civilization,' an outcome of the stresses and poor lifestyle choices of the members of modern societies, a sign that modern life is inherently damaging to health."[13]

The notion that cardiovascular conditions and diabetes are diseases of civilization or modernity is widely accepted by biomedical authorities. Steve Ferzacca writes of the "circumstantial" temporal perspective inherent in professional views of diabetes in Indonesia: "From the epidemiologic perspective, significations of insalubrious modernity and healthy tradition are measurable and coded in terms of human biology. Changes in body weight, life expectancy, food consumption patterns, levels of energy expenditure—important biological factors for the development of 'Western diseases'—index changing social and cultural forces. . . . Biological pathologies represent social and cultural pathologies related to change, and particularly related to the ambiguous shift from the traditional to the modern."[14] While such views on the etiological role of changing historical circumstances have overall currency among biomedical authorities, particular situations are also invoked by professionals in Uganda. Alice Lamwaka, clinical pharmacist and patron of the Gulu Diabetes Association, attributes the growing problem of Type 2 diabetes to greater longevity, malnutrition, overnutrition, hypertension, malaria, and HIV/AIDS and the drugs used to treat it. But most notably, she associates the rise of diabetes in northern Uganda with the insurgency and speaks of "Post-traumatic Stress Diabetes." In his Gulu speech, the minister of health picked up on this view: "What is causing diabetes in our people of northern Uganda, who were originally known to be a healthy population? The nearest scientific explanation could be stress, related to the over twenty years of insurgency and low socioeconomic status."[15]

Health workers in rural eastern Uganda agreed that NCDs were on the rise. One asserted that they were the real neglected tropical diseases. While some attributed this to changed eating habits and a few mentioned that prosperous people do not get enough exercise, they also considered other causes. Nurse Lucy, for example, pointed out that most diabetes patients in her rural area were not overweight. She thought there might be a link to HIV, but mainly she emphasized difficult life conditions: "The problem is stress because of school fees, extended families, low salary, the burden of looking after our old people." Her colleague, clinical officer Michael, mentioned several times that the pressure of work exacerbated his hypertension. Being in charge of the antiretroviral therapy (ART) clinic and going to so many workshops and meetings in that connection, in addition to his other duties at the understaffed hospital and his own private clinic, were too much.

Demotic Concerns

Demotic views expressed in rural eastern Uganda coincided to some extent with those of health professionals, but they reflected situated concerns even more explicitly—and some people were simply puzzled. Middle-aged and older informants spoke about the "new illnesses" of these days: "pressure" (hypertension, pronounced *plesha* in local languages), "sugar" (diabetes, called *sukari*), ulcer (*alusa*), cancer, and asthma. Particularly the first three were said to be increasing rapidly. Middle-aged and older rural people expressed some uncertainty about why this was so. Haji Habanga, a respected rural elder, expressed his puzzlement: "Pressure and diabetes are too much these last five years. Why? I used to think it was for the rich but now even poor people get it." Haji thought that pressure came from worries (many thoughts) and poverty. When I remarked that long ago people also had worries, he agreed, and said again, "We don't know the reason." He went on to speculate about why diseases of these days do not cure well, suggesting that maybe the medicine is no longer strong or maybe it is because of expired or fake medicine and corruption. His brother's son, the district education officer, joined the conversation and expressed the opinion, also held by others, that it had to do with changes in diet. Long ago, people had good, plentiful, and varied food including milk, chicken, and fruits. "But these days, unless you have money . . ." Haji's brother pointed out that those who did have money ate too much fatty food: "Meat has fat and you add in oil." One woman had heard from a visiting doctor that the new diseases were common because people no longer used the traditional salt made from plant ash (*omuherehe*—sometimes recommended to hypertensives as a replacement for salt). Others mentioned that people consumed too much cooking oil, sugar, soda drinks, and sweets from the shops. To this list Flora, a farmer and part-time tailor, added cold water from the refrigerator, expired items, and old bread and chapatis.

"The fatness of these days comes with sickness," observed one middle-aged woman, and the other five or six older people sitting around in the shade agreed. They gave examples of people in the neighborhood whose bodies were swollen and puffy and who must have pressure (though they had not been diagnosed by a health worker). Most of the less well-educated people who had an opinion on the cause of pressure said that it came from worry, grief, shock, and panic. They gave examples of how the unexpected loss of a close relative led to the onset of pressure. One made the connection to fat: "If you are fat and get thoughts [worries], the fat goes in your body and brings sickness." Diabetes was said by some to be caused by eating too much cooking oil, sugar, and sweets, while ulcers came from eating little and late and taking "dry food without any veg" (that is, starch dishes without sauce). But most people did not have very firm ideas about exactly what caused which specific disease.

Demotic views of etiology expressed by rural people and shared by many rural health workers can thus be summed up as one man did in Gulu: the "new diseases" are increasing because of not eating well and worrying. "Not eating well" covered a range of different things, but by and large diet was seen as a function of life conditions rather than a lifestyle choice.

Life Conditions and Body Ideals

The new public health enjoins care and cultivation of a particular kind of body.[16] Weight, body shape, muscular tone, and body mass index (BMI) have become indicators not only of health but also of virtue and attractiveness. In Uganda there are marked contrasts in body ideals, reflecting differences in class, education, generation, and rural or urban residence. In both rural and urban areas, there exists a common stereotype that Ugandans like people to be on the fat side: women should be plump and men should be solid. In the wake of the pandemic of "slim" disease (AIDS), people say, being slender is not good. Yet while some people do appreciate stout bodies, there are also alternative ideals, shaped by the media and by commercially promoted images of what is smart and modern.

"Heavy women with big bums are respected," said Lovisa, an urban middle-class Ugandan. She claims that her younger sister, who is fat, gets treated as a matron (they even kneel to greet her), while Lovisa is called "little girl" (kagirl) because she is slender. ("It's because I have a European husband," she explained; "He doesn't want me to be big. If I was not married to him I would probably be fat like everyone else in my family.") Keturah, the fashion editor of a major national newspaper, confirmed that a big bottom is considered attractive in women: "In Africa we like our bums. We don't want to lose that—rather the tummy." She said that especially rural people appreciate a big bum; wide hips show that a woman is capable of bearing children.

"Public opinion" refers to the big stomachs often characteristic of wealthy and influential men. As an urban university employee explained, "People listen to those who are rich, with big stomachs, not to poor men. So the public listens to your opinion. Politicians get big stomachs. Look at the vice president—his size increased a lot after he took office." The importance of wealth was emphasized by Lovisa, who remarked, "Women just like men with money—they don't mind about their body shape."

While a "big bum" and "public opinion" were supposed to be admirable, the picture was more complicated than that. A woman academic explained, and other informants agreed, that many urban women did not want to be big. "After childbearing and with busy schedules, women gain. It's not because they want to be big. It just happens. Maybe fatness is admired in rural areas, but not in the urban educated middle class. If someone is trim they ask, 'How do you do it?'" Television and newspapers show entertainers and other fashionable people who are slim or at least not heavy. The smart clothes are tight jeans and short tops. Young urban women try to keep trim, according to most of my urban informants. These days, "portable women" are appreciated; women should be light enough to lift. Keturah, the fashion editor, explained, "The trendsetters these days have no bum, no boobs, no tummy."

The appearance of fitness centers and commercial weight-loss programs in Kampala bears witness to the fact that at least some well-to-do city people are not satisfied with their body form. These are expensive and therefore only accessible to the elite. Yet their very existence suggests that the facile generalizations that Ugandans appreciate fat needs to be modified.

In rural eastern Uganda, pronounced fatness did not seem to be admired. People who were too fat could not work or walk easily, nor could they do "the work of the night," that is, play sex. What was admired was the wealth that allowed someone to be fat. The link between wealth and body substance was illustrated by a man who used to drive a bicycle taxi (bodaboda). At that time, he weighed seventy-six kilograms. "I was heavy then because I had the money to eat well. Now I am down to fifty-five [kilograms]."

Asking people about their weight was revealing. While a few urban elite families have weighing scales in their homes, most urbanites weigh themselves, if at all, for a small payment to the owner of a scale set out on a sidewalk, or at a health unit. In the rural areas, most health units have scales, and in principle pregnant women and HIV/AIDS patients are supposed to be weighed when they come for clinic. Others used the suspended weighing scales at the grinding mills, hanging on to the rope and hook meant for attaching a gunnysack of grain. In Butaleja District, informants said they weighed themselves on these scales at the trading center, as a standard against which to check the weight shown on the scales of traders who go round to homes to purchase cotton and maize. These people were less interested in how much they weighed than in whether the produce traders had rigged their scales.

Of fifteen people I asked around our home one morning, nine "knew their kilos," mostly from weighing themselves on produce scales. Those who did not know did not seem to care much. One friend said he had once weighed himself ten years ago. Another said he did not know, but maybe he weighed twenty kilos. When everyone exploded in laughter, he added, "If they roll me up and put me in a plastic sack, I can weigh fifteen kilos." Most poor men in the rural area wanted to gain weight. One farmer said that he weighs sixty-four kilos when he is heavy: "I would like to go to seventy to have energy for digging, walking, biking." Several men mentioned how they had lost weight because of worries, illness, and work. Difasi (a fifty-two-year-old farmer) said he weighed fifty-two kilos in May 2008 when a trader came to buy maize. He used to weigh sixty-nine but lost weight because of sickness and hard work. "When it decreases, you feel you're not normal. . . . Increase is good unless you have pressure." (He touches the back of his shoulder to show where one feels tension with stress and high blood pressure.)

By sharp contrast, the proprietor of Sleek and Slender, a health and fitness center in a posh area of Kampala, told how her clients (almost all women) start their program telling her how many kilos they want to lose. One whole wall of the reception is covered with before and after pictures showing dramatic loss of weight. The first two show the founder of the center herself. She, like most of her clients, was primarily concerned about her appearance, not her physical health. Women who have put on too much weight after having six or seven children want to slim down and look smart. Issues of depression and self-confidence were dealt with alongside weight loss. A combination of Christianity and popular psychology informed a holistic approach to sustainable lifestyle change and the achievement of a more attractive body shape. Epigraphs pinned on the wall gave messages about "doing something for yourself" and "feeling good about yourself."

Both the skinny poor rural men and the overweight elite urban women were concerned about their weight—although not primarily in relation to health promotion in the biomedical sense. They thought of weight in terms of wealth and strength, or smart appearance. To the extent that they spoke of a relation between weight and health, it was more linked to specific diseases: weight loss in connection with AIDS ("slim") and the inadvisability of weight gain for people with "sugar" or "pressure."

Eating

The new public health in the Global North promotes a plethora of diets both to avoid disease and to prevent deterioration of patients who develop hypertension and high blood sugar. In Uganda, advice on diet has long been given in schools and in health services, especially for pregnant women and mothers of small children. HIV patients are told when and what to eat. The media pour forth recommendations about eating. Yet the capacity to follow any dietary advice is shaped by position. Vernacular views and practices reflect social differences; people relate their eating patterns to their circumstances.

In modern rural Uganda, granaries are few and food self-sufficiency is a thing of the past. "Eating a healthy diet means you are able to buy everything. It means money so you can buy different things. Without money you eat the same. In school we learned about balanced diet, but people don't practice it." Fred, who made these assertions, was a rural, well-educated, unemployed schoolteacher and farmer. As he pointed out, schooled people have been exposed to the idea of a healthy diet with items from the different food groups. Other informants mentioned that they heard advice on the radio about how to eat: plenty of fruit and vegetables; less oil, fat, and salt; lots of water to drink. Moreover, many but not all people with diagnosed diabetes and hypertension were given instructions about diet. Yet for ordinary rural people, the concern was more about sufficient and good food than about eating according to the guidelines given in health education. That is to say, they saw healthy food in the broader sense of health as the good life. "Good eating brings health," said Manueli, a farmer in his late sixties, "and that means eating three times a day."

What Manueli meant was porridge in the morning and two proper meals of starch ("food") and relish ("veg," which also includes fish and meat). This was not always possible, as I found from daily checks with neighbors and acquaintances. Some informants took a minimal supper of "dry" tea (without milk) and roasted maize or groundnuts or a boiled sweet potato. Some had no money that day to buy food items they did not have from their own production. Some had not managed to get their grain ground for "food." In some households, the cook was too tired.

Just because people are not able to eat well all the time does not mean that they readily eat whatever is offered, however. Even in poor households, individuality is expressed in food preferences. Moses said that his fifteen-year-old daughter did not eat goat, mushrooms, offal, or the small dried fish called *mukene,* while all the other children loved mukene. His wife did not like maize meal (*posho*), while the children did. The elderly mama in our home did not eat millet, even though it is the traditional staple food of Bunyole. Manueli does not like rice, although most consider it an especially nice food.

While rural peasants were not starving, there was a universal feeling that their choices of what to eat were limited. They were constrained by not having money to buy what they could not produce themselves. City dwellers were exposed to a much greater variety of food items: well-stocked supermarkets for the elites and the more prosperous members of the "working class"; open-air markets, small shops, and the ubiquitous street vendors for everyone else. Recent dramatic increases in food prices have affected everyone, including the "working class." In a country where eating meat means eating well, it is striking to see what meat is available as street food in poorer areas of Kampala: boiled cow's head, hoof soup, or chunks of grilled intestine, throat, heart, and spleen (called *sala wano* ["cut here"] because the customer indicates how much he can afford). The cheapest parts of the animal find a market here.

The food item about which there were the strongest opinions and which in many ways mirrored social distinctions is cooking oil. Its production and consumption have increased enormously in Uganda; indeed, some Uganda-based producers are aiming to capture a regional African market. For many, being able to fry food is a luxury. In Bunyole, in eastern Uganda, it is called *obutu* (literally, "the nice little thing"). As Fred said, "In town, people eat better because they fry everything. In the village, people just boil their veg. Fried food tastes better. If meat is fried I can eat five pieces, but only two if it's boiled." The snacks bought by both urban and rural people are mostly fried in plenty of oil. This includes the older types such as *mandasi, sambusa,* chapati, and *kabalagala* and also newer items with catchy names. *Rolex* is a great favorite, consisting of a fried egg, rolled up in a fried chapati, sometimes with extras such as onions, tomatoes, and cabbage. Its cousin is *pisa* (pizza), a small fried chapati with a fried egg on top. Young men pointed out that oily snacks were more satisfying if you were hungry and did not have money.

Health concerns about oil are not entirely new. A colleague remembered that thirty-five years ago, girls in her secondary school believed that "oilies" (fried snacks) caused pimples. Today the talk shows on FM radio are full of warnings about the dangers of consuming too much oil and about the relative merits of various oils. The most prized of all is olive oil, the only one that is imported. As one radio message put it, "Olive oil is good for preparing food and drinking, anointing people in churches, [and] massaging patients who have high blood pressure and is also good for people with liver problems." Discerning people are convinced that some kinds of oil are better, and they can afford to buy them. Labels underscore the health benefits of "pure, healthy, natural, cholesterol-free" cooking oil. In Kampala, where large billboards advertise various brands of oil as being "healthy" or "good for the heart," one shopkeeper who sold both oil and deep-fried cassava used Kimbo and sunflower oil for his domestic consumption and stocked other cheaper types, in which he also fried the cassava, for his customers. He had heard on the radio and read in the newspaper that cottonseed and coconut oil "goes in the veins and clots." In small rural trading centers, people buy oil in tiny amounts (about one hundred milliliters), ladled out of large containers into plastic sacks or bottles they have brought. They may not know or care what kind of oil they get, as long as it is cheap. As one shopkeeper, who sold the inexpensive Rafiki brand produced by Mbale Soap Works, said dismissively, "People don't know the difference anyhow; it's all just *obutu.*"

Exercise

It is revealing that Ugandan languages do not have a word that accurately translates the English word *exercise.* Those who speak of doing physical activity for the sake of maintaining or strengthening the body, rather than for the sake of doing a piece of work or going somewhere, use the English word. A clinical officer at a rural hospital in eastern Uganda smiled as he told of the local term to describe what foreign visitors to the hospital did in the early morning: *ohuhola bisaizi. Ohuhola* means "to do"; *bisaizi* has *bi-* as the plural prefix for the root *-saizi,* from the English *exercise.* The concept and practice of exercise is spreading in Uganda, mainly in the middle class and in cities. For most rural and poor people, it is rather anomalous. Even those with salaried jobs that do not involve hard physical labor grew up in a world where tiring work was the norm from which people wanted relief. Several rural health workers who had been advised to exercise because of health conditions did so in privacy; one did calisthenics in her bedroom, so that not even her children could see her.

In the rural areas, work involves digging, carrying water, chopping wood, scrubbing clothes, and myriad other physically demanding chores. People walk if they have no bicycle or money to hire a bicycle taxi. The idea of tiring yourself if you do not have to seems strange. A rural health worker explained that the Lunyole term *ohwehalubirisa* ("to strain yourself") implies unnecessarily exerting oneself. The example was to walk if you could afford not to.

More educated and cosmopolitan people distinguished themselves from less sophisticated and enlightened people by their appreciation of exercise. Paul, a university student in the town of Mukono, said that he jogs once a week when he is there but never when he is home visiting his parents in the rural area. "We talk of exercise, but most people in the village don't know about it." As Wilburforce, a well-educated urbanite with his own consulting company, put it, "People want to show their wealth by driving or being driven. . . . People would wonder why you are walking." Yet a few people, such as himself, who could use a car nevertheless chose to walk to or from work. A university driver said with satisfaction that he often walks the five kilometers home in the evening "for exercise."

The elite people who are taking up walking as exercise (in contrast to walking to and from work, as poor people must) do so in the upmarket residential areas or on the Kololo airstrip or at the university sports ground, venues that are quieter and safer than walking along the busy roads. There are a few joggers, mainly young people and almost all male. But jogging and running are exceptional even in town; as one regular practitioner summed it up, "If they see you running, they think you're mad."

The practice of exercise, as something people with a lifestyle might do, is being promoted by commercial interests. The Kampala Marathon, sponsored by MTN, is well covered in the lifestyle sections of the national newspapers. Fitness centers, health clubs, and gyms are an increasingly prominent feature of urban life for wealthier Ugandans. The big international hotels have workout facilities, and fitness clubs are opening in the upscale shopping malls, as well as at the Makerere University campus. They are patronized by people who do not carry out strenuous activity in their daily lives. Some are referred by their doctors because of problems such as hypertension, heart conditions, and obesity. The manager of the health club at Hotel Africana spoke of providing "dosages of exercise." He said, "The club caters for all sorts of people; it is the money that throws you out [that is, excludes you]. A health club is like a clinic; if you don't attend, you die earlier. If you want to live longer and stay younger, attend the club daily."

Some NGOs are spearheading exercise as well, often to publicize their causes in a way that is enjoyable and healthy. The Gulu Diabetes Association, for example, has a traditional dance group that both encourages members to exercise and promotes interest in diabetes. NGOs increasingly use "walks" to demonstrate for their diseases or their campaigns. The kind of people who work for NGOs, including expatriates, are the kind who might regularly walk together for exercise. In northern Uganda, where NGOs are abundant, subscribers to the email list for the United Nations Organization for Coordination of Humanitarian Affairs (UNOCHA) organized long weekly walks and sent round photos of Ugandans and ex-pats smiling and wiping the sweat from their brows.

The Therapeutic Marketplace

In principle, treatment is free at government health facilities, including monitoring and medication of conditions such as hypertension and diabetes. In practice, equipment and medicines are very often lacking. Meters and strips for measuring blood glucose are hardly available in any government health unit. The main problem, according to the dispenser at a rural district hospital in eastern Uganda, was that drugs for diabetes and hypertension were expensive, so the hospital stocked few. Directly across from the rural hospital gate was a drug shop that stocked metformin and glibenclamide, the two oral hypoglycemics the hospital was supposed to provide, and seven kinds of hypertensives. It was from such outlets that people bought medicine when the public facilities ran out. The rich can buy medicine; the poor cannot; and those who are neither very rich nor very poor struggle to buy medicine when they can with the help of relatives and by forgoing other needs. In many ways, their situation resembles that of people with HIV before the rollout of free ART.[17]

In these circumstances, a particular therapeutic market is thriving, one that also catered to HIV-positive people before ART was common. In Kampala, and even in the rural area, nutritional supplements and remedies being marketed by international firms are claimed to promote health and alleviate chronic conditions of many types. The number of companies and range of products has expanded dramatically. Prominent in the field are Tianshi (Chinese), House of Health (South African), Swissgarde (South African), and Golden Neo-Life Diamite (South African). Other firms are Questnet, Forever Living, and Dynapharm. They are based on the multilevel marketing (MLM) strategy, whereby distributors pay to join, are rewarded for recruiting more distributors, and are encouraged to sell within their network and use the products themselves.[18]

The marketing material describes products with a wide range of claims: brain boosters for children sitting exams, anti-aging preparations, pills for weight loss and for potency, liver remedies for alcohol damage. Medicines to improve blood circulation and metabolism are common; there are many products for diabetes and high blood pressure. The material on Golden Neo-Life Diamite products uses phrases right out of the new public health: "Out of necessity, each of us must begin to actively promote our own well-being within our environment. Life has become a matter of risk management. We must educate ourselves and our children to recognize the risks and find ways to intervene before the damage is done. . . . We are entering into a new era in health care, an era where the responsibility for disease prevention and the state of our health rests largely in our own hands."

In addition to these international multilevel marketing enterprises, there are Uganda-based businesses and clinics that specialize in herbal medicines and techniques such as reflexology. They take a "lifestyle" approach to health, as do the MLM firms, and market "genuine natural products." The Genapo Holistic Health Information Centre is a good example. It is run by a medicinal chemist who sees her task as bridging the information gap between biomedicine and herbal medicine. She emphasizes that most diseases are due to eating habits and sedentary lifestyle, so that is where she starts her consultations with clients. She advises people living with HIV, diabetes, and high blood pressure about proper diet, which includes eating unprocessed foods, avoiding too much oil, and using olive oil and Moringa oil, which she sells in her clinic. On the shelves at her clinic-cum-shop were also four "Golden products" from Golden Neo-Life Diamite, suggesting overlap in these kinds of health business.

It was evident that in the city, and to some extent in the rural area, middle-class people were aware of, if not customers in, an emerging market in "lifestyle" health products. This new market features a discourse about the risks of modern life, stress, and diet; it targets diabetes, hypertension, and obesity. It overlaps with biomedicine and with public health discourses about diet and is by and large highly appreciated. However, these products, like those in the overlapping market for commercial "traditional" medicines, are expensive and thus accessible only to the more prosperous. While traditional healing practices and practitioners also provide an alternative to biomedical treatment of cardiovascular diseases and diabetes,[19] these new health commodities are more specifically targeted at cosmopolitan consumers.

The Media

The national English-language newspapers have articles and regular dedicated sections on health. Lifestyle, eating, exercise, and chronic diseases are featured here. Jane, the proprietor of Sleek and Slender, appreciated this coverage; she said that many of her clients were already well-informed by the time they contacted her.

Television also has regular programs on health and chronic diseases, often with biomedical experts providing advice. But the medium that reaches most people are the many FM radio stations, broadcasting in English and local languages. They have informative talks by experts and call-in programs during which people can ask their health questions. Chronic conditions, diet, exercise, and healthy lifestyle are well covered. The general pattern is that more orthodox biomedical information from physicians is offered on English-language television and radio, while alternative advice (about herbs, food supplements, reflexology, and Chinese medicine) is given on radio stations broadcasting in local languages. It is often promotional, ending in "Come to my clinic, we can treat that condition."

An example of this type of program is *Mulengera,* in Luganda, by health practitioners from Mukama Yawonya ("It Is God Who Heals") and Herbal Medicine Research. There was a talk about rest and trusting in God, which included the exhortation, "Don't overeat at supper. Eat very soft food that can be easily digested and exercise after. Most people live to eat instead of eating to live." Call-in questions after this talk included inquiries about genital warts, leg pain, hernia, gonorrhea, and the value of bathing in hot water in the evening. Two callers complained of sweating and were told that sweating may be due to high blood pressure: "Clogged veins cause one to sweat a lot because the blood is forcing itself to pass through clogged veins, which may result in high blood pressure. But we do reflexology to fight or treat high blood pressure."

One urban informant, Vincent, who had had his foot amputated because of diabetes and suffered from pressure, smiled when he said that he had become a herbalist by listening to the radio. He heard much good advice about drinking plenty of water, taking exercise, eating fruits, and using locally available plants for medicine. What had really helped him, he said, was not the hospital medicine but "these doctors on the radio." It was crushed garlic that finally healed the wound on his stump, and he took fresh lemon juice to clear his veins and bring down his blood pressure. He was listening mostly to programs in Luganda, where the experts were often people who had clinics offering "alternative" treatment and lifestyle advice, bridging "traditional" herbal medicine, food supplements, and biomedicine.

Biomedical science attempts to test different treatments to resolve questions of efficacy and establish the single therapy of choice. But the media present an ever-expanding field of differences—something for everyone—without ever determining which one is best. Clinics and products must distinguish themselves from their competitors. New advice on regimes of living keeps readers interested.

The Logic of Life Conditions

In the second decade of the twenty-first century, Ugandan government policy on the prevention and management of NCDs is still in its infancy. Given the extreme dependence of the health sector on donor funding and the problem of maintaining resources for AIDS treatment,[20] the donor-government axis may not be able to operationalize plans in the near future. More likely is an increase in the contributions of pharmaceutical companies. They have already made a start in that Novo Nordisk, with considerable publicity, provided free insulin for children in five African countries including Uganda in 2008. Quality Chemicals in Kampala, a daughter company of Cipla, which has started local production of metformin, supports a leading diabetologist to hold training sessions for health workers all around the country.

In the absence of a program that addresses all citizens, other forces are at work that appeal to particular publics. Lifestyle concerns are promoted by the media. Indeed, the lifestyle sections of the national newspapers are where advice about eating and exercise is to be found. They so clearly appeal to the "working class" that one is tempted to say that it is the "working class" that has a lifestyle or at least wants one. This is not just a matter of money. To be aware of diet and exercise marks one as not only prosperous but also enlightened. While rich men may have "public opinion" and their wives may be noted for "big bums," younger cosmopolitans are attracted by other body ideals, including "portability" and fitness. "Nutritionalism," Michael Pollan's term for the perception of food in terms of its measured nutritional value, and its companion "healthism," which assesses life's activities in terms of health, have made their entrance on the Ugandan scene.[21] Commercial interests pick up on these themes, promoting food products, fitness programs, and medicines to enhance health and prevent "lifestyle" diseases. Their reach too is partial; they interpellate those who have money and sophistication. They assume that people can make choices to take control of their lives and to live them differently. Although some voices from the lifestyle perspective speak of the "conditions" of modern life, they do so to call upon people to reflect and choose ways of managing them, as in the case of Golden Neo-Life Diamite products.

In contrast, the logic of the life conditions perspective emphasizes structural conditions that limit possibilities of choice. Implicating AIDS, insurgency, and displacement as causes of post-traumatic stress diabetes— or poverty, worry, and stress as factors bringing "pressure"—is to point to matters beyond one's immediate control. It is to say that people are victims of circumstances that have political and economic and biological bases. This is a muted perspective expressed by demotic voices and by a few activists. The logic of life conditions is used to explain etiology, one's ability to eat in a particular way, and a disinclination to perform unnecessary exercise on the part of people who do strenuous work. It is strongest and most convincing in relation to use of medicines, as Mr. Ajaliboye told us.

Yet to conclude that the "working class" has a lifestyle while poor people have life conditions would be too simple. First of all, these are not sharply bounded categories. Not all members of the "working class" are rich, and most interact frequently with their poorer relatives. Moreover, while poor people hardly read the newspapers, they hear FM radio with its messages about eating "soft" food and drinking water. Secondly, to assume that poor peasants have no scope for choice is to ignore likes and dislikes. There is widespread recognition of individual differences in "what your heart likes"—and dislikes. Perhaps this is why people seem to accept easily that this one has the disease of not eating salt and that one is not supposed to take sugar.

The new public health, according to Deborah Lupton, conceives of noncommunicable disease as an outcome of the stresses and poor lifestyle choices of the members of modern societies and as a sign that modern life is inherently damaging to health. On this point all of my informants agree, with some reservations about lifestyle choices. But more than being simply a generic product of contemporary life, noncommunicable diseases are an object for vernacular sociology. In their mirror, people reflect on the significance of social differences for prevention and management. Noncommunicable diseases also provide an excellent window onto the political economy of health care in contemporary Africa.

Notes

1. Abdhalah K. Ziraba, Jean Fotso, and Rhoune Ochako, "Overweight and Obesity in Urban Africa: A Problem of the Rich or the Poor?" *BMC Public Health* 9 (2009): 465–73.

2. The study was carried out over four weeks in late 2008 and one week in late 2009. In Butaleja District, rural eastern Uganda, where I had previously done long-term fieldwork, I repeatedly visited eight households to discuss health, the "new diseases," eating patterns, and physical activity. I also discussed these issues with staff at the local hospital, a health center, and two drug shops. In Kampala, I visited six households (three of them repeatedly) while pursuing the same topics. In addition, I interviewed three leading experts on NCDs, four proprietors of health businesses, and a journalist who specialized in lifestyle. In Gulu, I interviewed members of a patient group and their patron. I also had long conversations at their homes with ten people living with diabetes and/or hypertension. I gratefully acknowledge the collaboration of Dr. Jessica Jitta and Phoebe Kajubi, Child Health and Development Centre, Makerere University, and of Alice Lamwaka, Gulu University. The research was supported by a Copenhagen University faculty grant for research development in global health.

3. Abdallah S. Daar et al., "Grand Challenges in Chronic Non-communicable Diseases: The Top 20 Policy and Research Priorities for Conditions Such as Diabetes, Stroke and Heart Disease," *Nature* 450 (2007): 494–96.

4. WHO, "First NCDnet Global Forum," 2010, www.who.int/nmh/newsletter _apr2010.pdf.

5. See Abdesslam Boutayeb, "The Double Burden of Communicable and Non-communicable Diseases in Developing Countries," *Transactions of the Royal Society of Tropical Medicine and Hygiene* 100, no. 3 (2006): 191–99; Ama de-Graft Aikins et al., "Tackling Africa's Chronic Disease Burden: From the Local to the Global," *Globalization and Health* 6, no. 5 (2010).

6. Formation of a Uganda NCD Alliance, consisting of the Diabetes Association, the Heart Association, and the Cancer Society, is being supported by a modest grant from DANIDA, but it has not had much influence as yet. The Diabetes Association is the largest, though it is not represented in all parts of the country.

7. Charles Davison and George Davey Smith, "The Baby and the Bath Water: Examining Sociocultural and Free-Market Critiques of Health Promotion," in *The Sociology of Health Promotion: Critical Analyses of Consumption, Lifestyle and Risk*, ed. Robin Bunton, Sarah Nettleton, and Roger Burrows, 91–99 (London: Routledge, 1995).

8. Marie Kolling, Kirsty Winkley, and Mette von Deden, "'For Someone Who's Rich, It's Not a Problem': Insights from Tanzania on Diabetes Health-Seeking and Medical Pluralism among Dar es Salaam's Urban Poor," *Globalization and Health* 6, no. 8 (2010).

9. Charles L. Briggs, "Why Nation-States and Journalists Can't Teach People to Be Healthy: Power and Pragmatic Miscalculation in Public Discourses on Health," *Medical Anthropology Quarterly* 17, no. 3 (2003): 287–321.

10. Titus Serunjogi, "When You Eat Is Just as Important," *New Vision*, 22 November 2009, A4.

11. Martin O'Brien, "Health and Lifestyle: A Critical Mess? Notes on the Dedifferentiation of Health," in *The Sociology of Health Promotion: Critical Analyses of Consumption, Lifestyle and Risk*, ed. Robin Bunton, Sarah Nettleton, and Roger Burrows (London: Routledge, 1995), 192.

12. Ministry of Health, Republic of Uganda, *Health Sector Strategic Plan II: 2005/06–2009/2010*, vol. 1 (Kampala: Republic of Uganda, 2005), 46–47.

13. Deborah Lupton, *The Imperative of Health: Public Health and the Regulated Body* (London: Sage, 1995), 51, citing K. Figlio, "The Lost Subject of Medical Sociology," in *Sociological Theory and Medical Sociology*, ed. G. Scrambler (London: Tavistock, 1987), 79, 81.

14. Steve Ferzacca, "Chronic Illness and the Assemblages of Time in Multisited Encounters," in *Chronic Conditions, Fluid States: Chronicity and the Anthropology of Illness*, ed. Leonora Manderson and Caroline Smith-Morris (New Brunswick, NJ: Rutgers University Press, 2010), 172.

15. Speech by the Ugandan minister of health in Gulu on World Diabetes Day, 14 November 2009. The quotation is from a written copy of the speech given to me by the Patron of the Gulu Diabetes Association, Alice Lamwaka, one of the event organizers.

16. Dorothy Porter, *Health, Civilization and the State: A History of Public Health from Ancient to Modern Times* (London: Routledge, 1999), 297.

17. Susan Reynolds Whyte et al., "Treating AIDS: Dilemmas of Unequal Access in Uganda," in *Global Pharmaceuticals: Ethics, Markets, Practices*, ed. Adriana Petryna, Andrew Lakoff, and Arthur Kleinman, 240–62 (Durham, NC: Duke University Press, 2006).

18. See Detlev Krige, "Fields of Dreams, Fields of Schemes: Ponzi Finance and Multilevel Marketing in South Africa," *Africa* 82, no. 1 (2012): 69–92; Lyn Jeffery, "Placing Practices: Transnational Network Marketing in Mainland China," in *China Urban:*

Ethnographies of Contemporary Culture, ed. Nancy N. Chen et al., 23–42 (Durham, NC: Duke University Press, 2001).

19. Rhonda BeLue et al., "An Overview of Cardiovascular Risk Factor Burden in Sub-Saharan African Countries: A Socio-cultural Perspective," *Globalization and Health* 5, no. 10 (2009).

20. Peter Mugyenyi, "Flat-Line Funding for PEPFAR: A Recipe for Chaos," *Lancet* 374 (25 July 2009): 292.

21. Michael Pollan, *In Defense of Food: An Eater's Manifesto* (New York: Penguin Press, 2008).

EIGHT

Navigating "Global Health" in an East African City

RUTH J. PRINCE

DURING THE PAST FIFTEEN YEARS, THE CITY OF KISUMU IN WESTERN Kenya has become a center of global health interventions. Numerous international and donor country organizations and research groups run projects within the city and in the wider province focusing mainly on HIV. By 2008, an official total of 907 nongovernmental organizations (NGOs) and "community-based groups" with operations in Kisumu had been registered with the government, ranging from global organizations such as World Vision to national NGOs and local "self-help" groups that have mushroomed in response to Kenyan government and donor policies pushing for "community participation."[1] Since 2005, with funding from the United States Presidential Emergency Fund for AIDS Relief (PEPFAR) and the Global Fund to Fight AIDS, Tuberculosis and Malaria, free antiretroviral therapy (ART) has been rolled out through a network of new HIV clinics in government and NGO sites, which provide medicines, testing, counseling, and "care" to city residents. These transnational projects and programs draw material resources, organizations, technologies, expertise, and knowledge into Kisumu and its hinterlands. They superimpose an externally conceived grid of globalized interventions onto a city, the municipal infrastructure, public works, and public health services of which exhibit varying states of disrepair. As such, they produce an urban geography that is marked by juxtapositions between global and local, between intense activity and neglect, and, as I show below, between opportunity and exclusion.

This chapter examines the landscape of "global health" as it takes shape in Kisumu and explores its effects on practices and imaginations of public health and, more broadly, on imaginations of "development." Global HIV interventions have been described as introducing new biopolitical landscapes and "biosocialities," as well as new forms of governance and citizenship in Africa, as they focus on HIV-positive populations, bypassing state institutions and introducing globalized medical regimens and accompanying discourses of "positive living" and therapeutic "adherence."[2] Within these regimes, the ability to survive HIV is narrowed down to the responsibility of individuals who should "take control" of their own health. My concern is less with tracing the architecture of this apparatus of governmentality[3] and the possibilities and limitations of the "empowerment" it offers through global scripts and confessional technologies of "positive living," than with the question of how people in the city navigate these landscapes, how they live and work within them, and in so doing, produce something out of them. Global health interventions do not ignore the Kenyan state. They offer a grid of services, resources, and opportunities that interlock with government health services at key points. For many Kenyans, they are an improvement on the neglect and lack that characterized HIV medicine ten years ago. Yet they also produce what Susan Reynolds Whyte and colleagues call a "projectification" of health services, which has wider effects on social, political, and health structures.[4] These projects enact unequal relations of power, reinforced in the discourse of "donor" and "recipient," and they are unstable, driven by short-term funding cycles and working through a variety of often-precarious institutional "partnerships." Following how various actors—medical professionals and clinic staff, patients of HIV clinics, and "volunteer" health workers—navigate these spaces, I draw attention to the gaps left behind and opened up by the projectification of external intervention, as it touches only particular nodes and operates within circumscribed locations. These gaps are supposed to be filled by the informal networks that, promoted by NGOs and driven by urban poverty, take shape around self-help and community-based initiatives. As the ethnography reveals, the turn to "community" and "patient support" groups merely deflects responsibility for a more robust public health onto the poor and onto informal and unsustainable structures. Telling this story merely as a narrative of biopolitical and neoliberal change, however, may conceal and submerge other engagements with the public's health that emerge at the edges of these novel landscapes, as well as within overlapping and layered trajectories of public health practices in Kenya. I follow these frictions as globalized health resources and discourses, technologies, and expertise—embodied in the new HIV clinics and ART projects—intersect with local economies and livelihoods, aspirations, and imaginations in a city marked by poverty, marginalization, and insecurity.

Global Health and the Urban Landscape

Driven by resources from PEPFAR and the Global Fund, free HIV treatment programs were introduced in Kenya beginning in 2004. Located in Ministry of Health sites as well as NGOs, they offer HIV tests, counseling services, and basic health checks, as well as antiretroviral medicines, multivitamins, and prophylactic antibiotics. The aim is to provide comprehensive coverage, reaching all members of the public who need it.[5] By 2010, there were twenty-five HIV clinics (referred to as patient support centers, or PSCs) operating within Kisumu and sixty-four in Kisumu District, ranging from the large PSC attached to the provincial hospital, catering to over ten thousand patients, to small clinics run by local NGOs.[6]

For many Kenyans, the HIV clinics represent a form of "development" and are an example of what can be achieved, given international political will and adequate resources. Until very recently, members of the public, Ministry of Health staff, and medical professionals have struggled personally and professionally with the huge challenges of providing or accessing medical care in the absence of affordable antiretrovirals (ARVs).[7] Endowed with superior material resources—from adequate supplies of medicines to functioning laboratories and testing equipment to better-paid and motivated staff—the HIV clinics present a sharp contrast to much of the rest of the medical care and practice offered in government hospitals and health centers. Municipal public health services—still suffering from years of structural adjustment and privatization—are marked by stock-outs of medicines, underpaid and overworked staff, poor laboratory facilities, and overcrowded and under-resourced hospital wards. These differences are expressed in the buildings themselves; HIV clinics are newly painted or newly built. Some are covered with bright murals offering health education messages commissioned from local artists. They are nodal points for incoming flows of resources and expertise and are surrounded by activity, from the flows of patients and the density of staff to the rows of expensive vehicles with donor and NGO logos. These advantages are accentuated by their juxtaposition with the lack of resources and deteriorating material environment of public health services outside of HIV clinics and lead to a situation in which two practices of medicine exist side by side in the city.[8]

The operations of these globalized health interventions also contrast with the surrounding urban infrastructure—and lack of it. As in other African cities, the infrastructure that created Kisumu in the colonial and immediate postcolonial era—the electric power grid, the municipal water supply, the network of roads, the railway station, and the government-built urban housing estates—is today marked by disintegration, fragmentation, and decay. Power cuts are frequent, the extension of tapped and chlorinated water and a sewage system outside the central business district and the wealthy suburbs is patchy, and roads are in a constant state of disrepair and unable to support the large increases in traffic, while so-called informal settlements (characterized by semipermanent housing without water, sewage, and power connections) continue to grow. The absence of municipal rubbish collection, apart from in the central business district, is apparent in the rubbish that blows about the city's streets and informal settlements, accumulates in ditches, and forms a mountain, picked over by rag merchants and street children, behind Kisumu's new shopping malls. As is true elsewhere in urban Africa, the instability of urban infrastructures in Kisumu reflects wider experiences.[9] In the wake of the disintegration of formal-sector employment, public services, and municipal planning, urban residents struggle to find work in informal economies. It is not only the urban poor who must find a living in this way but also people who have lost their white-collar or public-sector jobs and youths who have formal education but are unable to find any formal employment.[10] In the past two decades, the HIV/AIDS epidemic compounded this situation, as many families faced the early death of breadwinners.

In this context, the pouring of external donor funds into HIV/AIDS interventions, together with the designation of Kisumu in 2001 as a UN "millennium" city, has had some positive effects on the urban economy. From being a small, dusty provincial town bypassed by most labor migrants on their way to Nairobi, and suffused with a sense of development having passed it by, Kisumu has become a hive of activity and a hub for NGOs, transnational funds, and donor-driven development.[11] Fifteen years ago, the occasional government or aid agency Land Rover could be seen on its streets. Today its roads are choked by the vehicles of NGO and disease-research projects and by the private cars of its growing middle class (many of them working for NGOS). In 2010 a new international airport was built by the Chinese to accommodate the mobility of aid, NGO, government, and business professionals. Supermarkets and shopping centers with Internet cafes, coffee shops, and ice-cream parlors cater to the growing salaried classes and an expatriate population. House rents in middle-class areas have skyrocketed as owners realize the potential of leasing property to NGOs and expatriate staff. All this creates an appearance of economic growth and fuels visions of development and a better life. It gives residents a sense that Kisumu is on the map. Middle-class residents told me that "things are improving in Kisumu," and even the young men offering bicycle taxis agreed: "Here in Kisumu we are moving ahead."[12]

Residents locate evidence of this "moving ahead" not only in the construction of new clinics and the proliferation of NGOs but also in the circulation of new vehicles on the road and the mushrooming of hotels, supermarkets, and bars. Young people with secondary school education and aspirations (if no employment) talk of the opportunities associated with what they call "exposure" to these globalized health interventions and their circulation of knowledge about HIV (and by extension, science), and of new ways of living, with their promise of a better life. "Exposure" implies learning new skills and knowledge as well as new ways of talking and acting that are promoted by NGOs; it points to ways of becoming, in local parlance, an "enlightened" and "empowered" person. Young people point to the circulation of knowledge associated with the world of global health, which materializes in posters, advertisements for jobs, and a growing "seminar" culture, organized largely by NGOs. Responding to this hunger for knowledge and skills, colleges have sprung up or expanded their operations and offer a range of courses tailored to the new economy of global health, from HIV counseling, public health, and community development to pharmacy, computing, and management, at all levels from certificates to diplomas and degrees. Those without means of paying for these courses can hope instead to get sponsored by NGOS offering workshops on HIV/AIDS issues, which provide participants with certificates and titles such as "community health worker," "peer mobilizer," and "HIV counsellor." If they are lucky, an HIV clinic or an NGO project may recruit them as a "volunteer." Across health interventions in Kenya, it is increasingly volunteers who conduct youth health education, persuade people to take HIV tests, counsel them, explain the regimen of antiretroviral medication, and "follow up" with patients in their homes. Volunteers are given some material compensation, which varies widely between organizations: some offer between one hundred and three hundred shillings for a day's work; others only a "lunch" allowance or transportation reimbursement. The access to new knowledge and the hope for a livelihood attracts not only young people aspiring to enter what people in East Africa call the "working class"—those lucky members of the population who have professional recognition and monthly salaries—but also others struggling to live in the informal economy, who, by embracing their HIV-positive status and becoming volunteers, position themselves in the patron-client relations that form around NGO projects and HIV clinics. Through a focus on "community participation," HIV interventions also encourage people to join self-help or community-based groups, and hundreds of these associations, from women's groups to patient groups, compete for the fluctuating opportunities and resources offered by NGOs.

For some residents of Kisumu, then, HIV interventions represent a vision of "development" and the opportunities it offers for the country, for the city, and for the individual. These interventions open up the city to globalized circulations of resources, medicines, knowledge, and expertise. They offer selected residents not only opportunities to access enclaves of privileged medical care and projects offering material support but also a sense of connection to the "global." Despite the inclusive rhetoric of participation, however, the incoming resources seem to benefit mainly the careers and lifestyles of salaried professionals and expatriates, while the "poor and positive" receive handouts of medicine and occasionally food.[13] Although millions of dollars have been spent on HIV/AIDS and, to a lesser extent, malaria and TB interventions, most people in Kisumu live in the expanding "informal" settlements, in housing with no sewage, water, or electricity. Most city dwellers are poor, and given the lack of employment and rising costs of food, they remain poor. Moreover, the seemingly solid infrastructure of intervention is undercut by a sense of fragility and transience. Uncertainties suffuse treatment regimes, from concerns about the future funding of "life-long" antiretroviral therapy by external donors (especially since the 2008 economic crisis) to the vulnerability of bodily health, as people struggle to find a livelihood. The landscape of "global health" in Kisumu appears as a confusing melange of institutions, projects, and resources that offer short-term, transient and unstable opportunities. This "projectification" of HIV/AIDS, together with the fact that intervention focuses on circumscribed "enclaves" or islands, reinforces and extends established patterns of what Julie Hearn, writing about structural readjustment in the 1990s, referred to as "NGO-led development" in Kenya.[14]

In the rest of the chapter, I follow the experiences, aspirations, and trajectories of medical staff, patients, and volunteers who live, work, or hope to gain a livelihood within this rather precarious landscape of intervention. I draw from interviews, conversations, and observations with staff members and volunteers working in HIV clinics attached to a public hospital, a government health center, and two NGOs in Kisumu and a health center outside the city, as well as with young people who describe themselves as "tarmacking"—or looking for work—in the city, who seek to attach themselves to NGOs and HIV clinics as volunteers. I also draw upon a long-term study of families living with HIV (most of them poor and without regular incomes), which I conducted together with a research assistant, Biddy Odindo, from November 2008 to November 2012. We visited these families regularly, to try to gain an understanding of their daily lives, their social networks (including churches, NGOs, and patient support groups), and their experiences with HIV clinics and other health services. The ethnographic research on which this chapter is based mostly took place from 2009 to 2010.[15]

The Projectification of Health Care

It is a typically busy morning in the HIV clinic run by Malaga, a small Catholic NGO that describes itself as a "leading humanitarian organization" working in Kisumu.[16] A steady stream of people enters the NGO's compound through metal gates that open onto one of the city's busy roads. Inside the hall are rows of benches filled with waiting people, and at the far end is a curtained-off arena where patients see health workers. Patients—or "clients," as they are referred to—show their clinic appointment cards to a clerk sitting behind a desk and then sit down to wait their turn. At the other side of the hall, three health workers are busy checking patients' vitals, while behind the curtains at the back, a nurse and a clinical officer see those who are unwell and write out prescriptions for ARVs, antibiotics, and multivitamins.

Opposite the community hall lies the NGO's small health clinic, recently painted with a large sign announcing the support of the U.S. "President's Emergency Plan for AIDS Relief" (PEPFAR). Set up by a Mill Hill Father in the 1970s, the NGO has conducted health work in the neighborhood for over twenty years, offering mainly maternal and child health services. In 1993 it set up an outpatient clinic. The clinic began offering HIV testing and counseling in 2001, but only when it began receiving funds from PEPFAR in 2007 did it set aside a separate building for HIV treatment and care. Smaller than the HIV clinics, or "patient support centers" (PSCs), located in the district and provincial hospitals, it is growing rapidly, as it has become one of six central city sites of ART provision.

Various organizations operate within the PSC. Betty has been nurse in charge of the Malaga health center since its beginnings as a small health clinic, but she is employed by the Ministry of Health. The four clerical assistants (who take patients' vitals, fill in medical files and enter records, and also follow up with patients at home) began their work as "volunteers"; they initially had no health training and were recruited from the clinic's HIV-positive patient support group. The NGO does not receive funds directly from PEPFAR; resources are channeled through another NGO, Family United Service, referred to as FUS (which was set up by an American university research group and receives PEPFAR funding to organize HIV "care and treatment" across government and NGO sites in the city). FUS pays the salaries of the clerical assistants, supports the volunteers, and sends a nurse and a clinical officer to work two days a week at Malaga's PSC. Medicines for "opportunistic infections" and for malaria and sexually transmitted disease are supplied by the state-run Kenya Medical Supply Agency (KEMSA), while FUS brings in supplies of antiretrovirals and HIV tests and takes laboratory samples to its own clinic in the city center. The PSC also runs a "Food by Prescription" program, funded by PEPFAR and distributed by the U.S. Agency for International Development (USAID), which provides sacks of nutritional flour supplements to "clients" deemed to be dangerously underweight. This coexistence of NGO and government structures, variously supported by external donors and funding agencies, is a common feature of PSCs. Yet while the density of these organizations has increased in recent years, such interaction has been a feature of government and NGO health work for decades, as the health workers I interviewed pointed out.

In a small government health clinic located in a market center outside the city, the nurse in charge, Sister Margaret, a woman in her midfifties, tells me about her work. Characterized by a continual maneuvering between government and donor research projects, NGOs, and private practice, her career is typical of that of health workers in Kenya, who struggle on low salaries to educate not only their children but also those of their extended families and thus must constantly look for extra income and pursue new opportunities. In the early 1990s, Sister Margaret was sent by the Ministry of Health to the health center. During that time of "structural adjustment," there were few resources; the laboratory had an old microscope and a lab technician who could do tests for malaria, but chemicals and equipment were rarely available, and electricity was intermittent. Supplies of basic medicines were also unreliable, and Sister Margaret sent most patients to the pharmacy she owned in the shopping center a few hundred meters down the road. Fed up with these working conditions, she left government service in 1996 to focus on her own private practice. Shortly afterwards, a northern university research group, together with a Kenyan parastatal institution, set up a district-level maternal health research project, and Sister Margaret was persuaded by the good salary, the opportunities for further training, and other perks to work for them. After three years, however, the project came to an abrupt end over concerns about accounting practices at the head office. Sister Margaret had to return to her government employment in the clinic. She continued to combine this with private practice, as it gave her much-needed additional income. In 2004, the clinic began offering HIV tests, and in 2006, with PEPFAR money, it began providing free ART. Since then, it has been built up considerably: in 2007, it received the first coat of paint it had seen in decades, a new wing was built to separate the PSC from other health services, and the supply of medicines from KEMSA became regular. A UK-based NGO provided funds for recruiting "volunteer" laypeople to provide HIV counselling and conduct HIV tests; it sent them on training seminars and supplied them with a small monthly remuneration.[17] Although the NGO's funds had dried up by 2008, leaving the volunteers with no remuneration, Sister Margaret encouraged them to continue working, hopeful that another donor would turn up.

Health workers involved with the new HIV clinics, like Sister Betty and Sister Margaret, were enthusiastic about the expansion of treatment. The ART programs enabled them to provide better care to patients:

"Medicines are available, supplies are reliable, there is more staff, and they are motivated," as Sister Betty told me, "and if you are not sure how to treat a patient you can call the hotline." This is a telephone number that connects medical professionals to expert HIV doctors, working for the American-run Global AIDS Program. The young clinical officer working at Malaga's PSC talked of the extra training he had received, and of his sense of "being connected."

Still, the interpenetration of government and nongovernmental organizations and projects also brought tensions. Health workers were sent on "refresher courses"—workshops that took place over a day or several days, during which they receive per diems—but access to places are limited and are hotly competed for. Moreover, health workers were acutely aware of the uneven salaries they received for doing the same work: PEPFAR-funded staff enjoyed higher salaries than did their Ministry of Health–employed counterparts. Those enjoying these privileged salaries tried to conceal them from their colleagues and were willing to talk to us about them only privately. The nurse in charge had to make difficult decisions, and her efforts to coordinate the various projects on offer and to channel opportunities to particular members of the staff created tensions.

Biopolitical Regimes and Relations?

HIV treatment programs enroll clients into new regimes of care: they must attend counseling sessions to learn about their HIV status, how to "live positively," and how to adhere to the medication. Such regimes are disciplining: they aim to make clients into "responsibilized" subjects who can take control of their health and lifestyle. Health workers are the vanguard of these regimes; nurses, counselors, and community health workers (CHWs) are expected to teach people about HIV, how to take ARVs regularly, eat a "balanced" diet, and avoid further infection; they must check clients' adherence to medication and chase up people who miss clinic appointments. They are instructed to give patients three chances and then expel them from the program: "If they default three times, they are out." The patronizing style of health worker interactions with patients does not necessarily indicate a lack of empathy, however. Health workers are well aware that few people living in the informal economy can afford a balanced diet. Ironically, the clinic's concern with diet renders issues of nutrition and, by extension, hunger, poverty, and the lack of a livelihood visible. Although health workers often admonished patients for failing to conform to the clinic regimes, they also recognized the associations of ill-health with poverty.

The disengagement and lack of motivation among health workers in African countries are often remarked upon. In Kisumu there was a sharp contrast, however, between patient experiences of medical staff in government hospital settings and non-HIV clinics—where people often complain about having to pay bribes to get anything done and about the indifference of staff to their suffering—and the kind of care that was being fostered in HIV clinics, where better resources, higher salaries, and training in "patient support" mean the working environment is more positive. Still, even in the large HIV clinics in Kisumu, which see thousands of HIV-positive clients every week, staff members are variously polite or abrupt and often professionally distant. In small clinics, such as Malaga, health workers saw clients regularly; they would bump into them on the streets while waiting for a minibus or when buying vegetables. They got to know something of their patients' lives and situations. They listened to their stories. "I just sympathized with her, that young mother! I just sympathized with her," Sister Betty told me, after seeing a patient who had "defaulted" and sending her for a second round of "adherence" classes. "She is alone—where is the husband!—She tells me she has not eaten today!" While ART programs focus heavily on "client education," health workers of all levels were well aware of the limited ability of many of their clients to conform to the expectations imposed by the medical regimen. Poverty and inadequate food, unstable and vulnerable family situations, poor housing, and open sewers made the focus on "knowledge" laughable. Betty wryly acknowledged that the provision of ART does not solve the problem of poverty; in fact, in heightening bodily needs for food and rest, in a context of high food prices and the struggle to find a daily living, ART may make patients more vulnerable.[18]

Health workers are members of the privileged "working class" in East Africa, yet only a thin line separates their lives from those of their patients. They face multiple claims on their incomes amid the expectations of extended family members, and they struggle to balance these ever-present obligations and responsibilities. In this context, the degree to which some health workers sought to help their patients beyond providing medical treatment is even more striking. Of course, I observed plenty of instances of bureaucratic indifference but also many of attentive care—which ranged from small gestures of kindness to giving particularly vulnerable patients material support. The CHWs were particularly involved with the patients they visited. Patients were more at ease with them, as many CHWs were openly HIV-positive themselves. CHWs visited patients who were either too ill to attend the clinic or had missed their appointments. Faced with the poverty of patients, even volunteer health workers, who had little income, sometimes put their hands in their own pockets and left something for the family they visited, particularly if the patient was a young mother, alone with children.

From the Clinic to the "Community": Navigating HIV and Health Crises

Outside Malaga's community hall, under the largest tree in the compound, one of the patient support groups attached to the HIV clinic holds its meetings. When Malaga began HIV testing and counselling back in 2000, the group was one of the first to be established in Kisumu. Its membership, of people who had been tested and were (at least within the group's boundaries) openly HIV positive, was initially small. Soon, however, the fact that group members—most of whom had no employment or regular income—received food parcels, flour, and sometimes even cash or mobile phone credit, as well as some opportunities to gain "training" in HIV issues, soon attracted other HIV-positive people. As observed elsewhere in East Africa, once an HIV-positive status opened up the possibility of material support and, later, medication, people's concerns about disclosing their status publicly became outweighed by the advantages (limited though they were) that an HIV-positive status conferred: vital material support in a unstable urban environment. HIV "patient support" and other self-help groups mushroomed in Kisumu, as people responded enthusiastically to the government- and donor-led turn toward "community-based" development.

Malaga support group meets every fortnight. Members "share" (using the English term) their problems, which include lack of income and the struggle to pay school fees, conflicts with in-laws, and worries about hospital and funeral expenses, as well as concerns about side effects of antiretrovirals, hunger, and the rising cost of food. Members come from all over the city. Many are simultaneously members of other support groups that are attached to other clinics and NGOs; in this way, they broaden their networks of contacts and sources of possible material support. On this morning, as the movement of people into and out of the clinic intensifies, the group listens to the request of one of its members:

BabaOdhis, a father of three, whose wife, Rose, has been very ill and has spent the past three weeks in the women's infectious disease ward of the provincial hospital. This is the second extended period that Rose has spent in the hospital in the past three months with what seems to be severe malaria. The first stay cost over five thousand shillings in ward fees, medicines, X-rays, and intravenous quinine (the equivalent of two months' income), and BabaOdhis was only able to cover it with money given by Rose's paternal aunt, a primary school teacher, and borrowed from neighbors and friends.[19] This time he and his relatives have no one to borrow money from, and no money left. Normally BabaOdhis keeps the family going with the income he gets from buying poor-quality secondhand clothes and resewing them—although even under "normal" circumstances, the family often manages only one meal in a day. During the previous weeks he has not managed to work. Addressing the chairperson of the group, BabaOdhis explains the situation and asks whether the group can give him some of the monthly "merry-go-round"—the money that each member contributes to a common pool.

By 2008, the privileged support that HIV-positive people had received from NGOs had mostly dried up. Occasionally there was news of an NGO distributing sacks of flour, but these events were few and far between. Instead, NGOs and the government were encouraging groups to apply to PEPFAR, through the government's National AIDS Control Council, for funding to start up "income-generating activities." Many groups—lacking the expertise to write such proposals or the funds to pay someone else to write them—could not "participate" in such ventures. Instead, they continued their credit-rotation activities—in which each member contributed a small sum at every meeting and then took turns receiving the proceeds. If a member needed the money urgently, though, an exception would be made in the normal order of credit rotation (this extended a practice of credit rotation that was common in other kinds of groups in both urban and rural life in Kenya). Not all groups, however, had successful "merry-go-rounds," as their members' contributions were too small and unreliable, and many groups disintegrated. BabaOdhis's group was more robust than many (which is partly why the group had persisted), as it was led by one of the NGO's volunteers, who had good connections.

After the meeting, BabaOdhis approached Pamela, a middle-aged widow who used to work as a "volunteer" counselor at the provincial hospital's HIV clinic, and asked her to persuade the nurse in charge of

the ward to waive some of Rose's fees. After three weeks on an intravenous drip, Rose's condition had stabilized and she wanted to go home,
but the hospital management would not let her leave until her fees had
been paid in full. This was a common practice, reinforced by guards
on the wards, which the hospital management was forced to adopt, as
many patients disappeared, leaving unpaid bills.

Luckily for BabaOdhis, the group decided to give him the "merry-go-
round," and Pamela agreed to go to the hospital and talk to the nurse.
The hospital management reduced Rose's fees, and with the money from
the support group, Rose was allowed to go home. The family managed
to get through this health crisis, through a combination of BabaOdhis's
care and network of contacts, the support of Rose's relatives, and the
support group's merry-go-round. However, with Rose too weak to find
work for many months, BabaOdhis struggled to earn enough to feed the
family. Sometimes they missed a meal, eating only the porridge made
with the fortified flour that Rose received from her PSC.

Another family we got to know was not even that lucky. It lost, in the
space of a year, both mother and child, soon after both had been initiated on ARVs. MamaAchieng', Jerome, and their two young daughters
had recently arrived in Kisumu from a small semiurban market. They
rented a room not far from that of BabaOdhis and Rose and tried to
get an income from making and selling *muhungala*, a low-grade charcoal made from mixing mud with charcoal. They had been rejected
by their church after MamaAchieng' had "disclosed" that she was HIV
positive—and had not joined a support group. Jerome refused to take
a test, and his wife dared not tell him that their youngest daughter was
positive. Soon after we met her, MamaAchieng' was admitted to hospital and, after three weeks of rapid deterioration, she died. Jerome was
left alone to care for the two girls. The health of the youngest daughter
was also deteriorating. She was on ARVs but hated taking them; she
became listless and lost her appetite. Her father took her again and
again to the PSC, where he was told to buy medicine "to add blood" and
advised to take his daughter to the hospital. Worried about paying the
fees, he delayed going. When he did eventually take his daughter there,
she died within a few hours.

This tragedy demonstrates how the new regimes of global health
represented by HIV clinics and their supply of free medication translate, or fail to translate, into better health. HIV clinics offer a package of
standardized care that cannot adequately deal with any deviation from

expected norms of antiretroviral responses. Episodes of severe malaria or other infections push patients into public hospital wards, where they do not enjoy privileged access to doctors, laboratory tests, and supplies of free medicines. The death of MamaAchieng' and her small daughter reveals the vulnerability of many families, as lack of income compounds HIV infection. Crucial to a family's ability to navigate across HIV clinics and hospital wards is its network of contacts. BabaOdhis drew upon family relationships, his membership in the patient support group, and his contacts with a volunteer health worker. Jerome and MamaAchieng' were new to Kisumu; they lacked such contacts and had no extended family in the city.

The importance of having the right contacts is underlined in the story of another family: Omondi (who worked as one of Malaga's clerical health officers) and Celestine (who was a community health worker at the HIV clinic in the government health center run by FUS, the American NGO) and their four children. Soon after finding out their HIV-positive status in 2005, Omondi and Celestine had become lay health "volunteers" at different HIV clinics in the city: Omondi at the provincial hospital, where he also got his HIV treatment, and Celestine at the FUS clinic. Three years later they became formally employed at these respective sites as community health workers, albeit on short-term contracts.[20] In 2010, when Celestine became seriously ill with tuberculosis, her employers, the American NGO running ART across several sites in the city, took her a private hospital in Kisumu, and paid her fees (which came to over fifty thousand shillings), on the understanding that her debt would be paid out of her monthly wages. Kenyan and American staff attached to the HIV clinic also helped her out with gifts of money.

For those who are struggling to live in the city—to find work and feed a family in the context of HIV infection and unemployment—accessing networks of material support from NGOs, often through patient support groups, is one means of survival. Another way of finding a living—albeit a precarious one—is becoming a "volunteer." This option is not available to everyone: you have to prove to those running the clinic that you are an "active" client who has taken on the "HIV gospel," as Omondi referred to it, and as more and more people are attracted to the clinic, competition is increasing. Volunteering rarely leads to a decent living—the trajectories of Omondi and Celestine, who managed to gain employment, are unusual. However, volunteering does open up new networks and contacts and new identities in the city. In the final section, I explore the trajectories and aspirations of some of these volunteers.

"We Are HIV Graduates": Volunteers in the Global Health Economy

Pamela was a widow in her forties. She lived with her last-born child, a teenager, and the three children of her deceased sister, in a rented room near Rose and BabaOdhis. Like them, she attended Malaga's patient support group and was a regular member at other support groups in the city. She discovered her status back in 2000, after losing her husband to AIDS and being forced by his family to leave their rural home. In 2001, a friend took her to one of the few clinics offering free HIV tests and treatment, as part of a pilot research study. Pamela became an active member of the clinic's "support group," and clinic staff presented her to an NGO that was looking for laypeople to train in HIV education. After that, she managed to attach herself as a "volunteer" to various NGO projects—providing advice about HIV and antiretroviral treatment, visiting patients in their houses and offering "home-based care." These projects never lasted for more than a few months, and as a volunteer Pamela gained little remuneration (one hundred to three hundred shillings a week, depending on the project; sometimes the money she was promised never materialized). Being under no illusions that her work as a CHW would lead to paid employment, she cobbled together a livelihood by combining volunteering with selling vegetables or fried food, the occasional support she received from NGOs (accessed through her membership in the patient support groups), and the intermittent gifts of money sent by her eldest son. Her income was extremely variable, and she was constantly on the verge of being thrown out of her room by her landlord. Her precarious situation was brought home to me when I bumped into her as she made her way home from an unsuccessful trip to an NGO at the other side of town, exhausted from the long walk. She had heard rumors that the organization was providing free sacks of flour, but she came back empty-handed. It is in this context that we can understand the value of the certificates that Pamela had collected and kept under lock and key in her bedside cabinet, framed copies of which were displayed on the walls of her room. These certificates attested to her participation in seminars and workshops. They did not offer formal qualifications, but they did provide evidence of what people in Kisumu refer to, in English, as "exposure" to the knowledge and skills promoted by the global health projects that have descended upon the city.

Pamela's work with HIV clinics and their "clients" was not easy. She spent her days walking in the hot sun to visit the people on the list provided by the clinic. Although she was given money to cover the cost of a bicycle taxi, she preferred to keep it and reach her destination on foot. Often she found that "clients" were not at home, and she had to go back later to find them. Some "clients" stop taking their medicine and, afraid of disapproval of the clinic staff, present themselves as new patients at another clinic. Some, afraid of the stigma associated with the HIV clinic, avoided her. It is particularly difficult for young women to be open about their HIV status, as, unlike Pamela, they are often dependent upon their male partners for economic support. Some people were suspicious of her motives and accused her of "eating" the benefits they believed she had access to from NGOs. She explained, "They feel that when you follow them to their house, there will be material benefits, and that you yourself gain from them. When they see you coming three times with empty hands, they feel you are wasting their time."

Still, Pamela was able to convert her HIV-positive status into a form of livelihood, even if it was unstable and uncertain. Volunteering also enabled her to navigate the often-confusing landscape of NGO projects and HIV clinics, and it gave her some status and a measure of respect and recognition. She knew a network of people working in HIV clinics and for NGO projects. Clinic staff appreciated her ability to navigate unfamiliar terrain that easily escapes bureaucratic procedures—the informal settlements and mobile lives of their inhabitants—while her neighbors appreciated her contacts with health workers at government and NGO facilities. She had managed to get her youngest son on a school sponsorship program run by the NGO World Vision. Volunteering also gave Pamela a sense of connection to something beyond her own neighborhood and, indeed, beyond Kisumu. She once showed me a smart black bag marked with the logo of an NGO and packed with still-unwrapped commodities, including soap and a towel. "Look at this!" she joked, "I have graduated! I'm at college! And people think I'm studying in America, I'm going to America!" Volunteers like Pamela often referred to themselves as "HIV graduates," drawing attention to the connection between volunteering and social mobility through their "exposure" to knowledge and to new ways of doing things (learned both in formal training through NGO-led workshops and in observing new ways of speaking, acting, and dressing). Yet Pamela's bag and its contents remained unused, perhaps because she feared that in displaying it she would become the object of heightened expectations and envy.

The pursuit of certificates, which give evidence of both "knowledge" and "exposure" to Kisumu's NGO world, are what motivated many of the young volunteers attracted to clinics, NGO projects, and community or self-help groups, who were, as they put it, "tarmacking" in the city—looking for employment. Many had secondary school education and nursed aspirations for what they termed "developing myself" and "moving ahead."[21] They hoped for formal employment, preferably in an office and for an NGO, and the knowledge and certificates that they could accrue through volunteering seemed to bring this goal a little closer. They came from families who had enjoyed social and geographical mobility over the previous two generations. Their fathers (and sometimes their mothers too) had been government civil servants— teachers, nurses, railway officers, or bureaucrats—until retiring or being retrenched, and their families had made great efforts to educate them as far as possible. Unlike their parents, however, they faced no easy path from education to employment. They came of age during or after the International Monetary Fund (IMF)–sponsored government retrenchments of the early 1990s and during a deepening employment crisis. The government employment enjoyed, for a while, by their parents provided no openings for them, and many (because of a lack of funds) had been unable to complete secondary school or college. Moreover, they belonged to a generation who had been children or came of age during the AIDS epidemic (which took hold in western Kenya in the late 1980s), and their lives had been intimately affected by it: many had lost parents and siblings to AIDS, and as families lost breadwinners, their education had been disrupted.

Given their frustrated aspirations for education and employment, the access to knowledge, training, and certificates offered by HIV projects in Kisumu was extremely attractive to these young people. Even if it involved walking in the heat and dust as "mobilizers" or "tracers" of patients, volunteering for HIV work offered the hope, if rarely the reality, of ending up with "office" work. Moreover, it associated one with the "working" classes, that is, with professional people, who are distinct from the majority of residents who must work in the "hot sun" (*juakali*) by the roadside. This distinction between office work and having to make a living in the juakali sector ran through many of the conversations I had with young volunteers about their motivations and hopes for the future. Actual experiences of volunteers, however, pointed to large gaps between the rhetoric of inclusion and opportunity and the realities of exclusion and insecurity. Many volunteers had spent months and even years volunteering, collecting various certificates, and applying for jobs, while supporting themselves through juakali work. Those who gained a foothold as volunteers in NGOs or HIV clinics often quickly lost it, as they navigated a landscape of tenuous projects, unstable flows of donor funds, uncertainty, and intense competition. Still, many of the volunteers I spoke to insisted that they were "moving ahead" and being "empowered": "Here I am getting exposed," explained one young woman, "and I am developing myself."

Developing Futures?

Juxtaposed with a struggling health system and faltering infrastructure, and in a city with few formal employment opportunities, global health interventions seem to offer not only (a limited form of) medical care but also opportunities for creating some kind of livelihood (or even, for some, a career) and a sense of a future. People's lives—their bodies and health, their hopes and future—have become intimately tied to these global assemblages of medicine, funding and expertise, and surveillance and care. Yet the intense forms of care—and control— emanating from the HIV clinic are temporally unstable, tied as they are to the "projectified" form that intervention takes. Moreover, they leave untouched the socioeconomic conditions that underlie exposure to disease and exacerbate ill-health. Such gaps are supposed to be filled by "the community" under the rubric of government and donor push for "community-based development."

The new ART programs add a further layer to health workers' experiences of negotiating and connecting public health practice and government employment with private practice, NGOs, and health research projects. For health workers they offer further opportunities for intertwining external funds and nongovernmental projects with national health services. However, this process is not without its tensions. First it exacerbates inequality in the provision of health care, as well-resourced HIV clinics stand alongside crumbling health-care infrastructures, producing enclaves of global medicine in a sea of "resource-poor" public health. One young intern on the hospital ward expressed his frustration with working there, "Because you know that just outside [that is, in the

HIV clinic], medicines are there, tests are there, but here, there is nothing!" Acutely aware of the differences between inside and outside HIV clinics, health workers at all levels of the hierarchy, as well as volunteers, compete to enter these globalized spaces of medical practice and to access projects. To gain access to medical care, to make a professional career, to gain new knowledge and skills, and to try to make a living, one has to maneuver oneself into these spaces, get "exposed," and grab whatever opportunities are available.

Second, global health interventions, organized through time-limited projects, deepen a sense of dependence. "What will we do when the donors/projects leave?" was a frequent question voiced by both health workers and patients. Dependent as they are on continued flows of donor funds, the new HIV clinics may ironically be a more ephemeral part of the urban infrastructure than the public hospital ward. It is this institutional precariousness layered upon the instability of urban lives that drives residents' desires for further knowledge, training, and certificates, and the constant search for contacts and positions as people struggle to navigate health crises, livelihoods, and futures in and beyond the "millennium" city. For those who don't succeed in entering these spaces, there is precious little insurance against the tragedy that Jerome experienced in losing his wife and child.

The temporal instability of this projectification of health and life in the city prompts some further questions. How do such interventions feed into and shape expectations of development and progress in Kisumu and beyond it? What kinds of futures *can* be imagined? For residents of the city, global health projects present a tangible form of development, which is evident in the newly built or repainted clinics, the fleets of shiny vehicles, and the circulation of Kenyan and expatriate professionals. Such development may be limited and circumscribed, and it fosters competition and inequality as much as solidarity. Still, it is attractive, partly because it offers a connection to what can be termed the "global," and partly because it represents a forward-moving trajectory, offering some kind of future, however vague that may be.[22] Pamela jokes about her journey to America, knowing full well this will never happen, while the younger volunteers hope against hope that, by "graduating" from volunteering, they will reach it. Development is not imagined here as a process encompassing the national collective but as an opportunity for individual social and geographic mobility. This process of self-transformation is captured in the expressions "I am developing myself" and "I am being empowered." Through projecting themselves into what they perceive to be spaces of personal transformation, volunteers hope to benefit from the trajectory of the "millennium" city and to partake of its hopeful future, even while the contours of this future remain unclear. However, few manage to gain a firm foothold in the global health economy and most people remain "tarmacking" in the city.

Despite the paradox between abundance and scarcity in the projectified landscape of global health in Kisumu, and despite the limitations of a public health that is focused on providing medicine to people in need of a livelihood, it is also clear that small movements and solidarities do emerge in this landscape of intervention, and that these are encouraged by the better conditions within HIV clinics. Whether these can lead to a more encompassing and sustained engagement with public health depends on making the resources available beyond HIV treatment and care, and thus on political will at both the national and international level.

Notes

1. See the 2007–8 report by the NGOs Coordination Board: www.ngobureau.or.ke /Publications/National%20Survey%20of%20NGOs%20Report.pdf. It shows that there are 117 NGOs with their headquarters in Kisumu and 790 operating in Kisumu but with their headquarters elsewhere. The survey staff could not physically locate or interview many of the smaller NGOs, raising questions about how they operate and indeed whether they still exist. See also www.kanco.org/KANCOmembers.php, which lists NGOs working in western Kenya.

2. Steve Robbins, "'Long Live Zackie, Long Live': AIDS Activism, Science and Citizenship after Apartheid," *Journal of Southern African Studies* 30 (2004): 651–72; Richard Rottenburg, "Social and Public Experiments and New Figurations of Science and Politics in Postcolonial Africa," *Postcolonial Studies* 12, no. 4 (2009): 423–40; Vinh-Kim Nguyen, *The Republic of Therapy: Triage and Sovereignty in West Africa's Time of AIDS* (Durham, NC: Duke University Press, 2011); Ruth J. Prince, "HIV and the Moral Economy of Survival in an East African City," *Medical Anthropology Quarterly* 26, no. 4 (2012): 534–56; Rebecca Marsland, "(Bio)sociality and HIV in Tanzania: Finding a Living to Support a Life," *Medical Anthropology Quarterly* 26, no. 4 (2012): 470–85.

3. Vinh-Kim Nguyen, "Government by Exception: Enrolment and Experimentality in Mass HIV Treatment Programs in Africa," *Social Theory and Health* 7, no. 3 (2009): 196–218.

4. Susan R. Whyte et al., "Therapeutic Clientship: Belonging in Uganda's Mosaic of AIDS Projects," in *When People Come First: Critical Studies in Global Health*, ed. João Biehl and Adriana Petryna, 140–65 (Princeton: Princeton University Press, 2013). The policies, politics, and practices associated with the move toward "global health"—such as vertical disease programs, drug donation projects, global health degrees, clinical tourism, and globalized medical research and scientific practice—are becoming objects of anthropological analysis. See, e.g., Craig R. Janes and Kitty Corbitt, "Anthropology and Global Health," *Annual Review of Anthropology* 38 (2009): 167–83; Johanna

Crane, "Unequal Partners: AIDS, Academia and the Rise of Global Health," *Behemoth* 3 (2010): 78–98; Ari Samsky, "Scientific Sovereignty: How International Drug Donation Programmes Reshape Health, Disease and the State," *Cultural Anthropology* 27, no. 2 (2012): 310–32; Lotte Meinert, Hanne O. Mogensen, and Jenipher Twebaze, "Tests for Life Chances: CD4 Miracles and Obstacles in Uganda," *Anthropology and Medicine* 16, no. 2 (August 2009): 195–209; Lisa Ann Richey, "Counselling Citizens and Producing Patronage: AIDS Treatment in South African and Ugandan Clinics," *Development and Change* 43, no. 4 (2012): 823–45.

5. Since early 2005, the free delivery of ART has been expanded, first in the city and later into rural areas, through government health facilities, private and mission hospitals, NGOs, and selected faith-based groups. See www.unaids.org/en/CountryResponses/Countries/kenya.asp. PEPFAR, the Global Fund, and (on a smaller scale) the Clinton Foundation and MSF (Médecins sans frontières/Doctors without Borders) fund the treatment. By September 2009, almost 300,000 people in Kenya were receiving ART (up from 10,000 in 2003); about a third of them lived in Nyanza Province. According to PEPFAR, by 2010, the numbers on ART had risen to 410,300, while 1,384,400 individuals were receiving "care and support" at HIV clinics. See www.aidskenya.org/Programmes/Treatment—Care-&-Support/ART, www.pepfar.gov/countries/kenya/index.htm. Other HIV/AIDS programs, such as prevention and provision for orphans, are supported by a wider range of institutions, including the World Bank.

6. In Kenya, PEPFAR provides funds to a host of "prime partners" (www.pepfar.gov/partners/103021.htm), which organize and monitor PSCs (e.g., Global AIDS Programme [GAP], Family Aids Care and Education Service [FACES], the Catholic Relief Services [CRS], Academic Model for the Prevention and Treatment of HIV/AIDS [AMPATH], and Liverpool VCT [LVCT]. See Philister A. Madiega et al., "'She's My Sister-in-Law, My Visitor, My Friend'—Challenges of Staff Identity in Home Follow-Up in an HIV Trial in Western Kenya," *Developing World Bioethics* 13, no. 1 (2011): 21–29.

7. Mary-Jo DelVecchio-Good et al., "Clinical Realities and Moral Dilemmas: Contrasting Perspectives from Academic Medicine in Kenya, Tanzania, and America," *Daedalus* 128, no. 4 (1999): 167–96; Susan Whyte et al., "Treating AIDS: Dilemmas of Unequal Access in Uganda," in *Global Pharmaceuticals: Ethics, Markets, Practices*, ed. Adriana Petryna, Andrew Lakoff, and Arthur Kleinman, 240–62 (Durham, NC: Duke University Press, 2006); Clare L. Wendland, *A Heart for the Matter: Journeys through an African Medical School* (Chicago: University of Chicago Press, 2010).

8. Clare Wendland and Noelle Sullivan present this contrast as one between the "global" and the "local": one part of medical practices operates at a "global" level (with state-of-the-art technology and facilities), while the other is resolutely "local." See Noelle Sullivan, "Enacting Spaces of Inequality," *Space and Culture* 15, no. 1 (2011): 57–67; Sullivan, "Mediating Abundance and Scarcity: Implementing an HIV/AIDS Targeted Project within a Government Hospital in Tanzania," *Medical Anthropology* 30, no. 2 (2011): 202–21; Claire L. Wendland, "Moral Maps and Medical Imaginaries: Clinical Tourism at Malawi's College of Medicine," *American Anthropologist* 114, no. 3 (2012): 108–22. Although this juxtaposition is extreme, the production of islands of "development" is not novel in Kenya, where NGO-led development has, particularly since the 1980s, been focused on projects that are geographically circumscribed and have not been scaled up to countrywide development. See Julie Hearn, "The NGO-isation of Kenyan Society: USAID and the Restructuring of Health Care," *Review of African Political Economy* 25 (1995): 89–100.

9. Kate Meagher, *Identity Economics: Social Networks and the Informal Economy in Nigeria* (Woodbridge, Suffolk, UK: James Currey, 2010).

10. James Ferguson, *Expectations of Modernity: Myths and Meanings of Urban Life on the Zambian Copperbelt* (Berkeley: University of California Press, 1999).

11. Angelique Haugerud, *The Culture of Politics in Modern Kenya* (Cambridge: Cambridge University Press, 1993); David W. Cohen and E.S.A. Odhiambo, *Siaya: The Historical Anthropology of an African Landscape* (Nairobi: Heinemann, 1989); Paul Wenzel Geissler and Ruth Jane Prince, *The Land Is Dying: Contingency, Creativity and Conflict in Kenya* (New York: Berghahn Books, 2010).

12. A similar picture of African towns being transformed as a whirl of NGOs and transnational organizations descend on them, fuelling an atmosphere of international development, has been observed in Mozambique. See James Pfeiffer, "International NGOs in the Mozambique Health Sector: The 'Velvet Glove' of Privatization," in *Unhealthy Health Policy: A Critical Anthropological Examination*, ed. Arachu Castro and Merrill Singer, 43–62 (Walnut Creek, CA: Altamira Press, 2004).

13. Prince, "HIV and the Moral Economy."

14. Hearn, "NGO-isation of Kenyan Society"; Whyte, Whyte, Meinert, and Twebaze, "Therapeutic Clientship."

15. I conducted sixty-four interviews with staff members and volunteers associated with two NGO-run and two government PSCs, including doctors, clinical officers (COs), nurses, nutritionists, pharmacists, counselors, clinic assistants, community health workers, "peer educators," and "follow-up" staff. I also observed clinic practice and accompanied health workers in visits to patients at home. In addition, I interviewed volunteers who had attached themselves to NGO-run "youth intervention" projects, and I visited various community-based organizations (CBOs), NGOs, patient support groups, and youth groups. The research was affiliated with the University of Maseno's Department of Sociology and Social Anthropology, and research permission was granted by the Ministry of Higher Education, Science and Technology.

16. All names are pseudonyms.

17. Their monthly remuneration was 3,000 shillings, about US$50 at the time.

18. Ippolytos Kalofenos, "All I Eat Is ARVs!" *Medical Anthropology Quarterly* 24, no. 3 (2010): 363–80; Prince, "HIV and the Moral Economy"; Marsland, "Value of HIV in Tanzania."

19. At the time, 5,000 shillings was about US$80.

20. In 2008, 11,000 shillings was approximately US$150.

21. Ann Swidler and Susan Cotts Watkins observe similar aspirations among volunteers in Malawi; see Swidler and Watkins, "'Teach a Man to Fish': The Sustainability Doctrine and Its Social Consequences," *World Development* 37, no. 7 (2009): 1182–96.

22. Michael Burawoy, "Manufacturing the Global," *Ethnography* 2, no. 147 (2001): 147–59.

NINE

The Archipelago of Public Health

Comments on the Landscape of Medical Research
in Twenty-First-Century Africa

P. WENZEL GEISSLER

ANTHROPOLOGISTS AND GEOGRAPHERS OF THE CONTEMPORARY world draw our attention to the spatial changes that accompany new economic forms, including transnational capital flows, direct investment, resource extraction and capital concentration, and connected political processes framed by denationalization and the progressive vitiation of the nation-state.[1] This has produced new landscapes, which intersperse contiguous territories with isolated enclosures—of investment, production, extraction—and which despite proliferating fictions of security are ruled by ephemerality and unpredictability for most of their inhabitants.

The novelty of this political-economic geography is evident by contrast to Thomas More's republic, a root source of the modern political imagination: an island, run by experts, who operate from the center outward, progressively integrating even the distant reaches of space into a concentric functional whole of mutually sustaining and enhancing production, reproduction, and administration, extending knowledge and responsibility to the far shores of Utopia's territory. This vision of a social, political-economic, historical whole entails a particular understanding of action, as expansive outward movement, appropriating space through work, back and forth between center and periphery, reflected in imaginaries of colonization and conquest, modernization and development, which (in more or less benevolent ways) envisaged the transformation of (all) space.

In the contemporary archipelago that (albeit always partially) replaces the vision of the island republic, action—political, economic, or scientific—takes on a different meaning. Rather than doggedly pushing forward—expanding the transformative reach of modernity, mid-twentieth-century style—effective action in this new landscape is a matter of short-circuiting the right nodes, establishing momentary and jumping connections across wider spaces, making the right moves to sustain networks, and entering compartments, containers of modern possibility, or exiting from spaces of abandon. This entails insulating enclosures and conduits, temporarily appropriating particular points or delimited spaces, but without the lasting claims and counterclaims entailed by historically rooted imagined communities like the nation-state.

Just as in earlier patterns of center and periphery upon which the trajectories of modernization and progress were played out, relations in this new geography (superimposed upon remnants of older topographic structures and directionalities) are asymmetrical. Inside and outside are not equivalent positions toward enclosures; and connections are initiated, controlled, and sustained from certain locations and positions of interest and ownership.

This reformulation of space, leading to new patterns and movements, is reiterated on diverse levels of scale: across the globe, in the stubbornly persistent framing of the nation-state, in our cities. And it operates across diverse domains of practice, which half a century ago were constituted in a different spatial-temporality: national frames of economic regulation and production are, for example, transcended by multinational corporations and foreign direct investment, export production zones, and other forms of exception; and policy and governance thrive in realms of nongovernmental globality, which at its benevolent pole takes the form of humanitarianism—epitomized by Médecins sans frontières and the UN refugee camp—and at its destructive pole that of global security policy, legitimizing the spaceless order of rendition, preemptive drone strikes, and surveillance (the poles being short-circuited by military "humanitarian interventions").[2]

Navigating the Archipelago

In charting these new spaces, it is important to acknowledge that these landscapes are neither unequivocal nor stable. While exclusion and inclusion, abandonment and control indeed are prominent features, these are not static structures of domination, but also spaces of opportunity and contestation. Exclusion relies upon inclusion, and who and what are included are not necessarily included in the same way. Exclusivity provokes desires, both of inclusion in an existing order, and of rupturing the enclosure, proposing alternative arrangements. Real-time links across unlikely distances, through transportation and communication technologies, connect some and disconnect others—oil pipelines through Fourth World marshlands. Bubbles are rarely impermeable. What operates as barriers protecting an enclosed space will also always occasion bridges and provoke tunnels and transgressions. And although the new ordering does often rely on mechanisms of spatial separation and violence, these do not exhaust the capacities of the landscape to reference other projects. Seemingly stable walls are erected on the accumulated historical traces of past inhabitation and struggles, established patterns of movement, and memories of past changes—and of failed hopes for change.[3] Thus, past vistas and vectors continue to define the landscape, and enable other movements, evoking past hegemonies or contesting hegemonic orders.

Geographies of Medical Science

The life sciences and medicine are not excluded from these geographical changes; indeed, it seems as if "life," as in the reckoning and protection of mere biological life and the technologies of maintaining, sheltering, or enhancing it, has obtained particular importance in the contemporary political-economic ordering.[4] This is especially marked in the large parts of the world where life is precarious, threatened by poverty and its pathological manifestations in the form of infectious diseases, hunger, and violence. In the absence of functioning national governments, or of resources for such governments to deploy, responses to these threats to human life rely especially in Africa often upon transnational interventions and collaborations, involving foreign governments, nongovernmental organizations, and industry and charity. Biopolitics, once associated with the nation-state, here takes new forms.

Charting this novel biopolitical space, Adriana Petryna, among others, focuses on the changing geography of multinational pharmaceutical production under the impact of the "outsourcing" of industry clinical trials.[5] Before this shift, pharmaceutical research had been primarily carried out within the framework of national regulation and health-care provision. Analogous to the outsourcing of industrial manufacturing to overseas export production zones—bounded territories of legislative and economic exception, relying on a hinterland of unlimited labor[6]—such research is now relocated in insular research sites (and legally insulated contract research organizations), dotted across low- and especially middle-income countries, which offer suitable study populations and pools of qualified but cheap scientific workers.

In a similar vein, the ethnography of nongovernmental transnational pharmaceutical interventions, ranging from the control of "neglected tropical diseases" to treatment and care for HIV/AIDS, reveals similar structures of long-distance flows of funding and expertise and enclosed treatment spaces, alongside generalized public health care—such as HIV patient support centers beside government hospitals and single-disease eradication programs parallel to national health systems.[7] At the same time, these ethnographies draw attention to countering movements to and unforeseen social productivity within these global pharmaceutical regimes, such as new local solidarities and political associations, as well as global activism.[8]

While the new geographies of private pharmaceutical industry have received extensive anthropological scrutiny, the contemporary order of *public* health science—research conducted by publicly employed scientists in public institutions and hospitals, using public funds (though usually not from the country in which the research is conducted), and aiming for public goods—has received less attention.[9] This omission is problematic, because the aims and practices of public health science are different from those of for-profit research—seeking treatments for diseases that mainly afflict the poor majority and that are thus of less interest to the pharmaceutical industry, and deploying government or charity resources to that end. Those who work with and fund public health research tend to be driven by different interests and motives—including presumably equity and justice. Thus, even though the public nature of such scientific work is currently under threat from the privatization of higher education and from the incursion of industry interests into public health and academic realms, one requires a clearer idea of what public science is in its own right, and what it should be, rather than subsuming it under a generalized critique of global (bio)economies.

In this chapter I begin charting emerging geographies of public health science, drawing upon studies of medical research in Africa over the past decade, and in particular one research station, where I have conducted long-term ethnographic fieldwork. Despite their different motivations, public health research institutions in Africa show geographical patterns—enclosures, exclusions, hopping connections, and ephemerality—that are strangely similar to the geography of commodity extraction and manufacturing, including of pharmaceuticals that I alluded to above. Yet these similarities cannot be explained in terms of capital accumulation or protection of profit interest. Instead, they may be partly economic effects of growing inequality (necessitating separations and securitization) and of state vitiation and corruption (requiring alternative control structures), partly driven by methodological changes in science itself (moving, for example, toward genomics and high-cost, rapid-turnover, automated apparatus), partly shaped by global regulatory mechanisms (such as the Federal Drug Agency [FDA] and the standardization of "good clinical practice" [GCP]), and further informed by new academic and managerial aesthetics and fashions.

Discerning and explaining such forms and patterns can only be a first step; more important is then to look at what they enable, and how people inhabit them and change their shapes. In the first part of the following discussion I will thus sketch pertinent forms of the archipelago of African public health science today around the case of one exemplary scientific field station. In the second part I take a look at the largest group of that research station's inhabitants—local, temporarily employed scientific staff—exploring their positions and movements within this landscape. While these observations cannot replace a proper ethnographic account, they serve as a caveat against simplified "critical" representations.

An Archipelago of Science

This is about a particular place of science:[10] a transnational medical research station that operates in and around a medium-sized African city, through a partnership between an African and a Northern, publicly funded research organization. The station is part of a larger national government scientific research institution that maintains several stations around the country, of which, however, only some are active, depending on the level of overseas funding they receive through "collaborations." This station is the largest in the country, comparable to about twenty similarly sized stations around Africa. While it thus is not average, it is typical for the contemporary formation of high-end medical research in Africa, and its scientific output has led to the development of new medical scientific knowledge and shaped public health policy across Africa.

Established thirty years ago, the station has annual core funding of around $25 million, provided by a key northern public health institution that conducts research in several African countries other than the one in which my exemplar station is located. Of the over 1,200 staff members (not accounting for volunteers who support field research activities, who also accrue some income from their work), a handful are expatriates, employed directly by the sponsoring government, while the majority are employees of the African national organization. Some of the latter are employed on permanent government contracts, while the vast majority is on short-term contracts funded through project grants by the overseas partner.

The research station runs numerous clinical trials and research projects in urban and rural areas, focused on developing and improving interventions against HIV and malaria. In the pursuit of cutting-edge scientific knowledge, it touches upon the lives of hundreds of thousands of people through data collection, monitoring, and surveillance and, not least, through the health benefits that it brings to almost everybody enrolled in its activities. The latter may take the form of trial-related health care and free treatment or of less systematic advice, support, and knowledge gleaned through informal association with medical personnel and exposure to research practices. As the region's largest employer (apart from civil service), its most influential producer of health-care knowledge, and a provider of care and treatment to many of its inhabitants, the research station is a prominent landmark, familiar to almost everybody in the area. Many people have applied for work there and even more would like to be participants in its research endeavors.

Arising from the collaboration between a major "northern" partner and an African national institution, the research station is also the material embodiment of the contemporary order of global health research. Despite its "capacity-building" efforts, it continues to rely on transfers of money, resources, and expertise from North to South, predominantly derived from public, government funds and some contributions from big charities and the pharmaceutical industry (mainly as drug donations). The African institutional host is formally associated with its national government but constituted as a "parastatal," that is, a corporation with independent accounts and the right to own physical and intellectual property. This allows it to directly engage in transnational partnerships, instead of channeling funds through government institutions (with the attendant problems of accountability and efficiency).[11] Formally constituted with the aim of seeking overseas collaboration, this parastatal would not be able to sustain significant medical research on its limited government allocation. Collaboration in this context entails the reinvigoration of members of the nation-state body by means of foreign funding, which creates bubbles of heightened activity in delimited sites and within the time limits of funding cycles and research outcomes (although often attracting series of consecutive projects).

The Atoll

The basic elements of this contemporary geography are reiterated across different levels of scale, as interconnected spatial enclosures, circulations between them, and vectors beyond them. The central node in this local version of the archipelago is the field station. This is located outside the city boundaries, in the semiurban countryside: a ten-acre compound with well-furnished offices, biosafety level 3 laboratories, and genome sequencing facilities. Partly on account of the valuable equipment concentrated here, the station is an enclosed space, protected by a concrete wall, CCTV cameras, and the staff of an international private security company. Access to the station is via two separate security gates, at each of which identity passes are required.

Inside the compound, the neat pavements, watered and trimmed lawns, freshly painted and cleaned buildings, and well-dressed young, cosmopolitan staff provide a pleasant environment that could be almost anywhere in the world. Outside the wall is African countryside: scattered homesteads among small maize fields and bush, traversed by roads flanked with the obligatory corrugated iron "hotels" and small shops. Because most of the research is conducted in designated study areas elsewhere, the surrounding countryside is largely untouched by the field station, except for the benefits of water supply and access to the staff clinic, and some economic activities servicing the station, such as rental housing and kiosks.

The station is the hub where the scientists and administrators have their offices, where meetings are held, major laboratory investigations are done, data are processed and analyzed, supplies and human resource matters are administered, and the station's large transport fleet is parked, fuelled, and maintained. Through independent satellite communication, the station is linked to the northern partner's headquarters, allowing for real-time communication and data sharing with distant centers of academic excellence and with international research consortia. In reference to its belonging to a different level of scale, the station is jokingly referred to, by local staff, by the name of the northern city in which the headquarters of the overseas collaborating partner is situated.

To conduct clinical work, the field station has built and maintains two clinical research centers, adjacent to major government hospitals. Although these are situated on government hospital land, they are distinctive custom-built facilities, protected enclaves that concentrate material resources and clinical and scientific capacity, and provide excellent working conditions to staff, as well as exceptionally good medical services to research participants. Like the main field station, their laboratory facilities are vastly superior to those of the adjacent hospitals (which they assist when resources allow, but which they cannot and should not replace). Their communication systems and drug supplies provide (nearly) seamless integration into global circuits of data and technology. Meanwhile, flows of information and resources across the immediate boundaries of the center into the government hospital and public health administration are limited, despite efforts to strengthen government facilities e.g. by provision of shared professional training. Like the HIV treatment centers described by Prince (this volume), these centers are also aesthetically demarcated from the surrounding architecture through their new, well-maintained, high-quality building materials, furnishing, and landscaping.

Within one rural government dispensary that has no unused spaces, custom-fitted maritime containers, furnished variously as clinic, office, or laboratory and deployed for the duration of a clinical trial, provide a mobile, miniature version of the research center.[12] While the mobility and temporariness of this deployable space of science are particularly obvious in this case, even the seemingly more solid edifices of the field station and research centers are temporary, dependent upon short funding cycles and threatened by political changes in the host country or overseas. Their apparently solid boundaries—and their deployment in a particular site—depend upon the continuity of sustenance from the overseas partner, refracting larger asymmetries into their geography.

The figure of the bubble, sustained by its boundaries, is reiterated in its smallest and most mobile form in the fleet of well-maintained and recognizable 4x4 vehicles, through which staff move between these compounds and into the field. These mobile units, which circulate across a territory of several hundred square kilometers, transporting staff and specimens, are the most visible material form of the research collaboration. Along main rural roads everybody knows them and associates them with both health and knowledge, and wealth: their well-kept shiny surfaces stand in stark contrast to the dusty landscape and most of the other cars in the village, and the foreign-embassy number plates (which were changed to national government plates after the end of our fieldwork) underlined their peculiar extraterritoriality. These cars are like traveling enclosures in their own right, linked through GPS monitoring and CCTV, through mechanics and drivers, to the research station. At the time of fieldwork, government regulations in principle prohibited transporting nonstaff local passengers (although the research management of course allowed for ad-hoc exceptions in medical and other emergencies), which made the cars hard to get into and thus particularly attractive to those outside, much like the research compounds themselves.

The creation of distinctive spatial compounds is not limited to the making of "insides," as in stations and centers. The "field" outside the enclosures is reshaped along similar spatial principles, creating bounded zones of scientific investigation, connected to the stations and centers and through them to the academic centers of excellence. This work of zoning pertains on a larger level of scale to the agreements between different overseas partners about their zones of influence, achieved through negotiation and strategic investment.[13] Within a given region, large organizations and trials similarly avoid complications by negotiating the boundaries of study areas and sometimes cooperating on recruitment, or standardizing recruitment procedures and participant identification (to avoid competition and prevent double recruitment, and attendant risks to participants).

The most efficient and costly way of demarcating territory and creating favorable conditions for valid scientific research is establishing areas of "demographic surveillance" (or "demographic surveillance systems" [DSS]), which today can be found across Africa. These are territories of up to several hundred square kilometers, with up to several hundred thousand inhabitants, in which all households are enumerated, mapped and regularly visited, and in which population vital statistics and sometimes morbidity data are routinely collected. To create such comprehensive surveillance, research programs invest about a million dollars per year. This work generates fine-grained observational data about health and illness comparable to the most developed countries, which can then be used to guide public health planning and policy; at the same time, this provides necessary background information for future clinical trials—for instance, on the prevalence of pathogens and incidence of infections, the efficacy of the infrastructure, and people's willingness to adhere to study procedures—and can thus attract cutting-edge global randomized controlled trials. DSS are also substantial apparatuses of governmentality that bestow a close interest on their denizens, often associated with some form of health care and other benefits. Against the backdrop of neglect by national government institutions that prevails outside the DS system, such attention and care are widely appreciated by recipients.

DSS zones produce new social relations and forms. Staff from the field station engage with locally recruited fieldworkers, as well as a large number of local "volunteers" (paid not a regular salary but remuneration for specific bits of work or information rendered). These workers—aided by maps, numbered homes and houses, GPS systems, hand-held computers, and local Wi-Fi hotspots—move around the area continuously, collecting specimens and survey data, visiting homes, maintaining contact with trial participants and "engaging community," distributing information, and resolving tensions. They create routine pathways, demarcate areas of activity for staff moving on bicycles or foot, and establish new grids and networks, associations, and modes of behavior.

Within the new geography of global health research, demographic surveillance areas function as sentinel sites that can pick up new health trends and as experimental laboratory spaces to try out new interventions. Their relationship to the territories around them is not that of center to periphery within an overall logic of expansion (as in the mid-twentieth-century developmentalist logic), but that of sample to sampling frame. And although meliorist, developmentalist narratives remain the background discourse of global health research, the effects of these zones on the surrounding spaces are at best indirect, mediated through scholarly publications, new pharmaceuticals and vaccines, and international policy processes.

The definite zoning of rural areas exemplified by DSS is more difficult within cities with their more mobile and heterogeneous inhabitants. In our case, urban study populations are instead drawn, in principle, from concentric areas defined by distance from the research center. Yet, most participants of the studies we observed came not from the general population of the city but from areas classified by town planners as "slums" (unplanned, located around the periphery of the planned city, and on average economically poorer). This was partly because of these areas' higher incidence of disease, and their population's greater need for quality diagnosis and care, which usually was provided by trials, as well as because of the density and accessibility of people in these areas. Not unlike the more obvious situation in the countryside, urban study populations thus belong to a particular social and geographical territory: unplanned high-density areas inhabited by comparatively poor people lacking vital infrastructure and employment. This social zoning is underlined by the use of the term *the community*, referencing local residential status, relatively low income and educational status, and adherence to customary practices. This urban "community" is further partitioned into distinct target groups of research and intervention, such as, for example, "HIV high-risk groups" such as prostitutes and young men, or HIV "discordant couples," which constitute bounded population subsets especially suitable for particular types of HIV prevention trials.

The landscape of research is shaped by enclosing (and excluding) boundaries, compounds and wastelands, and hopping real-time links in-between and beyond.[14] As a result of the combined fragmentation, or more precisely expatriation (carving out spaces from a larger whole and interconnecting these with similar entities elsewhere), and detemporalization (removing the clear-cut progressive and expansionist logic of older, modernist "public health" thinking), the ethnographer and, more significantly, public health workers, clinicians, and patients have difficulty making out an overarching whole or a directed long-term trajectory toward an improved future. Instead, this is a world of islands suspended in the present tense.

This geography is not limited to medical research; the field station is exemplary of wider trends in the public health landscape. As the chapter by Prince in this volume shows, HIV care and treatment (like research sustained through funds and pharmaceutical resources provided by overseas organizations) tends to create spatial distinctions similar to those described above—separate buildings, container deployments, parallel pharmacies and records systems, group-focused feeding programs, resulting experiences of in- and exclusion, and so forth—and similarly temporary economies of health care and of paragovernmental employment, dependent upon funding cycles, short-term contracts, and voluntarism.

Another domain of parallel medical-geographical change that provides the context of public health research is the progressive privatization of health care. African health care has been "privatized" for several decades (by reducing government spending and introducing user fees at public institutions, involving drug sellers in care, and so forth). More recently, global standard, high-quality health care has proliferated, located in well-equipped private hospitals that continuously enhance their technological possibilities and have become more visible through new buildings and publicity campaigns. While most people continue to rely on decaying government health services patched up with shifting overseas aid programs, a proportion of the new (though highly unstable) "middle classes" obtain private health insurance coverage through (usually short-term) employment with larger organizations and companies. They access, though only for the duration of their contracts and within tight limits of coverage, clinical and diagnostic services in the new health-care enclaves. This offers important services to some but excludes the majority. And it provides the latter with a manifest experience of exclusion that was less palpable only a decade ago (and that recalls a time when the city had segregated European and African hospitals). To most inhabitants of the emerging public health archipelago, billboards depicting caring and beautiful health-care personnel operating the latest MRI scanners and television advertisements promising dedicated cancer care make for an experience of potential connections that simultaneously evokes fear of exclusion and longings for inclusion, in much the same way as the medical research enclosures do.

Beyond the pursuit of health, this experience of desire and exclusion is also conveyed by the city itself. Newly built shopping centers have opened over the past decade at the perimeter of the planned city, adjacent to unplanned slums and, for that reason, surrounded by concrete walls and staffed with private security controlling access. These shopping centers contain commodities and entertainment that reference global connections and would satisfy most consumers' expectations. At the same time, they epitomize, for those excluded from their bounty, the growing violence of political-economic development; as potent symbols of contemporary im/possibilities they are poles of desire, and targets of resentment and aggression (brought to a desperate, awful, but not meaningless, extreme by "terrorist" attacks on Kenyan shopping malls). The same trend toward urban fragmentation and the spreading of walled enclaves is reflected around the city in gated housing communities in projected new suburbs, as well as in the establishment of export production zones on land around the new international airport. In this emerging urban topography, medical research enclaves are just one of the many kinds of "bubble" that the inhabitants of the city negotiate as they go about their daily lives.

Journeying the Archipelago

The institution of public health research described in the first part of this chapter is inhabited by a heterogeneous "trial community" consisting of local and expatriate scientists, administrators, and local staff ranging from doctors to fieldworkers; intermediaries such as community representatives, peer counsellors, and other "volunteers"; and the research participants, some of whom regularly enter the research enclaves, others being visited at home.[15] Each of these participates in the research endeavor with different resources and knowledge, different motivation and interests, making for a complex assemblage that defies simplified or antagonistic renderings, such as "researcher vs. researched," "local vs. outsider," "black vs. white." Below I focus on the largest group of these: temporary local staff. Working on short-term contracts with the local partner institution and paid by the overseas collaborator, these range from field workers with secondary school certificates, earning as little as $300 per month, to qualified doctors who can earn more than $2,000 per month (both being extremely good salaries by local standards).

While the map of the archipelago, roughed out above, foregrounds lines of enclosure and connection, boundaries and obstacles, focusing on inhabitation brings to light perspectives and movements, which indeed are regulated and sometimes obstructed by topographical features but also facilitated and orientated by the landscape. Boundaries (which on a map are rendered as stable, closed lines) can then be made, and remade, through practices of recognition and enforcement, as well as permeation and transgression. Boundaries are crossed, sometimes in regular ways, such as waiting at and legitimately passing gates, and sometimes irregularly, for example, when using the research lab to process a relative's blood sample or assisting a government medical colleague with a diagnostic test or drug. In the remainder of the chapter, I explore the trajectories of local scientific staff, following their movements from outside into the enclosure, in and out, and out again.

Looking from Outside

Everybody working with the research station had been familiar with its name and existence long before being employed by it. Staff members who joined the research teams after employment in the government hospitals or NGOs had often earlier worked alongside research staff or met these individuals through public health campaigns and policy meetings, and they had visited the buildings for seminars and training. Employees recruited from the countryside had often heard about research projects by virtue of living in a study area or through knowing study participants; all of them had observed the fleet of cars, with the collaboration's logo and distinct number plates, which had exponentially grown since the 1990s. These vehicles were experienced as objects of longing: "I was looking at these cars passing our village, but I never hoped that I someday could be inside one," as one junior staff member expressed a sentiment shared by many.

Vehicles reference multiple meanings. For most villagers, especially young people, a journey to the provincial city is a major, costly, and exciting undertaking. The rapid movements of the large 4×4 research vehicles, penetrating deeply into areas otherwise underserved by motorized transport and shuttling swiftly back and forth between the city and the remote "reserve," represent for them longed-for connections, that is, mobility away from the day-to-day experience of stasis, and to new experiences, knowledge and opportunity. This mobility, associated with medical endeavors, looks particularly attractive if one lives far from the nearest hospital and is without means of transport. The research vehicles are also attractive on account of their "beauty" and comfort, especially compared to crowded and dangerously fast local minibuses and motorbikes. The fact that drivers must not take additional passengers only adds to the exclusivity and desirability of these local manifestations of global medical research, which swiftly pass you as you wait for a minibus and may suddenly appear—as harbingers of opportunity or of health-related concerns—at the gate of your homestead.

As in most parts of the world, flashy cars reference money. The research station's vehicles are expensive 4×4s, of the brand preferred by wealthy and powerful people for their travel to the "upcountry" home. As a fieldworker commented, "People believe that inside [the research organization] there is a lot of money," adding with reference to his own career planning, "So I also wanted to get that money." Seen from outside—especially by aspiring rural youth yearning for education and employment—those traveling in a research car have made it. Disembarking from one of these cars, staff members remarked, made it impossible to convince study participants or even one's own relatives that one's salary was limited.

While money is universally attractive, its owners or dispensers are also often suspect in the eyes of those who do not have money. Most, especially rural, staff members recalled having heard rumors about medical research and the station prior to employment. These rumors take different forms, familiar from the historical and anthropological literature about medical research in Africa (notably the work of Luise White).[16] While these rumors rarely gain enough momentum to negatively affect research activities and are believed by only a few or only for brief moments, they point at the oddity and thus narrative productivity of research.

The explanatory gap in which such stories proliferate is partly due to the wealth evidenced by the cars and other resources; it is also caused by the unusual directionality of research work, deploying, by local standards, enormous resources to reach the doorstep of poor people, driving 4×4s to homes never before visited by a car—and all this to acquire small bodily specimens or answers to simple questions about everyday life issues like sex, childcare, or food.

Getting Inside

Despite some stories of envy and suspicion, for most people in the area, getting into (or, in local parlance, "being with") the research station is extremely attractive, not only as a source of income, but also as access to cutting-edge knowledge on medical issues and not least on HIV, which is one of the region's biggest health problems and, paradoxically, also accounts for its largest job market in interventions and research. While for most the only way to attain this status is to become a research participant, the desire and hope to gain employment in research is widespread, and few thrifty graduates of secondary schools, drivers, typists, and so forth have never applied for a position; as a study coordinator remarked, "Everyone wants to be employed [by research programs], so outsiders always flock in places where we advertise."

Because employment contracts are only up to one year (although people are often reemployed consecutively, sometimes for decades), positions are advertised frequently, both on the Internet and through printed advertisements that are posted in glass boxes outside the station's gates and in other public places. They are thus widely visible, triggering longings and applications. For less-skilled positions such as driver and fieldworker, it is not uncommon to have a hundred applications. Because most of these, unavoidably, are unsuccessful, rumors about irregularities in recruitment circulate. As a midlevel staff member summarized, disapprovingly, "People say that getting a job in [the field station] was very hard; they say you must know somebody inside." However, although the speaker continued that he had been lucky to hear about the job from "a friend inside" who gave him the advertisement, such perceptions may be driven more by the disappointment of people who applied for jobs, often many times, in vain, rather than being grounded in actual corruption or nepotism.

The feeling of "having to know someone" may also be fuelled by the fact that previous familiarity with health-related nongovernmental institutions and informal knowledge gleaned through such engagements are decisive advantages when applying for research employment. Such "exposure"—as it is locally referred to—is documented through thick portfolios of certificates from workshops and training, submitted by applicants, and evidenced through up-to-date vocabulary, self-confident manners, comportment, and dress. In other words, to become "working class" (see Whyte's and Prince's chapters in this volume) in an organization as attractive as the research station, which is the largest and most top-end employer around, it is almost a prerequisite that one already has a foot in that class.

Another important avenue to get "inside," in advance of job applications, are less formal, even more temporary ways of "being with" the research organization, either as research participants or as other types of "volunteers"—peer counsellors or recruiters, community advisers, and so forth—allowing one to gain experience and familiarize oneself with specific, rapidly shifting forms of knowledge and adequate ways of comportment, along with gaining some modest remuneration. While such attachments—especially research participation—do not commonly lead to formal employment, they form part of how the way inside is imagined by those who are still on the outside.

Being Inside

Those lucky enough to get a job and "enter research" experience a process of habituation to the inside environment. To start with, crossing boundaries—into the station and centers, between its parts, into vehicles, and so forth—has to be learned. Some staff had, prior to employment, visited the research station and experienced its stringent security procedures. The issuing of magnetic ID cards takes time, during which new staff are in an intermediary state, having to continuously negotiate security controls and access to transportation. These experiences, which are repeated whenever one forgets one's gate pass, inscribe the importance of external boundaries, as well as the privilege of being able to traverse them.

Once inside, many staff members recall a transition regarding personal appearance and habits. Those already inside have a distinct (and relatively more expensive) taste in dress and, for ladies, hairstyles. Intangible but no less important signs are vocabulary, accents, and bodily gestures, as well as preferred, or known, social venues and shopping places. "Being with" research involves adapting to these new ways, which is both enjoyable and thrilling and simultaneously potentially irritating as it challenges one's identity. As one junior female staff recalled, "I could hear my flip-flops in the staircase, among all these high heels; and [unlike other employed women] I refused wearing trousers. . . . I didn't like it. . . . And do you remember your habit of going [around in] bare feet and rolling up your trousers? Everybody was joking about it. You looked like a peasant. Now even you have improved yourself."

Cutting and Making Relations

The personal transformation into a "person of research," an insider, staff recalled, comes with changed social relations.[17] Kin and friendship relations outside work are affected by one's changed identity, which may entail raised status but also social distance. Staff commonly described tensions and ruptures arising from this. This alienation is partly an effect of material expectations provoked by the employment, which staff members were unable or unwilling to satisfy, and partly of the insights into matters of health, global connections, and international styles that insiders gain as part of their exposure and which create mutual distance from less-successful relatives and friends, or even spouses. Not infrequently, these tensions have a gendered aspect, because the research station provides well-paid, high-status employment to many young women, some of whom are married, while others prefer to have family on their own. While outright negative rumors—such as accusing staff members of evil deeds or corruption—do occur but are unusual, many especially junior workers recalled accusations by friends and family of "arrogance" or "selfishness" that negatively affected their social lives.

New social relations with work colleagues, inside, do not easily replace older social networks, partly because of marked managerial hierarchies but also because of the competitive relationships between staff on the same level, who would regularly compete for promotion, training opportunities, or new employment contracts. The culture of "looking good" among those inside also prevents too-open social contacts, as appearances can only be upheld up to some point. Thus, somewhat surprisingly, staff do not necessarily socialize with colleagues. As one fieldworker said, "Everywhere you go [in the city], you find [colleagues]. I am . . . careful about mixing my social and professional friends, so all the friendships I make at the workplace, they end at the gate, so outside there, I pick a new social life." Moreover, what from the outside may have looked like one unified space of difference vis-à-vis ordinary local life looks different from the inside; larger differences and separations are reflected by the social order inside. Inequalities and hierarchies shape work relations between different levels of staff, and between expatriate and local staff. Far from achieving the promise of unequivocal "being with," one discovers, once one is inside, that boundaries proliferate. The effort to negotiate entry gives way for struggles to get a little more inside, to rise in institutional hierarchies, and to gain access to requisite information and relations. At the same time, getting to know, through one's work, new people whom one would otherwise never have socialized with, on account of their educational status, class, or origins, is also exciting and rewarding, as this young technologist expressed, "Yah, I have exposure. I have met so many . . . people that I never knew that I could meet, in the world of [science], being with them, I have talked to them, I have shared with them. I have learned a lot."

Looking Out

Once inside, one discovers that the outside also looks different. Staff members described in different ways how what before was ordinary became strange, even unattractive or threatening, once they were employed. This applies to mundane aspects of everyday life, as well as to working conditions, as one study coordinator explained: "Being inside 'can cheat you' until you forget outside; you think that out there in the world, everything is like [research]; it makes you feel so comfortable . . . that it might even hamper your creativity in the African setup; you might start look[ing] at the world like a [foreigner]." What previously just was an area of the city, or a village, possibly including one's home spaces, becomes "the field" into which one ventures on "fieldwork" and which is inhabited by "the community"—a term that, as noted above, in this context connotes stable local attachments, as well as low economic and educational status. This re-envisaging of one's neighbors can entail some distancing, such as when, through the idiom employed at work, local medical and ritual practices are rendered as "traditional," common leisure life becomes "risk behavior," or when lamenting the apparently irrational "nonadherence" of research participants to research procedures—due to more-pressing everyday commitments—or their "ignorance" of basic medical-related knowledge. The more distanced perspective onto "the field" that results from adapting the epistemological distinction between researcher and research object means that doing fieldwork is a rather different experience from one's ordinary dealings with the same area and people (see also Brown's chapter in this volume).

Positioning oneself vis-à-vis a "community" also entails changing one's identity, especially for the majority of staff who without their employment would themselves pass as "community." Thus, a fieldworker recruited precisely because of his origins and ties in "the local community" becomes, once employed, someone who "represents community" toward more senior and expatriate staff, thereby attaining a position of distinction from ordinary community members in his relations with local people.

Venturing Out

Fieldwork, then, is often conceived of in terms of its "hardship." Visiting a research participant somewhere not far from one's own neighborhood or in the adjacent village, let alone walking or using a bicycle taxi (otherwise familiar modes of transportation for most staff members) may during fieldwork be considered a challenge. Unless particular circumstances preclude it—notably, the obligation to maintain confidentiality—the expectation would be to use the field stations' 4×4s to go to the field, even if only traveling within areas well serviced by public transportation. To rely on public transportation during fieldwork is considered inefficient and degrading, partly because higher levels of staff would not do this and because fieldwork entails a particular, independently mobile and enclosed mode of circulation.

This is supported by a well-developed discourse on "risks" among staff and the administration (wary of staff damage claims), evoking rabid dogs, allegedly hostile "community members," and nefarious rumors about researchers' evil deeds. These perceived risks of the field add to the sense of distance between staff members, in their role as fieldworkers, and otherwise familiar environments and people.

In some types of research—especially if HIV is involved—staff even venture into "the community" incognito, telling those who are not their research participants but their spouses, neighbors, or relatives that they are not HIV researchers but only "malaria people" or, more effectively, not researchers at all but church friends or in-laws. This practice of changed identity is necessary when dealing with stigmatized diseases and when legally obliged to maintain confidentiality, and it allows for closer, friendly relationships with some research participants, but at the same time it adds another layer of distance to the relationship between staff members and the world they live and work in.

Yet, while getting inside research thus may produce alienation from environments and populations that one otherwise belongs to, the experience of moving out and visiting a range of randomly chosen people across villages and urban spaces of research also broadens one's social field of vision to different realities and may produce changed sensitivities. As one nurse working among young women in poor areas of the city suggested, on account of the suffering and poverty that she had seen, "I have got a lot of experience from this study; it has actually made me know that human beings have different needs and everybody is unique."

Moving Out and On

Once people have been employed on temporary contracts for a while, especially if they are graduates or managed to obtain further education through their employment, they start to consider what previously seemed an enclosed section of their homely landscape—a bubble, a safe haven—as a conduit to elsewhere, a door into the world of the global. Often this is expressed through the metaphor of "graduating": "This place is just a high school; we are moving on. . . . Once we get through the high school we leave . . . and go to a different organization in a different capacity, we go very far out there; so this is a learning place, a school, until you get there." Staff members are keenly aware that working in a top research institution offers them access to the latest knowledge. In a city in which health interventions and research are a major motor of economic development, such exposure—to scientific facts and methods as well as working styles and "discipline"—is a marketable resource for moving ahead.

When asked for their future plans, many staffers articulated aspirations about moving out of the research station again, preferably up and on in life—to do a PhD with an overseas university or to join the world of international health policy. Above all, the expatriated life of the international expert—embodied by the overseas senior staff—fuelled dreams: "A professor gave us his experiences in going out . . . mhh, doing policy, . . . in different UN setups, . . . all over the world. . . . I got really inspired and I said, 'Yah, I want to be an international policy maker.'" By contrast, none of the staff members envisaged work for government institutions or public hospitals as a satisfactory next move. As one doctor employed for one trial said, "Government is frustrating for many, many reasons; you don't have things to work with . . . and if you are someone who is lazy and you just want to pass time . . . you can get away with it." The dream of making one's next move out of the enclosure into an exit, once and for all, from the local context and into the global realm of policy was nearly universal among staff. Yet few realistically hoped to achieve this, and they knew that they were more likely to move back to where they had come from, not up and away but down and out, back to "tarmacking," or seeking work. This alternative—losing the precarious security that employment brought about, the monthly paycheck and health insurance, the feeling of belonging to an important and recognized employer, and the opportunity to learn state-of-the-art knowledge—was a recurrent fear that clouded horizons and strained relations, when research projects ended or groups of staff "came up for contract renewal."

Everybody inside knew that at some point he or she would have to move out again. None of the staff dreamed of staying forever, or of rising through the ranks and gaining permanent employment. The realistic among them had a presentiment that moving out would mean back to local realities. Anticipating this, they maximized investment in future income possibilities, such as a small business, a rental property, and cash-cropping land, and most important, the education of their children in the best private schools they could afford. Eventually, the bubble of medical research would burst, hopefully to be replaced by another space of opportunity, another site through which to access— and possibly escape into—another world.

The unforeseen emergence and the equally surprising devaluation of such sites of possibility has a long tradition in postcolonial Africa, beginning with mission education and work and continuing through colonial clerical work and the military, railways, and migrant labor, on to participatory self-help groups and development projects in the later parts of the twentieth century. All of these offered, for some time and under particular circumstances, and only for some, hopes and opportunities for learning and personal advancement and local futures, through establishing linkages to distant places, which (with the exception of the brief period of postindependence nation building and apart from the partially transcendental nature of Christian hopes) were often located in the North.

However, this familiar pattern of shifting landscapes of opportunity has in recent decades been further fragmented, notably through the gradual replacement of ties to the nation-state by links to more diverse, distant and mobile larger entities and by the deterritorialization delineated earlier in this chapter. The process of enclosure, creating temporary hotspots rather than centralized and expansive networks (like the national educational systems, hospital referral chains and national railways of the past), also implies acceleration, as hotspots come and go, determined by forces beyond one's control. After decades of privatization and nation-state vitiation and complementary waves of nongovernmental and humanitarian interventions, the pattern of enclosure and dissolution, emergence, and reformation is an all-too-familiar trait of the twenty-first-century African landscape for the research staff to entertain dreams of certainty. Even if one temporarily gains access to the inside of modernity and its benefits, one's place there is never safe and lasting, as the spatial formation itself is not.

Living in the New Landscape of Public Health

Earlier in this chapter I map an "archipelago of medical research" around a transnational field station in Africa, marked by bounded enclosures carving up the territory between well-resourced interiors and impoverished and comparatively uncontrolled exteriors or interstices; the enclosed field station or research center serves as an exemplar of this spatial order, but also the "fields" of research, outside the enclosure, are similarly zoned. Between these islands of modern medical possibility, which are insulated but not completely set apart from their surroundings in political and economic terms, there exist hopping, often real-time, long-distance connections, embodied through data-sharing and communication technology, as well as more old-fashioned modes of financial transfers, equipment shipping, and expert travel and expatriate stationing. This landscape, although particularly striking and technologically advanced and based on health research, might be more generally representative of the changing territories of public health in Africa, and medical research enclaves thus might be characteristic of wider developments—a vanguard in social and political as well as in scientific terms.

The second part of my chapter emphasizes, in agreement with the introduction to this volume, that an anthropological examination of such seemingly obvious formations needs to take into account the diversity and movements of people within them: people who both respect and move across boundaries and reproduce them through discrete practices, or permeate and reshape them, see them from respectively inside and outside and, depending on this, see each other and thus identify and associate differently. Boundaries that when seen from above look un-equivocal are merely some of the lines of encounter and contestation found in any given landscape and engaged by its inhabitants.

The necessary critique of the emerging landscapes of exclusion—which proliferate across contemporary societies—requires an eye for practices of inhabitation, for contradictions and contestation. Struggles with and against tangible boundaries are enmeshed with separations—between classes, individuals, genders. And the inhabitants of these landscapes are in continuous communication with past lays of the land, half-forgotten or reluctantly remembered boundaries and conflicts—in this case, the sediments of imperial topographies and circulations, as well as those of postcolonial projects and hopes. The social processes arising from this diversity are less determined than the (perhaps) more clear-cut global economies of pharmaceutical production (or, by exten-sion, resource extraction and other novel forms of primary accumula-tion). This chapter, then, is only a first step, a sketch map of structures, complemented by few observations about inhabitation. It is offered to point at some areas and questions for future ethnographies of public health in Africa, which will go beyond the mere postulation of novel forms of encompassing order, or "regimes," to appreciate variegated movements within these: movements that also point beyond the order of the present, in the continued pursuit of public health.

Notes

I am very grateful to my colleagues—African and expatriate—who gave me generous access to their "research station" and freely shared their views and experiences with me. The directors of the collaboration also read, commented on, and corrected mistakes in earlier drafts of this chapter, which was extremely helpful. Thanks also to Ruth Prince, who offered me valuable advice during the conference that she organized in Cambridge (2007), where this material was originally discussed. The Wellcome Trust's support for this research is gratefully acknowledged.

1. See, for example, Doreen Massey, *World City* (Cambridge, UK: Polity Press, 2007); David Harvey, "Neoliberalism and the City," *Studies in Social Justice* 1, no. 1 (2007): 1–13. See also Theresa P. R. Caldeira, *City of Walls: Crime, Segregation, and Citizenship in São Paulo* (Berkeley: University of California Press, 2001); Aihwa Ong, *Neoliberalism as Ex-ception: Mutations in Citizenship and Sovereignty* (Durham, NC: Duke University Press, 2006); James Ferguson, *Global Shadows: Africa in the Neoliberal World Order* (Durham, NC: Duke University Press, 2006).

2. See Erica Bornstein and Peter Redfield, eds., *Forces of Compassion: Humanitarianism between Ethics and Politics* (Santa Fe, NM: School for Advanced Research Press, 2011); Ong, *Neoliberalism as Exception*; Aihwa Ong and Nancy Chen, *Asian Biotech: Ethics and Communities of Fate* (Durham, NC: Duke University Press, 2010); Michel Feher, ed., *Nongovernmental Politics* (New York: Zone Books, 2007); Bruce O'Neil, "Of Camps, Gulags and Extraordinary Renditions: Infrastructural Violence in Rumania," *Ethnography* 13(4) (2012):466–486.

3. Doreen Massey, "Landscape/Space/Politics: An Essay" (2011), http://thefutureoflandscape.wordpress.com.

4. See especially Nikolas Rose, *The Politics of Life Itself: Biomedicine, Power, and Subjectivity in the Twenty-First Century* (Princeton: Princeton University Press, 2006).

5. See, e.g., Adriana Petryna, *When Experiments Travel: Clinical Trials and the Global Search for Human Subjects* (Princeton: Princeton University Press, 2009).

6. See Aihwa Ong, "The Production of Possession: Spirits and the Multinational Corporation in Malaysia," *American Ethnologist* 15, no. 1 (1988): 28–41; Ong, *Neoliberalism as Exception*.

7. See, e.g., Susan Reynolds Whyte, ed., *Second Chances: Surviving AIDS in Uganda* (Durham, NC: Duke University Press, forthcoming).

8. See, e.g., Steven Robbins, *From Revolution to Rights in South Africa: Social Movements, NGOs and Popular Politics after Apartheid* (Woodbridge, UK: James Currey, 2008); Vinh-Kim Nguyen, "Government by Exception: Enrolment and Experimentality in Mass HIV Treatment Programs in Africa," *Social Theory and Health* 7, no. 3 (2009): 196–218; Ari Samsky, "'Since We Are Taking the Drugs': Labor and Value in Two International Drug Donation Programs," *Journal of Cultural Economy* 4, no. 1 (2011): 27–43; Melissa Parker, Tim Allen, Georgina Pearson, Rachel Flynn, and Nicholas Rees, "Border Parasites: Schistosomiasis Control among Uganda's Fisherfolk," *Journal of Eastern African Studies* 6, no. 1 (2012): 98–123; Ruth J. Prince, "HIV and the Moral Economy of Survival in an East African City," *Medical Anthropology Quarterly* 26, no. 4 (2012): 534–56; Ruth J. Prince, "The Politics and Anti-politics of HIV Interventions in Kenya," in *Biomedicine and Governance in Africa*, ed. Richard Rottenburg and Judith Zenker, 97–118 (Bielefeld, Germany: Transcript Verlag, 2012).

9. Except for the budding critique of "global health" on the largest level of scale, e.g., Johanna Crane, "Scrambling for Africa? Universities and Global Health," *Lancet* 377, no. 9775 (2011): 1388–90. See also, e.g., James Fairhead, Melissa Leach, and Mary Small, "Where Techno-Science Meets Poverty: Medical Research and the Economy of Blood in the Gambia, West Africa," *Social Science and Medicine* 63, no. 4 (2006): 1109–20; Melissa Leach and James Fairhead, *Vaccine Anxieties: Global Science, Child Health and Society*, Science in Society Series (London: Earth Scan, 2007); P. Wenzel Geissler, "Public Secrets in Public Health: Knowing Not to Know while Making Scientific Knowledge," *American Ethnologist* 40(1)(2013): 13–34.

10. It is also about a particular point in time: 2008. This is important, because the described structures change. For example, since the time of my fieldwork, the main funder's contribution to the overall budget has decreased, and collaborations were diversified; measures to protect research participants have been refined and standardized, a dedicated community liaison program was continuously expanded, and a corporate social responsibility program for the people of neighboring villages was created; key assets such as cars that previously had been owned by the northern partner were transferred onto government number plates. Seemingly static forms are thus undergoing continuous change.

11. See Geissler, "Public Secrets."

12. See Peter Redfield, "Vital Mobility and the Humanitarian Kit," in *Biosecurity Interventions: Global Health and Security in Question,* ed. Andrew Lakoff and Stephen Collier, 141–71 (New York: Columbia University Press, 2008), esp. 164.

13. Thus, across Africa, one can distinguish field territories and collaborative field stations predominantly associated with particular northern nations or one large institution—such as the Wellcome Trust, the U.K. Medical Research Council (MRC), the U.S. Centers of Disease Control and Prevention (CDC), the London or Liverpool School, or Harvard University, the University of California, or Columbia University.

14. Exemplars of these connections are increasingly widespread multisite clinical trials, which recruit and pool research participants from sites across the globe, controlling standards and analysis from a central locus in the Global North or in delocalized "consortia" and deploying advanced technologies to enable real-time data sharing and processing, for example, by entering field and laboratory-based data directly into mobile devices such as smartphones that link up with the centralized servers of particular clinical trials.

15. P. Wenzel Geissler and Catherine Molyneux, eds., *Evidence, Ethos and Experiment: The Anthropology and History of Medical Research in Africa* (New York: Berghahn Books, 2011).

16. These rumors associate research for example to "blood stealing," illicit or dangerous experimentation, devil worshipping, or assaults on fertility and reproduction. See, e.g., Luise White, *Speaking with Vampires: Rumor and History in Colonial Africa* (Berkeley: University of California Press, 2000); Fairhead, Leach, and Small, "Where Techno-Science Meets Poverty"; P. Wenzel Geissler and Robert Pool, "Popular Concerns with Medical Research Projects in Africa—a Critical Voice in Debates about Overseas Research Ethics," *Tropical Medicine and International Health* 11, no. 7 (2006): 975–82.

17. Lotte Meinert, "Cutting New Networks: Kin Relations and Research Relations in an ARV Study in Uganda," in *Para-states of Science: Ethnographic and Historical Perspectives on Life-Science, Government, and the Public in Twenty-First-Century Africa,* ed. P. Wenzel Geissler (Durham, NC: Duke University Press, forthcoming).

Bibliography

Adams, Vincanne, Thomas E. Novotny, and Hannah Leslie. "Global Health Diplomacy." *Medical Anthropology* 27, no. 4 (2008): 315–23.

Adome, Richard O., Susan Reynolds Whyte, and Anita Hardon, eds. *Popular Pills: Community Drug Use in Uganda.* Amsterdam: Het Spinhuis, 1996.

Aikins, Ama de-Graft, Nigel Unwin, Charles Agyemang, Pascale Allotey, Catherine Campbell, and Daniel Arhinful. "Tackling Africa's Chronic Disease Burden: From the Local to the Global." *Globalization and Health* 6, no. 5 (2010).

Akintola, Olagoke. "Gendered Home-Based Care in South Africa: More Trouble for the Troubled." *African Journal of AIDS Research* 5, no. 3 (2006): 237–47.

———. *Policy Brief: The Gendered Burden of Home-Based Care-Giving.* Durban: Health Economics and HIV/AIDS Research Division (HEARD), University of KwaZulu Natal, 2004.

Aldhous, Peter. "Counterfeit Pharmaceuticals: Murder by Medicine." *Nature* 434, no. 7030 (2005): 132–36.

Allen, Tim, and Melissa Parker. "Will Increased Funding for Neglected Tropical Diseases Really Make Poverty History?" *Lancet* 379, no. 9821 (2012): 1097–98.

Amin, Abdinasir A., and Gilbert O. Kokwaro. "Antimalarial Drug Quality in Africa." *Journal of Clinical Pharmacy and Therapeutics* 32, no. 5 (2007): 429–40.

Arendt, Hannah. *The Human Condition.* Chicago: University of Chicago Press, 1998.

Arora, Neeraj K. "Interacting with Cancer Patients: The Significance of Physicians' Communication Behaviour." *Social Science and Medicine* 57, no. 5 (2003): 791–806.

Askew, Kelly. *Performing the Nation: Swahili Music and Cultural Politics.* Chicago: University of Chicago Press, 2002.

Attisso, Michel. *Contrôle de la qualité des médicaments au Sénégal: Rapport de mission, 1–22 juillet 1969.* Edited by Organisation mondiale de la santé (World Health Organization). Geneva: OMS/WHO, 1970.

Atwood, Margaret. *Oryx and Crake.* London: Bloomsbury, 2003.

———. *The Year of the Flood.* London: Bloomsbury, 2009.

Ba, Babacar. "Communication à l'Assemblée nationale sur les produits pharmaceutiques." *Le point économique* 11 (1977): 34–39.

Baer, Hans A., Merrill Singer, and Ida Susser. *Medical Anthropology and the World System: A Critical Perspective.* Westport, CT: Bergin and Garvey, 1997.

Barber, Karin. *The Anthropology of Texts: Persons and Publics, Oral and Written Culture.* Cambridge: Cambridge University Press, 2007.

Bayart, Jean-François. "Africa in the World: A History of Extraversion." *African Affairs* 99 (2000): 239.

———. *The State in Africa: The Politics of the Belly*. London: Longman, 1993.

Bayart, Jean-François, Stephen Ellis, and Béatrice Hibou. *The Criminalisation of the State in Africa*. Indianapolis: Indiana University Press, 1999.

Beck, Ann. *A History of the British Medical Administration of East Africa, 1900–1950*. Cambridge, MA: Harvard University Press, 1970.

Beckmann, Nadine, and Janet Bujra. "The Politics of the Queue: The Politicisation of People Living with HIV/AIDS in Tanzania." *Development and Change* 41, no. 6 (2010): 1041–64.

BeLue, Rhonda, Titilayo A. Okoror, Juliet Iwelunmar, Kelly D. Taylor, Arnold N. Degboe, Charles Agyemang, and Gbenga Ogedegbe. "An Overview of Cardiovascular Risk Factor Burden in Sub-Saharan African Countries: A Socio-cultural Perspective." *Globalization and Health* 5, no. 10 (2009).

Berman, Bruce J. "Ethnicity, Patronage and the African State: The Politics of Uncivil Nationalism." *African Affairs* 97, no. 388 (1998): 305–41.

Biehl, João. "The Activist State: Global Pharmaceuticals, AIDS and Citizenship in Brazil." *Social Text* 22, no. 3 (2004): 105–32.

———. "Pharmaceutical Governance." In Petryna, Lakoff, and Kleinman, *Global Pharmaceuticals*, 206–39.

———. "Pharmaceuticalization: AIDS Treatment and Global Health Politics." *Anthropological Quarterly* 80, no. 4 (2007): 1083–1126.

———. *Will to Live: AIDS Therapies and the Politics of Survival*. Princeton: Princeton University Press, 2007.

Bierschenk, Thomas. "The Everyday Functioning of an African Public Service: Informalization, Privatization and Corruption in Benin's Legal System." *Journal of Legal Pluralism and Unofficial Law* 57 (2008): 101–39.

Blystad, Astrid, and Karen Marie Moland. "Technologies of Hope? Motherhood, HIV and Infant Feeding in Eastern Africa." *Anthropology and Medicine* 16, no. 2 (2009): 105–18.

Boddy, Janice. "Remembering Amal: On Birth and the British in Northern Sudan." In *Beyond the Body Proper: Reading the Anthropology of Material Life*, edited by Margaret Lock and Judith Farquhar, 315–29. Durham, NC: Duke University Press, 2007.

Boesten, Jelke. "Navigating the AIDS Industry: Being Poor and Positive in Tanzania." *Development and Change* 42, no. 3 (2011): 781–803.

Boesten, Jelke, Anna Mdee, and Frances Cleaver. "Service Delivery on the Cheap? Community-Based Workers in Development Interventions." *Development in Practice* 21, no. 1 (2011): 41–58.

Boffetta, Paolo, and D. Maxwell Parkin. "Cancer in Developing Countries." *CA: A Cancer Journal for Clinicians* 44, no. 2 (1994): 81–90.

Boni, Stefano. "'Brothers 30,000, Sisters 20,000; Nephews 15,000, Nieces 10,000': Akan Funeral Ledgers, Kinship and Value Negotiations, and Their Limits." *Ethnography* 11, no. 3 (2010): 381–408.

Bonneuil, Christophe. "Development as Experiment: Science and State Building in Late Colonial and Postcolonial Africa, 1930–1970." *Osiris* 15 (2000): 258–81.

Booth, Karen. *Local Women, Global Science: Fighting AIDS in Kenya.* Bloomington: Indiana University Press, 2004.

Bornstein, Erica, and Peter Redfield, eds. *Forces of Compassion: Humanitarianism between Ethics and Politics.* Santa Fe, NM: School for Advanced Research Press, 2011.

Boutayeb, Abdesslam. "The Double Burden of Communicable and Noncommunicable Diseases in Developing Countries." *Transactions of the Royal Society of Tropical Medicine and Hygiene* 100, no. 3 (2006): 191–99.

Briggs, Charles L. "Why Nation-States and Journalists Can't Teach People to Be Healthy: Power and Pragmatic Miscalculation in Public Discourses on Health." *Medical Anthropology Quarterly* 17, no. 3 (2003): 287–321.

Briggs, Charles L., and Clara Mantini-Briggs. *Stories in the Time of Cholera: Racial Profiling during a Medical Nightmare.* Berkeley: University of California Press, 2003.

Brown, Hannah. "Hospital Domestics: Care Work in a Kenyan Hospital." *Space and Culture* 15 (2012): 18–30.

———. "Living with HIV/AIDS: An Ethnography of Care in Western Kenya." Doctoral thesis, University of Manchester, 2010.

Brown, Theodore M., Marcos Cueto, and Elizabeth Fee. "The World Health Organization and the Transition from 'International' to 'Global' Public Health." *American Journal of Public Health* 96, no. 1 (2006): 62–72.

Brudon, Pascale, Miloud Kaddar, Dominique Ben Abdallah, A. Diaw, Michel Etchepare, A. Diouf, El Hadj Sy, F. Sy, R. Sylla, and Jeanne Maritoux. *Le secteur pharmaceutique privé au Sénégal: Dynamiques de développement et effets sur l'accès aux médicaments essentiels.* Série de recherche no. 23. Geneva: World Health Organization, 1997.

Burawoy, Michael. "Manufacturing the Global." *Ethnography* 2, no. 2 (2001): 147–59.

Burton, Andrew, and Michael Jennings. "The Emperor's New Clothes? Continuities in Governance in Late Colonial and Early Postcolonial East Africa." *International Journal of African Historical Studies* 40, no. 1 (2007): 1–25.

Buse, Kent, and Gill Walt. "An Unruly Melange? Coordinating External Resources to the Health Sector; A Review." *Social Science and Medicine* 45, no. 3 (1997): 449–62.

Caldeira, Theresa P. R. *City of Walls: Crime, Segregation, and Citizenship in São Paulo.* Berkeley: University of California Press, 2001.

Caudron, J. M., N. Ford, M. Henkens, C. Mace, R. Kiddle-Monroe, and J. Pinel. "Substandard Medicines in Resource-Poor Settings: A Problem That Can No Longer Be Ignored." *Tropical Medicine and International Health* 13, no. 8 (2008): 1062–72.

Chabal, Patrick, and Jean-Pascal Daloz. *Africa Works: Disorder as Political Instrument.* London: James Currey, 1999.

Charsley, Simon. *The Princes of Nyakyusa.* Nairobi: East African Publishing House, 1969.

Cisse, Mamadou. "Luttre contre le paludisme: Le traitement graduit à partir du 1er mai." *Le soleil,* 27 April 2010, www.lesoleil.com.

Clark, Elizabeth J. "Chemotherapy and the Issue of Patients' Rights." In *Psychosocial Aspects of Chemotherapy in Cancer Care: The Patient, Family, and Staff,* edited by Robert DeBellis, George A. Hyman, Irene B. Seeland, Austin H. Kutscher, Alison Kimberg, Mary-Ellen Sigel, and Lillian G. Kutscher, 43–52. New York: Haworth Press, 1987.

Cohen, David W., and E.S.A. Odhiambo. *Siaya: The Historical Anthropology of an African Landscape.* Nairobi: Heinemann, 1989.

Collins, David, Grace Njeru, and Julius Meme. *Hospital Autonomy in Kenya: The Case of Kenyatta National Hospital; Data for Decision Making Project.* Boston: Harvard School of Public Health, 1996.

Collins, David, Grace Njeru, Julius Meme, and William Newbrander. "Hospital Autonomy: The Experience of Kenyatta National Hospital." *International Journal of Health Planning and Management* 14, no. 2 (1999): 129–53.

Comaroff, Jean. "Beyond Bare Life: AIDS, (Bio)Politics, and the Neoliberal Order." *Public Culture* 19, no. 1 (2007): 197–219; reprinted in Dilger and Luig, *Morality, Hope and Grief,* 21–42.

———. *Body of Power, Spirit of Resistance.* Chicago: University of Chicago Press, 1985.

———. "The Diseased Heart of Africa: Medicine, Colonialism, and the Black Body," in *Knowledge, Power, and Practice: The Anthropology of Medicine and Everyday Life,* edited by Shirley Lindenbaum and Margaret Lock, 305–27. Berkeley: University of California Press, 1993.

Comaroff, Jean, and John L. Comaroff. "Home-Made Hegemony: Modernity, Domesticity, and Colonialism in South Africa." In *African Encounters with Domesticity,* edited by Karen Tranberg Hansen, 37–74. New Brunswick, NJ: Rutgers University Press, 1992.

———. "Millennial Capitalism: First Thoughts on a Second Coming." *Public Culture* 12, no. 2 (2000): 291–343.

———. "Occult Economies and the Violence of Abstraction: Notes from the South African Postcolony." *American Ethnologist* 26, no. 2 (1999): 279–303.

Comaroff, John L., and Jean Comaroff. *Ethnography and the Historical Imagination.* Boulder, CO: Westview Press, 1992.

———. *Of Revelation and Revolution.* Vol. 2, *The Dialectics of Modernity on a South African Frontier.* Chicago: University of Chicago Press, 1997.

Cooper, Frederick. *Africa since 1940: The Past of the Present.* Cambridge: Cambridge University Press, 2002.

———. *Decolonization and African Society: The Labor Question in French and British Africa.* Cambridge: Cambridge University Press, 1996.

———. "The Dialectics of Decolonization: Nationalism and Labour Movements in Postwar French West Africa." In Cooper and Stoler, *Tensions of Empire,* 406–35.

————. *Struggle for the City: Migrant Labor, Capital, and the State in Urban Africa*. London: Sage, 1983.

Cooper, Frederick, and Randall M. Packard. Introduction to *International Development and the Social Sciences: Essays on the History and Politics of Knowledge*, edited by Frederick Cooper and Randall M. Packard, 1–44. Berkeley: University of California Press, 1997.

Cooper, Frederick, and Ann Laura Stoler, eds. *Tensions of Empire: Colonial Cultures in a Bourgeois World*. Berkeley: University of California Press, 1997.

Cooper, Melinda. *Life as Surplus: Biotechnology and Capitalism in the Neoliberal Era*. Seattle: University of Washington Press, 2008.

Crane, Johanna. "Adverse Events and Placebo Effects: African Scientists, HIV, and Ethics in the 'Global Health Sciences.'" *Social Studies of Science* 40, no. 6 (2010): 843–70.

————. "Scrambling for Africa? Universities and Global Health." *Lancet* 377, no. 9775 (2011): 1388–90.

————. "Unequal Partners: AIDS, Academia and the Rise of Global Health." *Behemoth* 3 (2010): 78–98.

Curtin, Philip. "Medical Knowledge and Urban Planning in Colonial Tropical Africa." In Feierman and Janzen, *Social Basis of Health and Healing in Africa*, 235–55.

Daar, Abdallah S., P. A. Singer, D. L. Persad, S. K. Pramming, D. R. Matthews, R. Beaglehole, A. Bernstein, et al. "Grand Challenges in Chronic Noncommunicable Diseases: The Top 20 Policy and Research Priorities for Conditions Such as Diabetes, Stroke and Heart Disease." *Nature* 450 (2007): 494–96.

Dahou, Tarik, and Vincent Foucher, eds. *Sénégal, 2002–2004: L'alternance et ses contradictions*. Politique africaine 96. Paris: Karthala, 2004.

Davison, Charles, and George Davey Smith. "The Baby and the Bath Water: Examining Sociocultural and Free-Market Critiques of Health Promotion." In *The Sociology of Health Promotion: Critical Analyses of Consumption, Lifestyle and Risk*, edited by Robin Bunton, Sarah Nettleton, and Roger Burrows, 91–99. London: Routledge, 1995.

DelVecchio Good, Mary-Jo, Byron J. Good, Cynthia Schaffer, and Stuart E. Lind. "American Oncology and the Discourse on Hope." *Culture, Medicine and Psychiatry* 14, no. 1 (1990): 59–79.

DelVecchio Good, Mary-Jo, Ester Mwaikambo, Erastus Amayo, and James M' Imunya Machoki. "Clinical Realities and Moral Dilemmas: Contrasting Perspectives from Academic Medicine in Kenya, Tanzania, and America." *Daedalus* 128, no. 4 (1999): 167–96.

De Witte, Marleen. "Money and Death: Funeral Business in Asante, Ghana." *Africa* 73, no. 4 (2003): 531–59.

Diallo, Ndiouga. "(13) Programme de distribution des antipaludiques au Sénégal." In *E-med: Le forum francophone sur les médicaments essentiels*, edited by ReMed, 5 January 2009, www.essentialdrugs.org/emed/archive/200901/.

Diaw, Fara. "Dr Emmanuel Sarr, pharmacien: '20% des officines dans la tourmente . . .'" *Le soleil*, 19 May 2004, www.lesoleil.sn.

Dieng, Abdoulaye. "(3) Sénégal: Saisie de médicaments d'une valeur de plus de deux millions de francs." In *E-med: Le forum francophone sur les médicaments essentiels,* edited by ReMed, 19 May 2008, www.essentialdrugs.org/emed /archive/200805/.

Dilger, Hansjörg. "Doing Better? Religion, the Virtue-Ethics of Development, and the Fragmentation of Health Politics in Tanzania." *Africa Today* 56, no. 1 (2009): 89–110.

Dilger, Hansjörg, Abdulaye Kane, and Stacey Langwick, eds. *Medicine, Mobility and Power in Global Africa: Transnational Health and Healing.* Bloomington: Indiana University Press, 2012.

Dilger, Hansjörg, and Ute Luig, eds. *Morality, Hope and Grief: Anthropologies of AIDS in Africa.* New York: Berghahn Books, 2010.

Diop, Momar-Coumba. "Introduction: Du 'socialisme' au 'libéralisme'; Les légitimités de l'état." In *Sénégal: Trajectoires d'un état,* edited by Momar-Coumba Diop, 13–38. Dakar: CODESRIA, 1992.

Diop, Pape. "Société: Pharmacies clandestines; Touba, plaque tournante du traffic de médicaments." *Info 7,* 11 January 2001. In *Dossier pharmacie.* On file, Centre de documentation, Bibliothèque nationale du Sénégal, Dakar.

Diop, Talla. "(4) Programme de distribution des antipaludiques au Sénégal à 150 fcfa pour les enfants et 300 fcfa pour les adultes." In *E-med: Le forum francophone sur les médicaments essentiels,* edited by ReMed, 18 December 2008, www.essentialdrugs.org/emed/archive/200812/.

Diouf, Makhtar. "La crise et l'ajustement." *Politique africaine* 45 (1992): 62–85.

Diouf, Mamadou. "Le clientélisme, la 'technocratie' et après?" In *Sénégal: Trajectoires d'un état,* edited by Momar-Coumba Diop, 223–78. Dakar: CODESRIA, 1992.

Durham, Deborah. "Love and Jealousy in the Space of Death." *Ethnos* 67, no. 2 (2002): 155–80.

Durham, Deborah, and Frederick Klaits. "Funerals and the Public Space of Sentiment in Botswana." *Journal of Southern African Studies* 28, no. 4 (2002): 777–96.

Ecks, Stephen. "Pharmaceutical Citizenship: Antidepressant Marketing and the Promise of Demarginalization in India." *Anthropology and Medicine* 12, no. 3 (2005): 239–54.

Edelman, Marc, and Angelique Haugerud. "Introduction: The Anthropology of Development and Globalization." In *The Anthropology of Development and Globalization: From Classical Political Economy to Contemporary Neoliberalism,* edited by Marc Edelman and Angelique Haugerud, 1–74. Malden, MA: Blackwell Publishing, 2005.

Ellison, James G. "Transforming Obligations, Performing Identity: Making the Nyakyusa in a Colonial Context." PhD thesis, University of Florida, 1999.

Elyachar, Julia. *Markets of Dispossession: NGOs, Economic Development and the State in Egypt.* Durham, NC: Duke University Press, 2005.

E-med. "Forum pharmaceutique de Dakar." In *E-med: Le forum francophone sur les médicaments essentiels,* edited by ReMed, 2001, www.essentialdrugs.org/emed.

Epstein, Helen. *The Invisible Cure: Africa, the West, and the Fight against AIDS.* New York: Farrar, Straus and Giroux; London, Penguin Books, 2007.

Evans-Pritchard, Edward E. *Witchcraft, Oracles and Magic among the Azande.* 1937. Oxford: Clarendon Press, 1973.

Fairhead, James, Melissa Leach, and Mary Small. "Where Techno-Science Meets Poverty: Medical Research and the Economy of Blood in the Gambia, West Africa." *Social Science and Medicine* 63, no. 4 (2006): 1109–20.

Fall, Abdou Salam, Babacar Gueye, Djiby Diakhate, Omar Saip Sy, Abdoulaye Dieye, Sémou Ndiaye, Yaya Bodian, and Abdoulaye Sakho. "Gouvernance et corruption dans le système de santé au Sénégal: Rapport provisoire." Edited by Forum Civil/CRDI, 2004.

Fanon, Frantz. *Black Skin, White Masks.* New York: Grove, 1967.

Farmer, Paul. *AIDS and Accusation: Haiti and the Geography of Blame.* Berkeley: University of California Press, 1992.

———. *Infections and Inequalities: The Modern Plagues.* Berkeley: University of California Press, 1999.

———. *Pathologies of Power: Health, Human Rights and the New War on the Poor.* Berkeley: University of California Press, 2005.

Fassin, Didier. "Another Politics of Life Is Possible." *Theory, Culture and Society* 26, no. 5 (2009): 44–60.

———. "Du clandestin à l'officieux: Les réseaux de vente illicite des médicaments au Sénégal." *Cahiers d'études africaines* 25, no. 2 (1985): 161–77.

———. "Humanitarianism: A Nongovernmental Government." In *Nongovernmental Politics,* edited by Michel Feher, 149–60. New York: Zone Books, 2007.

———. "La vente illicite des médicaments au Sénégal: Économies 'parallèles,' état et société." *Politique africaine* 23 (1986): 123–30.

———. *When Bodies Remember: Experiences and Politics of AIDS in South Africa.* Berkeley: University of California Press, 2007.

Fassin, Didier, and Jean-Pierre Dozon, eds. *Critique de la santé publique: Une approche anthropologique.* Paris: Editions Balland, 2001.

Fassin, Didier, and Maria Pandolfi. *Contemporary States of Emergency: The Politics of Military and Humanitarian Interventions.* New York: Zone Books, 2010.

Faye, El Hadji Massiga. "Marché illicite du médicament, cambriolages: Les pharmaciens baissent rideau." *Le soleil,* 30 April 2008, www.lesoleil.sn.

Faye, Mame Marie. *L'immolation par le feu de la petite fille du Président Wade: Crimes, trahisons et fin du régime libéral.* Paris: L'Harmattan, 2008.

Feher, Michel. "The Governed in Politics." In *Nongovernmental Politics,* edited by Michel Feher, 12–27. New York: Zone Books, 2007.

———, ed. *Nongovernmental Politics.* New York: Zone Books, 2007.

Feierman, Steven. "Colonizers, Scholars, and the Creation of Invisible Histories." In *Beyond the Cultural Turn: New Directions in the Study of Society and Culture,* edited by Victoria E. Bonnell and Lynn Hunt, 182–216. Berkeley: University of California Press, 1999.

———. "Healing as Social Criticism in the Time of Colonial Conquest." *African Studies* 54, no. 1 (2010): 73–88.

———. "On Socially Composed Knowledge: Reconstructing a Shambaa Royal Ritual." In *In Search of a Nation: Histories of Authority and Dissidence in Tanzania,* edited by James L. Giblin and Gregory H. Maddox, 14–32. Athens: Ohio University Press, 2005.

———. *Peasant Intellectuals: Anthropology and History in Tanzania.* Madison: University of Wisconsin Press, 1990.

———. "Struggles for Control: The Social Roots of Health and Healing in Modern Africa." *African Studies Review* 28 (1985): 73–147.

———. "When Physicians Meet: Local Medical Knowledge and Global Public Goods." In *Evidence, Ethos and Experiment: The Anthropology and History of Medical Research in Africa,* edited by P. Wenzel Geissler and Catherine Molyneux, 171–96. New York: Berghahn Books, 2011.

Feierman, Steven, and John M. Janzen, eds. *The Social Basis of Health and Healing in Africa.* Berkeley: University of California Press, 1992.

Ferguson, James. *The Anti-politics Machine.* Cambridge: Cambridge University Press, 1991.

———. *Expectations of Modernity: Myths and Meanings of Urban Life on the Zambian Copperbelt.* Berkeley: University of California Press, 1999.

———. "Formalities of Poverty: Thinking about Social Assistance in Neoliberal South Africa." *African Studies Review* 50, no. 2 (2007): 71–86.

———. *Global Shadows: Africa in the Neoliberal World Order.* Durham, NC: Duke University Press, 2006.

———. "The Uses of Neoliberalism." *Antipode* 41, no. 1 (2009): 166–84.

Ferguson, James, and Akhil Gupta. "Spatializing States: Toward an Ethnography of Neoliberal Governmentality." *American Ethnologist* 29, no. 4 (2002): 981–1002.

Ferzacca, Steve. "Chronic Illness and the Assemblages of Time in Multisited Encounters." In *Chronic Conditions, Fluid States: Chronicity and the Anthropology of Illness,* edited by Leonora Manderson and Caroline Smith-Morris, 157–74. New Brunswick, NJ: Rutgers University Press, 2010.

Fisher, William F. "Doing Good? The Politics and Anti-politics of NGO Practices." *Annual Review of Anthropology* 27 (1997): 439–64.

Foley, Ellen E. *Your Pocket Is What Cures You: The Politics of Health in Senegal.* New Brunswick, NJ: Rutgers University Press, 2010.

Fondation Chirac. "Accès à une santé et à des médicaments de qualité." www.fondationchirac.eu/programmes/acces-aux-medicaments/ (accessed 12 October 2012).

Foucault, Michel. "Governmentality." In Michel Foucault, *Power,* 201–22. Vol. 3 of *Essential Works of Foucault, 1954–1984,* edited by James D. Faubion. New York: New Press, 2000 (1994); London: Penguin, 2002 (1978).

———. "Governmentality." In *The Foucault Effect: Studies in Governmentality,* edited by Graham Burchell, Colin Gordon, and Peter Miller, 87–104. Hemel Hempstead, UK: Harvester Wheatsheaf, 1991.

————. *The History of Sexuality*. Vol. 1, *An Introduction*. Translated by Robert Hurley. 1978. Reprint, London: Penguin, 1990.

————. *The History of Sexuality*. Vol. 3, *The Care of the Self*. Translated by Robert Hurley. 1986. Reprint, London: Penguin, 1990.

————. "Space, Knowledge and Power." In *The Foucault Reader: An Introduction to Foucault's Thought*, edited by Paul Rabinow, 239–56. London: Penguin, 1991.

Franklin, Sarah, and Margaret Lock. *Remaking Life and Death: Toward an Anthropology of the Biosciences*. Santa Fe, NM: School of American Research Press; Oxford: James Currey, 2003.

Gable, Eric. "The Funeral and Modernity in Manjaco." *Cultural Anthropology* 21, no. 3 (2006): 385–415.

Garrett, Laurie. "The Challenge of Global Health." *Foreign Affairs* 86, no. 1 (2007): 14–38.

Geest, Sjaak van der, and Kaja Finkler. "Hospital Ethnography: Special Issue." *Social Science and Medicine* 59, no. 10 (2004): 1995–2001.

Geest, Sjaak van der, and Susan R. Whyte, eds. *The Context of Medicines in Developing Countries: Studies in Pharmaceutical Anthropology*. Dordrecht: Kluwer, 1998.

Geest, Sjaak van der, Susan R. Whyte, and Anita Hardon. "The Anthropology of Pharmaceuticals: A Biographical Approach." *Annual Review of Anthropology* 25 (1996): 153–78.

Geissler, P. Wenzel. "Kachinja Are Coming! Encounters around Medical Research Work in a Kenyan Village." *Africa* 75, no. 2 (2005): 174–202.

————. "Parasite Lost: Remembering Modern Times with Kenyan Government Medical Scientists." In *Ethos, Evidence and Experiment: The Anthropology and History of Medical Research in Africa*, edited by P. Wenzel Geissler and Catherine Molyneux, 297–332. New York: Berghahn Books, 2011.

————. "Public Secrets in Public Health: Knowing Not to Know while Making Scientific Knowledge." *American Ethnologist* 40, no. 2 (2013): 13–34.

Geissler, P. Wenzel, Ann Kelly, Babatunde Imoukhuede, and Robert Pool. "'He Is Now Like a Brother, I Can Even Give Him Some Blood': Relational Ethics and Material Exchanges in a Malaria Vaccine 'Trial Community' in the Gambia." *Social Science and Medicine* 67 (2008): 696–707.

Geissler, P. Wenzel, Lotte Meinert, Ruth J. Prince, Catherine Nokes, Jens Aagaard-Hansen, and John H. Ouma. "Self-Treatment by Kenyan and Ugandan Schoolchildren and the Need for School-Based Education." *Health Policy and Planning* 16, no. 4 (2001): 362–71.

Geissler, P. Wenzel, and Catherine Molyneux, eds. *Evidence, Ethos and Experiment: The Anthropology and History of Medical Research in Africa*. New York: Berghahn Books, 2011.

Geissler, P. Wenzel, K. Nokes, Ruth J. Prince, R. A. Odhiambo, Jens Aagaard-Hansen, and John H. Ouma. "Children and Medicine: Self-Treatment of Common Illnesses among Luo School Children in Western Kenya." *Social Science and Medicine* 50 (2000): 1771–83.

Geissler, P. Wenzel, and Robert Pool. "Popular Concerns with Medical Research Projects in Africa—a Critical Voice in Debates about Overseas Research Ethics." *Tropical Medicine and International Health* 11, no. 7 (2006): 975–82.

Geissler, P. Wenzel, and Ruth J. Prince. *The Land Is Dying: Contingency, Creativity and Conflict in Western Kenya.* New York: Berghahn Books, 2010.

———. "Purity Is Danger: Ambiguities of Touch around Sickness and Death in Western Kenya." In *Morality, Hope and Grief: Anthropologies of AIDS in Africa,* edited by Hansjörg Dilger and Ute Luig, 240–69. New York: Berghahn Books, 2010.

Gerrets, Rene. "International Health and the Proliferation of 'Partnerships': Unintended Boosts for State Institutions in Tanzania?" In *Para-states of Science: Ethnographic and Historical Perspectives on Life-Science, Government, and the Public in Twenty-First-Century Africa,* edited by P. Wenzel Geissler. Durham, NC: Duke University Press, forthcoming.

Geschiere, Peter. *The Modernity of Witchcraft, Politics and the Occult in Postcolonial Africa.* Charlottesville: University of Virginia Press, 1997.

———. *The Perils of Belonging: Autochthony, Citizenship and Exclusion in Africa and Europe.* Chicago: University of Chicago Press, 2009.

Gibbon, Peter. "Structural Adjustment and Structural Change in Sub-Saharan Africa: Some Provisional Conclusions." *Development and Change* 27, no. 4 (1996): 751–84.

Gibbon, Sahra, and Carlos Novas. *Biosocialities, Genetics and Social Sciences.* London: Routledge, 2008.

Global Fund. "Program Grant Agreement." In *Senegal: Program to Reinforce the Fight against Malaria.* Http://portfolio.theglobalfund.org/en/Grant/Index /SNG-405-G03-M (accessed 13 October 2012).

———. "Program Grant Agreement between the Global Fund . . . and the Ministry of Health of the Government of the Republic of Senegal." www .theglobalfund.org/grantdocuments/4SNGM_813_0_ga.pdf.

———. "Senegal." Grantportfolio.http://portfolio.theglobalfund.org/en/Grant /List/SNG (accessed 13 October 2012).

Graboyes, Melissa. "Fines, Orders, Fear . . . and Consent? Medical Research in East Africa, c. 1950s." *Developing World Bioethics* 10, no. 1 (2010): 34–41.

Green, Carolyn. *Handbook on Access to HIV/AIDS-Related Treatment: A Collection of Information, Tools and Other Resources for NGOs, CBOs and PLWHA Groups.* Geneva: UNAIDS / World Health Organization / International HIV/AIDS Alliance, 2003.

Green, Maia. "Making Development Agents: Participation as Boundary Object in International Development." *Journal of Development Studies* 46, no. 7 (2010): 1240–63.

———. "Participatory Development and the Appropriation of Agency in Southern Tanzania." *Critique of Anthropology* 20, no. 1 (2000): 67–89.

Grøn, Lone, Cheryl Mattingly, and Lotte Meinert. "Kronisk Hjemmearbejde: Sociale håb, dilemmaer og konflikter i hjemmearbejdsnarrativer i Uganda, Danmark og USA." *Tidsskrift for forskning i sygdom og samfund,* no. 9 (October 2008): 71–95.

Gueye, Maimouna. "Entretien avec . . . Dr Mamadou Ndiadé (président de l'Ordre des pharmaciens) et Dr Aboubakrine Sarr (président du Syndicat des pharmaciens): 'Dire que des pharmaciens ne sont pas impliqués dans le marché illicite du médicament est une contrevérité.'" *Le soleil*, 8 May 2007, www.lesoleil.sn.

―――."Partenariat public-privé: Les pharmaciens demandent leur implication dans les programmes de santé." *Le soleil*, 27 April 2007, www.lesoleil.sn.

Gupta, Akhil. *Postcolonial Developments: Agriculture in the Making of Modern India.* Durham, NC: Duke University Press, 1998.

Habermas, Jürgen. *The Structural Transformation of the Public Sphere: An Inquiry into a Category of Bourgeois Society.* Translated by Thomas Burger. Cambridge, MA: MIT Press, 1989.

Hansen, Thomas Blom, and Finn Stepputat, eds. *States of Imagination: Ethnographic Explorations of the Postcolonial State.* Durham, NC: Duke University Press, 2001.

Hardon, Anita, and Hansjörg Dilger. "Global AIDS Medicines in East African Health Institutions." In "AIDS Treatment in East Africa," special issue, *Medical Anthropology* 30, no. 2 (2011): 136–57.

Harvey, David. *A Brief History of Neoliberalism.* Oxford: Oxford University Press, 2005.

―――. "Neoliberalism and the City." *Studies in Social Justice* 1, no. 1 (2007): 1–13.

Haugerud, Angelique. *The Culture of Politics in Modern Kenya.* Cambridge: Cambridge University Press, 1993.

Hayden, Cori. "A Generic Solution? Pharmaceuticals and the Politics of the Similar in Mexico." *Current Anthropology* 48, no. 4 (2007): 475–95.

Heald, Suzette. "It's Never as Easy as ABC: Understandings of AIDS in Botswana." *International Journal of African AIDS Research* 1 (2002): 1–10.

Hearn, Julie. "The 'Invisible' NGO: US Evangelical Missions in Kenya." In "Christian and Islamic Non-governmental Organisations in Contemporary Africa," special issue, *Journal of Religion in Africa* 32, no. 1 (2002): 32–60.

―――. "The NGO-isation of Kenyan Society: USAID and the Restructuring of Health Care." *Review of African Political Economy* 25 (1985): 89–100.

Hill, Martin J. D. *The Harambee Movement in Kenya: Self-Help, Development and Education among the Kamba of Kitui District.* London School of Economics Monographs on Social Anthropology 64. London: Athlone Press, 1991.

Hobsbawm, Eric. "The Future of the State." *Development and Change* 27, no. 2 (1996): 267–78.

Hoffman, Frederick L. *Mortality from Cancer throughout the World.* Newark, NJ: Prudential Press, 1916.

Hsu, Elisabeth. "'The Medicine from China Has Rapid Effects': Chinese Medicine Patients in Tanzania." *Anthropology and Medicine* 9, no. 3 (2002): 291–313.

Human Rights Watch. *Needless Pain: Government Failure to Provide Palliative Care for Children in Kenya.* New York: Human Rights Watch, 2010.

————. "*They Do Not Own This Place*": Government Discrimination against *"Non-indigenes" in Nigeria.* New York: Human Rights Watch, 2006.

Hunt, Nancy Rose. *A Colonial Lexicon: Of Birth Ritual, Medicalization and Mobility in the Congo.* Durham, NC: Duke University Press, 1999.

————. "Condoms, Confessors, Conferences: Among AIDS Derivatives in Africa." *Journal of the International Institute* 4, no. 3 (1997): 15–17.

————. "'Le Bébé en Brousse': European Women, African Birth Spacing, and Colonial Intervention in Breast Feeding in the Belgian Congo." In Cooper and Stoler, *Tensions of Empire,* 287–321.

Hürbst, Viola. "Assisted Reproductive Technologies in Mali and Togo: Circulating Knowledge, Mobile Technologies." In Dilger, Kane, and Langwick, *Medicine, Mobility and Power in Global Africa,* 162–89.

Iliffe, John. *The African AIDS Epidemic: A History.* Oxford: James Currey, 2006.

————. *East African Doctors: A History of the Modern Profession.* Cambridge: Cambridge University Press, 1998.

Janes, Craig R. "Going Global in Century XXI: Medical Anthropology and the New Primary Health Care." *Human Organization* 63, no. 4 (2004): 457–71.

Janes, Craig R., and Kitty Corbitt. "Anthropology and Global Health." *Annual Review of Anthropology* 38 (2009): 167–83.

Janzen, John M. "Ideologies and Institutions in Pre-colonial Western Equatorial African Therapeutics." In Feierman and Janzen, *Social Basis of Health and Healing in Africa,* 195–211.

————. *The Quest for Therapy: Medical Pluralism in Lower Zaire.* Berkeley: University of California Press, 1978.

Jeffery, Lyn. "Placing Practices: Transnational Network Marketing in Mainland China." In *China Urban: Ethnographies of Contemporary Culture,* edited by Nancy N. Chen, Constance D. Clark, Suzanne Z. Gottschang, and Lyn Jeffery, 23–42. Durham, NC: Duke University Press, 2001.

Jennings, Michael. "'A Very Real War': Popular Participation in Development in Tanzania during the 1950s and 1960s." *International Journal of African Historical Studies* 40, no. 1 (2007): 71–95.

Kaleeba, Noerina, with Sundanda Ray. "We Miss You All: AIDS in the Family." In *HIV and AIDS in Africa: Beyond Epidemiology,* edited by Ezekeil Kalipeni, Susan Craddock, Joseph Oppong, and Jayati Ghosh, 259–78. Oxford: Blackwell, 2004.

Kalofenos, Ippolytos. "All I Eat Is ARVs!" *Medical Anthropology Quarterly* 24, no. 3 (2010): 363–80.

Kalusa, Walima T. "Language, Medical Auxiliaries, and the Re-interpretation of Missionary Medicine in Colonial Mwinilunga, Zambia, 1922–51." *Journal of Eastern African Studies* 1, no. 1 (2007): 57–78.

Kaly, Eugene. "Accès aux médicaments: Abdou Fall pour une stratégie nationale de promotion de génériques de qualité." *Le soleil,* 14 December 2006, www.lesoleil.sn.

Kane, Aline. "(7) Programme de distribution des antipaludiques au Sénégal." In *E- med: Le forum francophone sur les médicaments essentiels,* edited by ReMed, 19 December 2008, www.essentialdrugs.org/emed/archive/200812/.

———. "Re: Wade dit niet à Serign Bara." In *E-med: Le forum franco-phone sur les médicaments essentiels*, edited by ReMed, 3 August 2009, www .essentialdrugs.org/emed/archive/200908/.

Kasili, E. D. "Leukemia in Kenya." MD thesis, University of Nairobi, 1979.

Kelly, Ann. "The Progress of the Project: Scientific Traction in the Gambia." In *Differentiating Development: Beyond an Anthropology of Critique*, edited by Tom Yarrow and Soumhya Venkatesan, 65–83. New York: Berghahn Books, 2012.

Kenyatta National Hospital. *Strategic Development Plan, 2005–2010.* Nairobi: Kenyatta National Hospital, 2005.

King, Nikolas B. "Security, Disease, Commerce: Ideologies of Postcolonial Global Health." *Social Studies of Science* 32, no. 5/6 (2002): 763–89.

Kipnis, Andrew. "Neoliberalism Reified: Suzhi Discourse and Tropes of Neoliberalism in the People's Republic of China." *Journal of the Royal Anthropological Institute* 13, no. 2 (2007): 383–400.

Kipp, Walter, Denis Tindyebwa, Edna Karamagi, and Tom Rubaale. "How Much Should We Expect? Family Caregiving of AIDS Patients in Rural Uganda." *Journal of Transcultural Nursing* 18, no. 4 (2007): 358–65.

Klaits, Frederick. *Death in a Church of Life: Moral Passion in a Time of AIDS.* Berkeley: University of California Press, 2010.

———. "Faith and Intersubjectivity of Care in Botswana." *Africa Today* 56, no. 1 (2009): 3–19.

———. "The Widow in Blue: Blood and the Morality of Remembering in Botswana." *Africa* 75, no. 1 (2005): 46–62.

Kleinman, Arthur. *Patient and Healers in the Context of Culture: An Exploration of the Borderland between Anthropology, Medicine, and Psychiatry.* Berkeley: University of California Press, 1980.

Knowles, James, Abdo S. Yazbeck, Steven Brewster, and Bineta Ba. "The Private Sector Delivery of Health Care: Senegal." Major Applied Research Paper no. 16, edited by the United States Agency for International Development. Washington, DC: USAID, 1994.

Kolling, Marie, Kirsty Winkley, and Mette von Deden. "'For Someone Who's Rich, It's Not a Problem': Insights from Tanzania on Diabetes Health-Seeking and Medical Pluralism among Dar es Salaam's Urban Poor." *Globalization and Health* 6, no. 8 (2010).

Konrad, Monica. *Narrating the New Predictive Genetics: Ethics, Ethnography and Science.* Cambridge: Cambridge University Press, 2005.

Krige, Detlev. "Fields of Dreams, Fields of Schemes: Ponzi Finance and Multilevel Marketing in South Africa." *Africa* 82, no. 1 (2012): 69–92.

Kusiak, Pauline. "Instrumentalized Rationality, Cross-Cultural Mediators, and Civil Epistemologies of Late Colonialism." *Social Studies of Science* 20, no. 10 (2010): 1–32.

Lachenal, Guillaume. "Le médecin qui voulut être roi: Médecine coloniale et utopie au Cameroun." *Annales HSS* 1 (January–February 2010): 121–56.

Laclau, Ernesto. *On Populist Reason.* London: Verso, 2005.

Lakoff, Andrew. "The Problem of Securing Health." In *Biosecurity Interventions: Global Health and Security in Question,* edited by Andrew Lakoff and Stepher J. Collier, 7–32. New York: Columbia University Press, 2008.

Lal, Priya. "Self-Reliance and the State: The Multiple Meanings of Development in Early Post-colonial Tanzania." *Africa* 82, no. 2 (2012): 205–19.

Lancet. "What Has the Gates Foundation Done for Global Health?" Editorial. 373 (2009): 1577.

Langwick, Stacey A. "Articulate(d) Bodies: Traditional Medicine in a Tanzanian Hospital." *American Ethnologist* 35, no. 3 (2008): 428–39.

———. *Bodies, Politics and African Healing: The Matter of Maladies in Tanzania.* Bloomington: Indiana University Press, 2011.

———. "Devils, Parasites and Fierce Needles: Healing and the Politics of Translation in Southern Tanzania." *Science, Technology and Human Values* 32, no. 1 (2007): 1–30.

Last, Murray. "The Importance of Knowing about Not Knowing: Observations from Hausaland." In Feierman and Janzen, *Social Basis of Health and Healing in Africa,* 393–407.

———. "Understanding Health." In *Culture and Global Change,* edited by Tim Allen and Tracey Skelton, 72–86. London: Routledge, 1999.

Latour, Bruno. "From Realpolitik to Dingpolitik or How to Make Things Public." In *Making Things Public: Atmospheres of Democracy,* edited by Bruno Latour and Peter Weibel, 14–41. Cambridge, MA: MIT Press, 2005.

Leach, Melissa, and James Fairhead. *Vaccine Anxieties: Global Science, Child Health and Society.* Science in Society Series. London: Earth Scan, 2007.

Leopold, Mark. *Inside West Nile: Violence, History and Representation on an African frontier.* Oxford: James Currey, 2005.

Lewis, Joanna. *Empire State-Building: War and Welfare in Kenya, 1925–52.* Oxford: James Currey, 2000.

Li, Tania Murray. *The Will to Improve: Governmentality, Development and the Practice of Politics.* Durham, NC: Duke University Press, 2007.

Linsell, C. A. "Cancer Incidence in Kenya, 1957–63." *British Journal of Cancer* 21, no. 3 (1967): 464–73.

Livingston, Julie. *Debility and the Moral Imagination in Botswana.* Bloomington: Indiana University Press, 2005.

———. "Productive Misunderstandings and the Dynamism of Plural Medicine in Mid-century Bechuanaland." *Journal of Southern African Studies* 33, no. 4 (2007): 801–10.

Lock, Margaret. *Twice Dead: Organ Transplants.* Berkeley: University of California Press, 2007.

Lock, Margaret, and Vinh-Kim Nguyen, *The Anthropology of Biomedicine.* Oxford: Blackwell, 2010.

Lorber, Judith. "Good Patients and Problem Patients: Conformity and Deviance in a General Hospital." *Journal of Health and Social Behavior* 16, no. 2 (1975): 213–225.

Luedke, Tracy J., and Harry G. West, eds. *Borders and Healers: Brokering Therapeutic Resources in Southeast Africa*. Bloomington: Indiana University Press, 2005.

Lupton, Deborah. *The Imperative of Health: Public Health and the Regulated Body*. London: Sage, 1995.

Lyons, Maryinez. *The Colonial Disease: A Social History of Sleeping Sickness in Northern Zaire, 1900–1940*. Cambridge: Cambridge University Press, 1992.

MacCormack, Carol. "Health Care and the Concept of Legitimacy in Sierra Leone." In Feierman and Janzen, *Social Basis of Health and Healing in Africa*, 426–36.

Madiega, Philister A., Gemma Jones, Ruth J. Prince, and P. Wenzel Geissler. "'She's My Sister-in-Law, My Visitor, My Friend'—Challenges of Staff Identity in Home Follow-Up in an HIV Trial in Western Kenya." *Developing World Bioethics* 13, no. 1 (2011): 21–29.

Makina, Anesu. "Caring for People with HIV: State Policies and Their Dependence on Women's Unpaid Work." *Gender and Development* 17, no. 2 (2009): 309–19.

Malowany, Maureen. "Unfinished Agendas: Writing the History of Medicine of Sub-Saharan Africa." *African Affairs* 99 (2000): 325–49.

Mamdani, Mahmood. *Citizen and Subject: Contemporary Africa and the Legacy of Late Colonialism*. Princeton: Princeton University Press, 1996.

Markovitz, Irving Leonard. *Leopold Sedar Senghor and the Politics of Negritude*. London: Heinemann, 1969.

Marks, Shula. "What Is Colonial about Colonial Medicine? And What Happened to Imperialism and Health?" *Social History of Medicine* 10, no. 2 (1997): 205–19.

Marks, Shula, and Neil Andersson. "Industrialization, Rural Health and the 1944 National Health Services Commission in South Africa." In Feierman and Janzen, *Social Basis of Health and Healing in Africa*, 131–62.

Marres, Noortje. "Issues Spark a Public into Being." In *Making Things Public: Atmospheres of Democracy*, edited by Bruno Latour and Peter Weibel, 208–17. Cambridge, MA: MIT Press, 2005.

Marsland, Rebecca. "(Bio)sociality and HIV in Tanzania: Finding a Living to Support a Life." *Medical Anthropology Quarterly* 26, no. 4 (2012): 470–85.

———. "Community Participation the Tanzanian Way: Conceptual Contiguity or Power Struggle?" *Oxford Development Studies* 34, no. 1 (2006): 65–79.

———. "The Modern Traditional Healer: Locating 'Hybridity' in Modern Traditional Medicine, Southern Tanzania." *Journal of Southern African Studies* 33, no. 4 (2007): 751–65.

Marsland, Rebecca, and Ruth J. Prince. "What Is Life Worth? Biomedical Intervention, Survival and the Politics of Life." *Medical Anthropology Quarterly* 24, no. 4 (December 2012): 453–69.

Masquelier, Adeline. "Behind the Dispensary's Prosperous Façade: Imagining the State in Rural Niger." *Public Culture* 13, no. 2 (2001): 267–91.

———. "Public Health or Public Threat: Polio Eradication Campaigns, Islamic Revival and the Materialization of State Power in Niger." In Dilger, Kane, and Langwick, *Medicine, Mobility and Power in Global Africa*, 213–40.

Massey, Doreen. *World City*. Cambridge, UK: Polity Press, 2007.

Mattingly, Cheryl, Lone Grøn, and Lotte Meinert. "Chronic Homework in Emerging Borderlands of Healthcare." *Culture, Medicine, and Psychiatry* 35, no. 3 (2011): 347–75.

Maxon, Robert. "The Kenyatta Era, 1963–78: Social and Cultural Changes." In *Decolonization and Independence in Kenya: 1940–93*, edited by Bethwell A. Ogot and William R. Ochieng', 110–47. Athens: Ohio University Press, 1995.

Maxon, Robert M., and Peter Ndege. "The Economics of Structural Adjustment." In *Decolonization and Independence in Kenya, 1940–93*, edited by Bethwell A. Ogot and William R. Ochieng', 151–86. London: James Currey, 1995.

Mbaye, Assane. "Vente illicite des médicaments: L'Ordre des pharmaciens riposte et contre attaque." *Sud quotidien*, 24 July 2009, www.sudonline.sn.

Mbembe, Achille. "Provisional Notes on the Postcolony." *Africa* 62, no. 1 (1992): 3–37.

Mbembe, Achille, and Janet Roitman. "Figures of the Subject in Times of Crisis." *Public Culture* 7 (1995): 323–52.

McNeil, Donald G. "At Front Lines, AIDS War Is Falling Apart." *New York Times*, 9 May 2010.

Meagher, Kate. *Identity Economics: Social Networks and the Informal Economy in Nigeria*. Woodbridge, UK: James Currey, 2010.

Meinert, Lotte. "Cutting New Networks: Kin Relations and Research Relations in an ARV Study in Uganda." In *Changing States of Science: Ethnographic and Historical Perspectives on Government, Citizenship and Medical Research in Contemporary Africa*, edited by P. Wenzel Geissler. Durham, NC: Duke University Press, forthcoming.

———. *Hopes in Friction: Schooling, Health and Everyday Life in Uganda*. Charlotte, NC: Information Age Publishing, 2009.

———. "Usund Viden? Sundhedsundervisning og medicinsk praksis blandt itesobørn i Uganda." *Tidsskriftet Antropologi* 38 (1998): 65–78.

———. "The Work of the Virus: The Cutting and Creation of Kin Relations in an ART Project." In *Science and the Para-state: Ethnographic and Historical Perspectives on Life-Science, Government, and the Public in 21st Century Africa*, edited by P. Wenzel Geissler. Durham, NC: Duke University Press, forthcoming.

Meinert, Lotte, Hanne O. Mogensen, and Jenipher Twebaze. "Tests for Life Chances: CD4 Miracles and Obstacles in Uganda." *Anthropology and Medicine* 16, no. 2 (2009): 195–209.

Meinert, Lotte, Michael Whyte, Susan R. Whyte, and Betty Kyaddondo. "Faces of Globalisation." *Folk* 45 (2003): 105–24.

Meyer, Birgit. *Translating the Devil: Religion and Modernity among the Ewe in Ghana*. Edinburgh: Edinburgh University Press, 1999.

Ministry of Health, Kenya. *AIDS in Kenya: Trends, Interventions and Impact.* 7th ed. Nairobi: Republic of Kenya, 2005.

———. *Home-Based Care for People Living with HIV/AIDS: National Home-Based Care Programme and Service Guideline.* Nairobi: National AIDS/STD Control Programme, 2002.

———. *Home-Based Care for People Living with HIV/AIDS: Home Care Handbook; A Reference Manual for Home-Based Care for People Living with HIV/AIDS in Kenya.* 2nd ed. Nairobi: National AIDS/STD Control Programme, 2006.

———. *Reversing the Trends: The Second National Health Sector Strategic Plan of Kenya—NHSSP II—2005–2010.* Nairobi: Ministry of Health, 2005.

Ministry of Health, Republic of Uganda. *Health Sector Strategic Plan II: 2005/06–2009/2010,* vol. 1. Kampala: Republic of Uganda, 2005.

———. *Implementation Guidelines for the Home Based Management of Fever Strategy.* 1st ed. Kampala, Uganda: Ministry of Health / UNICEF / BASICS / DISH, 2002.

Mitchell, Timothy. *Rule of Experts: Egypt, Techno-Politics, Modernity.* Berkeley: University of California Press, 2002.

Miyakazi, Hirokazu. *The Method of Hope: Anthropology, Philosophy, and Fijian Knowledge.* Palo Alto, CA: Stanford University Press, 2004.

Mkandawire, Thandika. "Thinking about Developmental States in Africa." *Cambridge Journal of Economics* 25, no. 3 (2001): 289–314.

Mol, Annemarie. *The Body Multiple.* Durham, NC: Duke University Press, 2005.

———. *The Logic of Care: Health and the Problem of Patient Choice.* London: Routledge, 2008.

Mol, Annemarie, Ingunn Moser, and Jeanette Pols, eds. *Care in Practice: On Tinkering in Clinics, Homes and Farms.* New Rockford, ND: Transcript, 2010.

Møller, M.C.R. "A Living Corpse: Rethinking AIDS Stigma, AIDS Medicines and a Human Longing for Recognition in Southeastern Uganda." Master's thesis, Department of Anthropology and Ethnography, Aarhus University, 2008.

Molyneux, Maxine. "The 'Neoliberal Turn' and the New Social Policy in Latin America: How Neoliberal, How New?" *Development and Change* 39, no. 5 (2008): 775–97.

moniteur africain du commerce et de l'industrie, Le. "Produits pharmaceutiques: Un marché en rapide expansion." 519, no. 9 (September 1971): 8.

Monnais, Laurence. *Médicaments coloniaux: Distribution, circulation et consommation de produits pharmaceutiques au Viêt Nam, 1905–1940.* Paris: Indes Savantes, forthcoming 2013.

Moore, Donald S. "The Crucible of Cultural Politics: Reworking 'Development' in Zimbabwe's Eastern Highlands." *American Ethnologist* 26, no. 3 (1999): 654–89.

Moore, Henrietta L. *Feminism and Anthropology.* Cambridge, UK: Polity, 1988.

Morris, Rosalind C. "Rush/Panic/Rush: Speculations on the Value of Life and Death in South Africa's Age of AIDS." *Public Culture* 20 (2008): 199–231.

Mosse, David. *Cultivating Development: An Ethnography of Aid Policy and Practice.* London: Pluto Press, 2005.

Mugyenyi, Peter. "Flat-Line Funding for PEPFAR: A Recipe for Chaos." *Lancet* 374 (25 July 2009): 292.

Mulemi, Benson A. *Coping with Cancer and Adversity: Hospital Ethnography in Kenya.* Leiden: African Studies Center, 2010.

———. "Patients' Perspectives on Hospitalization: Experiences from a Cancer Ward in Kenya." *Anthropology and Medicine* 15, no. 2 (2008): 117–31.

Mur-Veeman, Ingrid, Irmgard Eijkelberg, and Cor Spreeuwenberg. "How to Manage the Implementation of Shared Care: A Discussion of the Role of Power, Culture and Structure in the Development of Shared Care Arrangements." *Journal of Management in Medicine* 15, no. 2 (2001): 142–55.

Mutongi, Kenda. *Worries of the Heart: Widows, Family and Community in Kenya.* Chicago: University of Chicago Press, 2007.

Mutuma, Geoffrey Z., and Anne Ruggut-Korir. *Cancer Incidence Report: Nairobi, 2000–2002.* Nairobi: Nairobi Cancer Registry, Kenya Medical Research Institute, 2006.

NASCOP. *Kenya AIDS Incidence Survey 2007 Preliminary Report.* Nairobi: National AIDS and STI Control Programme, 2007.

National Malaria Control Programme. *Plan of Action for Accelerated Implementation of Malaria Control in Tanzania.* Dar es Salaam: Ministry of Health, United Republic of Tanzania / World Health Organization, 1999.

Navarro, Vicente. "Neoliberalism and Its Consequences: The World Health Situation since Alma Ata." *Global Social Policy* 8 (2008): 152–55.

Ndegwa, Stephen N. "Civil Society and Political Change in Africa: The Case of Non-governmental Organizations in Kenya." *International Journal of Comparative Sociology* 35, no. 1/2 (1994): 19–36.

Nelson, Jenenne P. "Struggling to Gain Meaning: Living with Uncertainty of Breast Cancer." *Advances in Nursing Science* 18, no. 3 (1996): 59–76.

Ngabission, Noel Ngouo. "Tout savoir sur . . . l'industrie pharmaceutique." *Jeune Afrique* 612, no. 30 (September 1972): 51–65.

Ngubane, Harriet. *Body and Mind in Zulu Medicine.* London: Academic Press, 1977.

Nguyen, Vinh-Kim. "Antiretroviral Globalism, Biopolitics, and Therapeutic Citizenship." In Ong and Collier, *Global Assemblages,* 124–44.

———. "Government by Exception: Enrolment and Experimentality in Mass HIV Treatment Programs in Africa." *Social Theory and Health* 7, no. 3 (2009): 196–218.

———. *The Republic of Therapy: Triage and Sovereignty in West Africa's Time of AIDS.* Durham, NC: Duke University Press, 2011.

Nguyen, Vinh-Kim, Cyriaque Y. Ako, Pascal Niamba, Aliou Sylla, and Issoufou Tiendrébéogo. "Adherence as Therapeutic Citizenship: Impact of the

History of Access to Antiretroviral Drugs on Adherence to Treatment." *AIDS* 21, no. 5 (2007): 31–35.

Niang, Issa. "Vol dans les pharmacies: Des pertes estimées à plus de 21 millions en 2007." *Walf Fadjiri,* 30 April 2008, www.walf-groupe.com/.

Nichter, Mark. *Global Health: Why Cultural Perceptions, Social Representations and Biopolitics Matter.* Tucson: University of Arizona Press, 2008.

Niehaus, Isak P. "Death before Dying: Understanding AIDS Stigma in the South African Lowveld." *Journal of Southern African Studies* 33, no. 4 (2007): 845–60.

Nnko, Soori, Betty Chiduo, Flora Wilson, Wences Msuya, and Gabriel Mwaluko. "Tanzania: AIDS Care—Learning from Experience." *Review of African Political Economy* 86 (2000): 547–57.

Nshakira N., M. Kristensen, F. Ssali, and S. R. Whyte. "Appropriate Treatment of Malaria? Use of Anti-malarial Drugs for Children's Fevers in District Medical Units, Drug Shops and Homes in Eastern Uganda." *Tropical Medicine and International Health* 7, no. 4 (2002): 309–16.

O'Brien, Donal Cruise. "Le sens de l'état au Sénégal." In *Le Sénégal contemporain,* edited by Momar-Coumba Diop, 501–6. Paris: Karthala, 2002.

O'Brien, Martin. "Health and Lifestyle: A Critical Mess? Notes on the Dedifferentiation of Health." In *The Sociology of Health Promotion: Critical Analyses of Consumption, Lifestyle and Risk,* edited by Robin Bunton, Sarah Nettleton, and Roger Burrows, 189–202. London: Routledge, 1995.

Ogden, Jessica, Simel Esim, and Caren Grown. "Expanding the Care Continuum for HIV/AIDS: Bringing Carers into Focus." *Health Policy and Planning* 21, no. 5 (2006): 333–42.

Ogot, Bethwell A. *Politics and the AIDS Epidemic in Kenya, 1983–2003.* Kisumu: Anyange Press, 2004.

Okeke, Iruka N. *Divining without Seeds: The Case for Strengthening Laboratory Medicine in Africa.* New York: Cornell University Press, 2011.

Olivier de Sardan, Jean-Pierre. "A Moral Economy of Corruption in Africa." *Journal of Modern African Studies* 37, no. 1 (1995): 25–52.

Ombongi, Kenneth. "The Historical Interface between the State and Medical Science in Africa: Kenya's Case." In *Ethos, Evidence and Experiment: The Anthropology and History of Medical Research in Africa,* edited by P. Wenzel Geissler and Catherine Molyneux, 353–72. New York: Berghahn Books, 2011.

O'Neil, Bruce. "Of Camps, Gulags and Extraordinary Renditions: Infrastructural Violence in Rumania." *Ethnography* 13, no. 4 (2012): 466–86.

Ong, Aihwa. *Neoliberalism as Exception: Mutations in Citizenship and Sovereignty.* Durham, NC: Duke University Press, 2006.

———. "The Production of Possession: Spirits and the Multinational Corporation in Malaysia." *American Ethnologist* 15, no. 1 (1988): 28–41.

Ong, Aihwa, and Nancy Chen. *Asian Biotech: Ethics and Communities of Fate.* Durham, NC: Duke University Press, 2010.

Ong, Aihwa, and Stephen Collier, eds. *Global Assemblages: Technology, Politics, and Ethics as Anthropological Problems.* Malden, MA: Blackwell Publishing, 2005.

Onyango, J. F., and I. M. Macharia. "Delays in Diagnosis, Referral and Management of Head and Neck Cancer Presenting at Kenyatta National Hospital, Nairobi." *East African Medical Journal* 83, no. 4 (2006): 85–91.

Orner, Phyllis. "Psychosocial Impacts on Caregivers of People Living with AIDS." *AIDS Care* 18, no. 3 (2006): 236–40.

Othieno-Abinya, N. A., L. Nyabola, H. O. Abwao, and P. Ndege. "Post-surgical Management of Patients with Breast Cancer at the Kenyatta National Hospital." *East African Medical Journal* 79, no. 3 (2002): 156–62.

Packard, Randall. "Industrialization, Rural Poverty, and Tuberculosis in South Africa, 1850–1950." In Feierman and Janzen, *Social Basis of Health and Healing in Africa,* 104–30.

———. "Visions of Postwar Health and Development and Their Impact on Public Health Interventions in the Developing World." In *International Development and the Social Sciences: Essays on the History and Politics of Knowledge,* edited by Frederick Cooper and Randall Packard, 93–115. Berkeley: University of California Press, 1997.

———. *White Plague, Black Labour: Tuberculosis and the Political Economy of Health and Disease in South Africa.* Berkeley: University of California Press, 1989.

Parker, Melissa, Tim Allen, Georgina Pearson, Rachel Flynn, and Nicholas Rees. "Border Parasites: Schistosomiasis Control among Uganda's Fisherfolk." *Journal of Eastern African Studies* 6, no. 1 (2012): 98–123.

Parker, Melissa, and Ian Harper. "The Anthropology of Public Health." *Journal of Biosocial Science* 38, no. 1 (2006): 1–5.

Parkhurst, Justin O. "The Crisis of AIDS and the Politics of Response: The Case of Uganda." *International Relations* 15, no. 6 (2001): 69–87.

———. "The Ugandan Success Story? Evidence and Claims of HIV1 Prevention." *Lancet* 360, no. 9326 (2002): 78–80.

Parkhurst, Justin O., and Louisiana Lush. "The Political Environment of HIV: Lessons from a Comparison of Uganda and South Africa." *Social Science and Medicine* 59, no. 9 (2004): 1913–24.

Parkin, David. *The Cultural Definition of Political Response: Lineal Destiny among the Luo.* London: Academic Press, 1978.

Parkin, D. Maxwell, Freddy Sitas, Mike Chirenje, Lara Stein, Raymond Abratt, and Henry Wabinga. "Part I: Cancer in Indigenous Africans—Burden, Distribution, and Trends." *Lancet Oncology* 9, no. 7 (2008): 683–92.

Petersen, Kristin. "AIDS Policies for Markets and Warriors: Dispossession, Capital and Pharmaceuticals in Nigeria." In Dilger, Kane, and Langwick, *Medicine, Mobility and Power in Global Africa,* 138–62.

Petryna, Adriana. "Ethical Variability: Drug Development and Globalizing Clinical Trials." *American Ethnologist* 32 (2005): 183–97.

———. *Life Exposed: Biological Citizens after Chernobyl.* Princeton: Princeton University Press, 2002.

———. *When Experiments Travel: Clinical Trials and the Global Search for Human Subjects.* Princeton: Princeton University Press, 2009.

Petryna, Adriana, and Arthur Kleinman. "The Pharmaceutical Nexus." In Petryna, Lakoff, and Kleinman, *Global Pharmaceuticals*, 1–32.

Petryna, Adriana, Andrew Lakoff, and Arthur Kleinman, eds. *Global Pharmaceuticals: Ethics, Markets, Practices.* Durham, NC: Duke University Press, 2006.

Pfeiffer, James. "Condoms and Social Marketing: Pentecostalism and Structural Adjustment in Mozambique." *Medical Anthropology Quarterly* 18, no. 1 (2004): 77–103.

———. "International NGOs and Primary Health Care in Mozambique: The Need for a New Model of Collaboration." *Social Science and Medicine* 56 (2003): 726–37.

———. "International NGOs in the Mozambique Health Sector: The 'Velvet Glove' of Privatization." In *Unhealthy Health Policy: A Critical Anthropological Examination,* edited by Arachu Castro and Merrill Singer, 43–62. Walnut Creek, CA: Altamira Press, 2004.

Pfeiffer, James, and Mark Nichter. "What Can Critical Medical Anthropology Contribute to Global Health?" *Medical Anthropological Quarterly* 22 (2008): 410–15.

Pigg, Stacy Leigh. "Inventing Social Categories through Place: Social Representations and Development in Nepal." *Comparative Studies in Society and History* 34, no. 3 (1992): 491–513.

Pollan, Michael. *In Defense of Food: An Eater's Manifesto.* New York: Penguin Press, 2008.

Pool, Robert. *Dialogue and the Interpretation of Illness: Conversations in a Cameroon Village.* Oxford: Berg, 1994.

Porter, Dorothy. *Health, Civilization and the State: A History of Public Health from Ancient to Modern Times.* London: Routledge, 1999.

———. *The History of Public Health and the Modern State.* Wellcome Institute Series in the History of Medicine. Amsterdam: Editions Rodopi, 1994.

President's Malaria Initiative. "Malaria Operational Plan: Year Four—Fiscal Year 2010 Senegal." 2010. http://pmi.gov/countries/mops/fy10/senegal_mop-fy10.pdf.

Prince, Ruth J. "HIV and the Moral Economy of Survival in an East African City." *Medical Anthropology Quarterly* 26, no. 4 (2012): 534–56.

———. "The Politics and Anti-politics of HIV Interventions in Kenya." In *Biomedicine and Governance in Africa,* edited by Paul Wenzel Geissler, Richard Rottenburg, and Judith Zenker. Bielefeld, Germany: Transcript Verlag, 2012.

———. "Public Debates about Luo Widow Inheritance." In *Christianity and Public Culture in Africa,* edited by Harri Englund, 109–30. Athens: Ohio University Press, 2011.

Prince, Ruth J., with Rijk van Dijk and Philippe Denis. Introduction to "Engaging Christianities: Negotiating HIV/AIDS, Health and Social Relations in East and Southern Africa." *Africa Today* 56, no. 1 (2009): v–xviii.

quotidien, Le. "Entretien avec . . . Cheikh Oumar Dia, président de l'Ordre des pharmaciens au Sénégal." 22 July 2009, www.lequotidien.sn.

———. "Vendredi, jour de grève des pharmacies: Une ordonnance contre l'insécurité et la démission de l'état." 22 July 2009, www.lequotidien.sn.

Rabinow, Paul. *Artificiality and Enlightenment: From Sociobiology to Biosociality; Essays on the Anthropology of Reason.* Princeton: Princeton University Press, 1996.

Rabinow, Paul, and Nikolas Rose. "Biopower Today." *BioSocieties* 1, no. 2 (2006): 195–217.

Ranger, Terence. "Godly Medicine: The Ambiguities of Medical Mission in Southeastern Tanzania, 1900–1945." In *The Social Basis of Health and Healing in Africa,* edited by Steven Feierman and John M. Janzen, 256–82. Berkeley: University of California Press, 1992.

Redfield, Peter. "Doctors, Borders, and Life in Crisis." *Cultural Anthropology* 20, no. 3 (2005): 328–61.

———. "Vital Mobility and the Humanitarian Kit." In *Biosecurity Interventions: Global Health and Security in Question,* edited by Andrew Lakoff and Stephen Collier, 147–71. New York: Columbia University Press, 2008.

Reich, Michael. "Public-Private Partnerships for Public Health." *Nature Medicine* 6, no. 6 (2000): 617–20.

———. "Reshaping the State from Above, from Within, from Below: Implications for Public Health." *Social Science and Medicine* 54, no. 11 (2002): 1669–75.

ReMed. "ReMed s'engage contre le marché illicite des médicaments." www.remed.org/html/marche_illicite_de_medicaments.html (accessed 13 October 2012).

Renne, Elisha. *The Politics of Polio in Northern Nigeria.* Bloomington: Indiana University Press, 2010.

République du Sénégal. "Convention d'établissement entre le gouvernement du Sénégal . . . et la société 'Soffin'" [c. 1972]. In *Dossier pharmacie.* On file, Centre de documentation, Bibliothèque nationale du Sénégal, Dakar.

———. "Note à la très haute attention de M. le PM sur l'évolution du secteur de la santé de 2000 à 2010." Formerly available at www.sante.gouv.sn, accessed 10 October 2010.

———, Ministère du plan, du développement et de la coopération technique. "Propositions de planification dans les domaines de l'hygiène et de la santé publique," Dakar, 1961, document Br 5097 C, Archives nationales, Section Outre Mer, Aix en Provence, France.

Richey, Lisa Ann. "Counselling Citizens and Producing Patronage: AIDS Treatment in South African and Ugandan Clinics." *Development and Change* 43, no. 4 (2012): 823–45.

Robbins, Steven. *From Revolution to Rights in South Africa: Social Movements, NGOs and Popular Politics after Apartheid.* Woodbridge, UK: James Currey, 2008.

———. "Humanitarian Aid beyond 'Bare Survival': Social Movement Responses to Xenophobic Violence in South Africa." *American Ethnologist* 36, no. 4 (2009): 637–50.

———. "'Long Live Zackie, Long Live': AIDS Activism, Science and Citizenship after Apartheid." *Journal of Southern African Studies* 30 (2004): 651–72.

Robson, Elsbeth. "Invisible Carers: Young People in Zimbabwe's Home-Based Healthcare." *Area* 32, no. 1 (2000): 59–69.

Roitman, Janet. *Fiscal Disobedience: An Anthropology of Economic Regulation in Central Africa.* Princeton: Princeton University Press, 2005.

Rono, Joseph Kipkemboi. "The Impact of Structural Adjustment Programmes on Kenyan Society." *Journal of Social Development in Africa* 17, no. 1 (2002): 81–98.

Rosaldo, Michelle Zimbalist. "Woman, Culture and Society: A Theoretical Overview." In *Woman, Culture and Society,* edited by Michelle Zimbalist Rosaldo, Louise Lamphere, and Joan Bamberger, 17–42. Stanford: Stanford University Press, 1974.

Rose, Nikolas. "The Death of the Social? Re-figuring the Territory of Government." *Economy and Society* 25, no. 3 (1996): 327–56.

———. "The Politics of Life Itself." *Theory, Culture and Society* 18, no. 6 (2001): 1–30.

———. *The Politics of Life Itself: Biomedicine, Power, and Subjectivity in the Twenty-First Century.* Princeton: Princeton University Press, 2007.

———. *Powers of Freedom: Reframing Political Thought.* Cambridge: Cambridge University Press, 1999.

Rose, Nikolas, and Carlos Novas. "Biological Citizenship." In Ong and Collier, *Global Assemblages,* 439–63.

Rosen, George. *A History of Public Health: Expanded Edition.* Baltimore, MD: John Hopkins University Press, 1993.

Rottenburg, Richard. "Social and Public Experiments and New Figurations of Science and Politics in Postcolonial Africa." *Postcolonial Studies* 12, no. 4 (2009): 423–40.

Routley, Laura. "NGOs and the Formation of the Public: Grey Practices and Accountability." *African Affairs* 111, no. 442 (2012): 116–34.

Rudé, George. *The Crowd in History.* London: Serif, 2005.

Sahlins, Marshall. *Islands of History.* Chicago: University of Chicago Press, 1987.

Samba, Ebrahim Malick. "Message sur la vente illicite des médicaments." www.remed.org/message_samaba-OMS-Afro-1.rtf (accessed 13 October 2012).

Samsky, Ari. "Scientific Sovereignty: How International Drug Donation Programmes Reshape Health, Disease and the State." *Cultural Anthropology* 27, no. 2 (2012): 310–32.

———. "'Since We Are Taking the Drugs': Labor and Value in Two International Drug Donation Programs." *Journal of Cultural Economy* 4, no. 1 (2011): 27–43.

Sanders, Todd. "Reconsidering Witchcraft: Postcolonial Africa and Analytic (Un)certainties." *American Anthropologist* 105, no. 2 (2003): 338–52.

Sane, Idrissa. "Sénégal: Vente illicite de médicaments à Keur Serigne-Bi—Les vendeurs acceptent de se conformer à l'interdiction." *Le soleil*, 29 July 2009, www.lesoleil.sn.

Sansom, Clare, and Geoffrey Mutuma. "Kenya Faces Cancer Challenge." *Lancet Oncology* 3, no. 8 (2002): 456–58.

Sarr, Aboubakrine. "Indignation." *Sud Online*, 23 July 2008, www.sudonline.sn.

Sassen, Saskia. "Globalization or Denationalization?" *Review of International Political Economy* 10, no. 1 (2003): 1–22.

Schneider, Leander. "Colonial Legacies and Postcolonial Authoritarianism: Connects and Disconnects." *African Studies Review* 49, no. 1 (2006): 93–118.

Schumaker, Lyn. "Slimes and Death-Dealing Dambos: Water, Industry and the Garden City on Zambia's Copperbelt." *Journal of Southern African Studies* 34, no. 4 (2008): 823–40.

Scott, James C. *Seeing Like a State: How Certain Schemes to Improve the Human Condition Have Failed.* New Haven, CT: Yale University Press, 1998.

SEDE. *Possibilités d'implantation d'une usine de fabrication de produits pharmaceutiques au Sénégal.* Paris: Ministère du plan et de l'industrie, 1969.

Seely, Jennifer. "A Political Analysis of Decentralisation: Co-opting the Tuareg Threat in Mali." *Journal of Modern African Studies* 39, no. 3 (2001): 499–524.

Semboja, Joseph, and Ole Therkildsen, eds. *Service Provision under Stress in East Africa: The State, NGOs and People's Organizations in Kenya, Tanzania and Uganda.* Copenhagen: Centre for Development Research; Nairobi: East African Educational Publishers, 1995.

Serunjogi, Titus. "When You Eat Is Just as Important." *New Vision*, 22 November 2009, A4.

Setel, Philip W., Milton Lewis, and Maryinez Lyons, eds. *Histories of Sexually Transmitted Diseases and HIV/AIDS in Sub-Saharan Africa.* London: Greenwood Press, 1999.

Sherr, Kenneth, Antonio Mussa, Baltazar Chilundo, Sarah Gimbel, James Pfeiffer, Amy Hagopian, and Stephen Gloydl. "Brain Drain and Health Worker Distortions in Mozambique." *PLoS One* 7, no. 4 (2012), www.ncbi.nlm.nih.gov/pmc/articles/PMC3338796/.

Shipton, Parker. *The Nature of Entrustment: Intimacy, Exchange and the Sacred in Africa.* New Haven, CT: Yale University Press, 2007.

Shivji, Issa G. *Silences in NGO Discourse: The Role and Future of NGOs in Africa.* Nairobi: Pambazuka Press / Fahamu Books, 2007.

Shore, Cris, and Susan Wright. "Policy: A New Field of Anthropology." In *Anthropology of Policy: Critical Perspectives on Governance and Power,* edited by Cris Shore and Susan Wright, 3–34. London: Routledge, 1997.

Smith, James H. *Bewitching Development: Witchcraft and the Reinvention of Development in Neoliberal Kenya.* Chicago: University of Chicago Press, 2008.

soleil, Le. "5e réunion de l'Ordre des pharmaciens: 100 millions pour la 'Maison du pharmacien.'" 4 July 2005, www.lesoleil.sn.

SONEPI. *Perspectives de l'industrie pharmaceutique au Sénégal: Problèmes et solutions.* Dakar: Ministère du développement industriel, 1970.

Southall, Roger. "Re-forming the State? Kleptocracy and the Political Transition in Kenya." *Review of African Political Economy,* no. 79 (1999): 93–108.

Star, Susan Leigh, and James R. Griesemer. "Institutional Ecology, 'Translations' and Boundary Objects: Amateurs and Professionals in Berkeley's Museum of Vertebrate Zoology, 1907–39." *Social Studies of Science* 19, no. 3 (1989): 387–420.

Stewart, Sheelagh. "Happy Ever After in the Marketplace: Non-government Organisations and Uncivil Society." *Review of African Political Economy* 24, no. 71 (1997): 11–34.

Streefland, Pieter. "Public Health Care under Pressure in Sub-Saharan Africa." *Health Policy* 71, no. 3 (2005): 375–82.

Street, Alice, and Simon Coleman. "Introduction: Real and Imagined Spaces." *Space and Culture* 15, no. 1 (2012): 4–17.

Sullivan, Noelle. "Enacting Spaces of Inequality." *Space and Culture* 15, no. 1 (2011): 57–67.

———. "Mediating Abundance and Scarcity: Implementing an HIV/AIDS Targeted Project within a Government Hospital in Tanzania." *Medical Anthropology* 30, no. 2 (2011): 202–21.

Sunder Rajan, Kaushik. *Biocapital: The Constitution of Postgenomic Life.* Durham, NC: Duke University Press, 2006.

Swidler, Ann, and Susan Cotts Watkins. "'Teach a Man to Fish': The Sustainability Doctrine and Its Social Consequences." *World Development* 37, no. 7 (2009): 1182–96.

Taylor, Shelley E. "Hospital Patient Behavior, Reactance, Helplessness or Control?" In *Interpersonal Issues in Health Care,* edited by Howard S. Friedman and M. Robin DiMatteo, 209–32. Paris: Academic Press, 1982.

Thomas, Barbara P. *Politics, Participation and Poverty: Development through Self-Help in Kenya.* Boulder, CO: Westview Press, 1985.

Thomas, Lynn M. *Politics of the Womb: Women, Reproduction and the State in Kenya.* Berkeley: University of California Press, 2003.

Tilley, Helen. *Africa as a Living Laboratory: Empire, Development and the Problem of Scientific Knowledge, 1870–1950.* Chicago: University of Chicago Press, 2011.

Tsing, Anna Lowenhaupt. *Friction: An Ethnography of Global Connection.* Princeton: Princeton University Press, 2005.

Turner, Victor. *The Forest of Symbols: Aspects of Ndembu Ritual.* Ithaca, NY: Cornell University Press, 1967.

———. *The Ritual Process: Structure and Anti-structure.* Chicago: Aldine Publishing, 1969.

Turshen, Meredeth. *Privatizing Health Services in Africa.* New Brunswick, NJ: Rutgers University Press, 1999.

Uganda National Drug Authority. National Drug Policy and Authority Statute. Entebbe: Government Printer, 1994.

United States Pharmacopeial Convention. "PQM: Promoting the Quality of Medicines in Developing Countries." www.usp.org/global-health-impact-programs/promoting-quality-medicines-pqmusaid (accessed 13 October 2012).

U.S. Pharmacopoeia. "USP in Developing Countries." www.usp.org/worldwide/.

Van Damme, Wim, Katharina Kober, and Guy Kegels. "Scaling Up Antiretroviral Treatment in Southern African Countries with Human Resource Shortage: How Will Health Systems Adapt?" *Social Science and Medicine* 66, no. 10 (2008): 2108–21.

Vaughan, Megan. *Curing Their Ills: Colonial Power and African Illness.* Oxford: Polity Press, 1991; Stanford: Stanford University Press, 1992.

———. "'Divine Kings': Sex, Death and Anthropology in Inter-war East/Central Africa." *Journal of African History* 49 (2008): 383–401.

Waite, Gloria. "Public Health in Precolonial East-Central Africa." In Feierman and Janzen, *Social Basis of Health and Healing in Africa,* 212–31.

Walf Fadjiri. "Poursuite des activités de Keur Serigne Bi: Wade dit Niet à Serigne Bara." 1 August 2009, www.walf-groupe.com/.

Wane, Almamy Mamadou. *Le Sénégal entre deux naufrages? Le Joola et l'alternance.* Paris: L'Harmattan, 2004.

Warner, Michael. *Publics and Counterpublics.* New York: Zone Books, 2002.

Watts, Michael. "Development and Governmentality." *Singapore Journal of Tropical Geography* 24, no. 1 (2003): 6–34.

Weidle, Paul J., Nafuna Wamai, Peter Solberg, Cheryl Liechty, Sam Sendagala, Willy Were, Jonathan Mermin, Kate Buchacz, Prosper Behumbiize, Ray L. Ransom, and Rebecca Bunnell. "Adherence to Antiretroviral Therapy in a Home-Based AIDS Care Programme in Rural Uganda." *Lancet* 386, no. 4 (2006): 1587–94.

Wendland, Claire L. *A Heart for the Matter: Journeys through an African Medical School.* Chicago: University of Chicago Press, 2010.

———."Moral Maps and Medical Imaginaries: Clinical Tourism at Malawi's College of Medicine." *American Anthropologist* 114, no. 3 (2012): 108–22.

West, Harry G. *Ethnographic Sorcery.* Chicago: University of Chicago Press, 2007.

———. *Kupilikula: Governance and the Invisible Realm in Mozambique.* Chicago: University of Chicago Press, 2005.

White, Luise. *Speaking with Vampires: Rumor and History in Colonial Africa.* Berkeley: University of California Press, 2000.

WHO. *Community Home-Based Care: Action Research in Kenya, September–October 2000.* Geneva: World Health Organization, 2001.

———. *Community Home-Based Care in Resource-Limited Settings: A Framework for Action.* Geneva: World Health Organization, 2002.

———. *Continuity and Change: Implementing the Third WHO Medicines Strategy, 2008–2013.* Geneva: World Health Organization, 2009.

———. "First NCDnet Global Forum." 2010. www.who.int/nmh/newsletter_apr2010.pdf.

————. *Impact Brochure*. Geneva: World Health Organization / Interpol, 2008. www.who.int/impact/FinalBrochureWHA2008a.pdf.

————. *Key Elements in HIV/AIDS Care and Support*. Geneva: World Health Organization / UNAIDS, 2000.

————. *Scaling Up Home Based-Management of Malaria: From Research to Implementation*. Geneva: WHO / HTM / MAL, 2004.

Whyte, Susan Reynolds. "Going Home? Burial and Belonging in the Era of AIDS." *Africa* 75, no. 2 (2005): 154–72.

————. "Medicines and Self-Help: The Privatisation of Health Care in Eastern Uganda." In *Changing Uganda: The Dilemmas of Structural Adjustment and Revolutionary Change*, edited by H. B. Hansen and M. Twaddle, 130–48. London: James Currey, 1991.

————. "Pharmaceuticals as Folk Medicine: Transformations in the Social Relations of Health Care in Uganda." *Culture, Medicine and Psychiatry* 16 (1992): 163–86; reprinted in *The Art of Medical Anthropology: Readings*, edited by Sjaak van der Geest and A. Rienks, 319–34. Amsterdam: Het Spinhuis Publishers, 1998.

————. "The Power of Medicines in East Africa." In *The Context of Medicines in Developing Countries: Studies in Pharmaceutical Anthropology*, edited by Sjaak van der Geest and Susan R. Whyte, 217–33. Dordrecht: Kluwer, 1988.

————. *Questioning Misfortune: The Pragmatics of Uncertainty in Eastern Uganda*. Cambridge: Cambridge University Press, 1997.

————, ed. *Second Chances: Surviving AIDS in Uganda*. Durham, NC: Duke University Press, forthcoming.

Whyte, Susan Reynolds, Sjaak van der Geest, and Anita Hardon. "Pharmacists as Doctors: Bridging the Sectors of Health Care." In *Social Lives of Medicines*, by Susan Whyte, Sjaak van der Geest, and Anita Hardon, 91–103. Cambridge: Cambridge University Press, 2002.

Whyte, Susan Reynolds, Michael A. Whyte, and Betty Kyaddondo. "Health Workers Entangled: Confidentiality and Certification." In Dilger and Luig, *Morality, Hope and Grief*, 80–101.

Whyte, Susan R., Michael A. Whyte, Lotte Meinert, and Betty Kyaddondo. "Treating AIDS: Dilemmas of Unequal Access in Uganda." In Petryna, Lakoff, and Kleinman, *Global Pharmaceuticals*, 240–62.

Whyte, Susan Reynolds, Michael A. Whyte, Lotte Meinert, and Jenipher Twebaze. "Therapeutic Clientship: Belonging in Uganda's Projectified Landscape of AIDS Care." In *When People Come First: Critical Studies in Global Health*, edited by João Biehl and Adriana Petryna, 140–65. Princeton: Princeton University Press, 2013.

Wilson, Monica. *Communal Rituals of the Nyakyusa*. Oxford: Oxford University Press, 1959.

————. *Good Company: A Study of Nyakyusa Age Villages*. Oxford: Oxford University Press, 1951.

————. *Rituals of Kinship among the Nyakyusa*. Oxford: Oxford University Press, 1957.

Wipper, Audrey. "The Maendeleo Ya Wanawake Movement in the Colonial Period: The Canadian Connection, Mau Mau, Embroidery and Agriculture." *Rural Africana* 29 (1975): 197–201.

————. "The Maendeleo Ya Wanawake Organization: The Co-optation of Leadership." *African Studies Review* 18, no. 3 (1975): 99–120.

Wolf, Angelika. "Health Security on the Move: Biobureaucracy, Solidarity and the Transfer of Health Insurance to Senegal." In Dilger, Kane, and Langwick, *Medicine, Mobility and Power in Global Africa*, 92–114.

Worboys, Michael. "The Colonial World as Mission and Mandate: Leprosy and Empire, 1900–1940." *Osiris* 15 (2000): 190–206.

World Bank. *The Challenge of Development*. World Development Report 1991. Oxford: World Bank and Oxford University Press, 1991.

————. *Investing in Health*. World Development Report 1993. Oxford: World Bank and Oxford University Press, 1993.

Wright, Marcia. *German Missions in Tanganyika, 1891–1941: Lutherans and Moravians in the Southern Highlands*. Oxford: Clarendon Press, 1971.

Wringe, Alison, Fabian Cataldo, Nicola Stevenson, and Ade Fakoya. "Delivering Comprehensive Home-Based Care Programmes for HIV: A Review of Lessons Learned and Challenges Ahead in the Era of Antiretroviral Therapy." *Health Policy and Planning* 25, no. 5 (2010): 352–62.

Yar, Majid. "The Other Global Drugs Crisis: Assessing the Scope, Impacts and Drivers of the Trade in Dangerous Counterfeit Pharmaceuticals." *International Journal of Social Inquiry* 1, no. 1 (2008): 151–66.

Yarrow, Tom. "Life/History: Personal Narratives of Development amongst NGO Workers and Activists in Ghana." *Africa* 78, no. 3 (2009): 334–58.

Yarrow, Tom, and Soumhya Venkatesan. "Anthropology and Development: Critical Framings." In *Differentiating Development: Beyond an Anthropology of Critique*, edited by Tom Yarrow and Soumhya Venkatesan, 1–22. New York: Berghahn Books, 2012.

Young, Allan. "The Relevance of Traditional Medical Cultures to Modern Primary Health Care." *Social Science and Medicine* 17, no. 16 (1983): 1205–11.

Zahra. "Le président de l'Ordre des pharmaciens sur la vente illicite de produits pharmaceutiques à Keur Serigne Bi: 'L'état peut fermer "Keur Serigne-Bi" s'il le veut.'" Nettali.net, 25 June 2009.

Ziraba, Abdhalah K., Jean Fotso, and Rhoune Ochako. "Overweight and Obesity in Urban Africa: A Problem of the Rich or the Poor?" *BMC Public Health* 9 (2009): 465–73..

Contributors

HANNAH BROWN is a lecturer in the Department of Anthropology at the University of Durham. Her most recent research was an ethnographic study of health management in western Kenya, based on fieldwork undertaken in 2011. This work explores issues around governance, bureaucracy, work, the state, and global health interventions. She is also currently working on a monograph, *Domains of Care: Living with HIV/AIDS in Western Kenya*, which brings together aspects of this research with earlier fieldwork concerned with the intersections between gendered care work, domestic economies of care, and institutional responses to HIV.

P. WENZEL GEISSLER teaches social anthropology at the Institute of Social Anthropology, University of Oslo. His research explores the practice of scientific research and collaboration in Africa, combining ethnography and history. His most recent books are the monograph *The Land Is Dying* (2010; with Ruth Prince), and *Evidence, Ethos and Experiment: The Anthropology and History of Medical Research in Africa* (2011; edited with Catherine Molyneux).

MURRAY LAST is a professor emeritus in the Department of Anthropology, University College London. He specializes in both the precolonial history of Muslim northern Nigeria and the ethnography of illness and healing. In 1967 he published *The Sokoto Caliphate* (London: Longmans Green); it has since been published in Hausa as *Daular Sakkwato*. In 1986 he edited (with G. L. Chavunduka) *The Professionalisation of African Medicine* (Manchester: Manchester University Press for the International African Institute). He has published over a hundred articles on northern Nigeria and continues to visit there each year. He was editor of the International African Institute's journal, *Africa*, from 1986 to 2001.

REBECCA MARSLAND is a lecturer in social anthropology at the University of Edinburgh. She is currently completing a book entitled *The*

Words of the People that addresses questions about tradition, morality, and public health, which have been debated by the Nyakyusa in southwestern Tanzania since the 1930s. Other publications have dealt with traditional medicine, development, and HIV/AIDS.

LOTTE MEINERT is a professor of anthropology in the Department of Culture and Society at Aarhus University, Denmark. She carries out anthropological research in Uganda on issues related to health, education, human security, and land. Her current research projects are on *Changing Human Security: Recovery after Armed Conflict in Northern Uganda; Cultural Epidemics and Social Contagion* (EPICENTER); and *Governing Transitions in Northern Uganda: Trust and Land.* Her publications include the monograph *Hopes in Friction: Schooling, Health and Everyday Life in Uganda* (Information Age Publishing, 2009) and *Time Objectified: Ethnographies of Global Youth,* edited with Anne Line Dalsgaard, Martin Demant Frederiksen, and Susanne Højlund (Temple University Press, 2013). She is participating in a book project with Susan Reynolds Whyte and other colleagues titled *Second Chances: Surviving AIDS in Uganda* (to be published by Duke University Press).

BENSON A. MULEMI is a senior lecturer in the Department of Social Sciences at the Catholic University of Eastern Africa in Nairobi, Kenya. He has served as a visiting lecturer at the Institute of Anthropology, Gender and African Studies, University of Nairobi, Institute for Peace Studies and International Relations at Hekima College, Nairobi, and the Institute of Tropical Medicine and Infectious Diseases at the Jomo Kenyatta University of Agriculture and Technology and Kenya Medical Research Institute in Nairobi. His research interests include hospital ethnography, ethnographies of health and livelihood, and ethnography of human albinism and livelihood of affected people in East Africa. He has published articles in medical anthropology and African ethno-medicine and contributed to *African Folklore: An Encyclopedia, The Oxford Encyclopedia of African Thought, Encyclopedia of Religion and Psychology, and "Orafrica,"* among other publications.

RUTH J. PRINCE is senior research associate at the Department of Social Anthropology, University of Cambridge, and research fellow at the Institute of Anthropology, University of Oslo. She is currently pursuing a project on East African doctors. *The Land Is Dying: Contingency,*

Creativity and Conflict in Kenya (with P. Wenzel Geissler) explores people's attempts, in the face of the AIDS epidemic, land pressure, and urban unemployment, to engender "growth" across different domains of everyday and ritual practice, ranging from caring for children and relatives to funeral ritual and land transactions.

NOÉMI TOUSIGNANT is a research associate with the Anthropologies of African Biosciences research group in the Department of Archeology and Anthropology at the University of Cambridge. Her current research focuses on scientific capacity, moral and political subjectivity, memory, and public health in Senegal. She is currently writing a book on the history and ethnography of toxicology in postcolonial Senegal.

SUSAN REYNOLDS WHYTE, a professor in the Department of Anthropology, University of Copenhagen, carries out anthropological research in East Africa on social efforts to secure well-being under adverse circumstances. Her publications deal with misfortune and uncertainty, the social lives of medicines, disability, and changing kinship practices. With colleagues she is currently completing a book entitled *Second Chances* on the first generation of AIDS survivors in Uganda.

Index

AIDS. *See* HIV/AIDS

AIDS Support Organization, The (TASO), 122, 123, 124–25, 138n21, 153

Alma Ata conference, 21, 153

antiretroviral therapy (ART), 1, 6, 29–31, 38; in Kenya, 141, 157n7, 208, 216, 218, 226, 229n5; in Uganda, 121–22, 124, 130, 133, 134–36, 192

antiretrovirals (ARVs), 121–22, 124, 125, 136, 145, 210

ART. *See* antiretroviral therapy

ARVs. *See* antiretrovirals

asthma, 192

Bamako Initiative, 23, 74n1, 104, 114n44

Barber, Karin, 83

Benn, Hilary, 153

Biehl, João, 31, 135

biopolitics, 2, 7, 8, 15, 135, 209–10, 217, 233

biosociality, 30, 120, 135, 209

blood-stealing, 13, 255n16

Botswana, 28, 121

Briggs, Charles L., and Clara Mantini-Briggs, 81

Bush, George W., 29

Cameroon, 22

cancer, 2, 39, 162–81, 188, 192

cardiovascular diseases, 162, 188, 191, 202

CBOs. *See* community-based organizations

Centers for Disease Control and Prevention (CDC), 123–24, 255n13

chemotherapy, 164, 166–67, 169–71, 176–77

cholera, 80, 84

Christianity, 13, 16–17, 25, 66–68, 84, 90

chronic lung disease, 188

citizenship, 8–9, 20, 96–97, 101, 102–3, 110–11, 120–21, 135, 209

colonial health practices, 5–6, 7, 10, 12–13, 15–18, 66–68, 88–89, 122–23

Comaroff, Jean and John, 13

community-based organizations (CBOs), 2, 26, 140, 143–47, 150–55, 158n19, 208, 213

community home-based care (CHBC). *See* home-based care

"community participation," 20, 21, 26, 33, 148, 213

Congo, 13, 22

contraception, 21, 24

Cooper, Frederick, 18

corruption, 22, 25, 56, 58, 64–65, 106–7, 192, 235, 247

crowds vs. publics, 83–85

decentralization, 57–58, 59

demographic surveillance systems, 239–40

developmentalism, 18–21, 23, 30, 31, 56, 81, 240; in Senegal, 97, 99, 101–2

diabetes, 2, 39, 187–88, 191–93, 200, 202, 204

diarrhea, 21

diet, 39, 189–90, 192–93, 196–98, 202, 217

Diouf, Abdou, 102, 104

Doctors without Borders. *See* Médecins sans frontières

drug donation, 14, 32, 33, 34, 228–29n4, 236

drugs. *See* pharmaceutical issues

Durham, Deborah, 77

dystopias, 14

E-med, 98, 108

Ellison, James, 88

epidemics, 16, 17, 19, 63, 66

Evans-Pritchard, Edward, 11–12

exercise, 198–200

Farmer, Paul, 43n45, 49n153

Fassin, Didier, 103–4

Fanon, Franz, 13

Feierman, Steven, 15, 87, 94n42, 132

Ferguson, James, 8, 34

Ferzacca, Steve, 191

fieldwork, 248–49

Foucault, Michel, 7, 13, 120, 134, 143, 155

Fowler, Alan, 27

funerals: in Botswana, 83, 95n53; in Tanzania, 76–80, 82–83, 88, 90, 92, 93n17